MORE 4U!

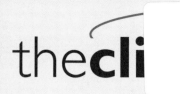 the**cli**

MW00570103

This Clinics series is available online.

Here's what you get:

■ Full text of EVERY issue from 2002 to NOW

■ Figures, tables, drawings, references and more

■ Searchable: find what you need fast

Search | All Clinics ▼ | for | | GO

■ Linked to MEDLINE and Elsevier journals

■ E-alerts

INDIVIDUAL SUBSCRIBERS

LOG ON TODAY. IT'S FAST AND EASY.

Click **Register** and follow instructions

You'll need your account number

Your subscriber account number is on your mailing label

BOUGHT A SINGLE ISSUE? Sorry, you won't be able to access full text online. Please subscribe today to get complete content by contacting customer service at 800 645 2452 (US and Canada) or 407 345 4000 (outside US and Canada) or via email at elsols@elsevier.com.

NEW!

Now also available for INSTITUTIONS

ELSEVIER

Works/Integrates with MD Consult
Available in a variety of packages: Collections containing 14, 31 or 50 Clinics titles
Or Collection upgrade for existing MD Consult customers

Call today! 877-857-1047 or e-mail: mdc.groupinfo@elsevier.com

Bennett

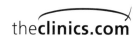

CHILD AND ADOLESCENT PSYCHIATRIC CLINICS OF NORTH AMERICA

Child Psychiatry and the Media

GUEST EDITORS
Eugene V. Beresin, MD, and
Cheryl K. Olson, SD

CONSULTING EDITOR
Melvin Lewis, MBBS, FRCPsych, DCH

CONSULTING EDITOR (ACTING)
Andrés Martin, MD, MPH

July 2005 • Volume 14 • Number 3

SAUNDERS

An Imprint of Elsevier, Inc.
PHILADELPHIA   LONDON   TORONTO   MONTREAL   SYDNEY   TOKYO

W.B. SAUNDERS COMPANY
A Division of Elsevier Inc.

Elsevier, Inc. • 1600 John F. Kennedy Boulevard • Suite 1800 • Philadelphia, Pennsylvania 19103-2899

http://www.theclinics.com

CHILD AND ADOLESCENT PSYCHIATRIC CLINICS
OF NORTH AMERICA
July 2005
Editor: Sarah E. Barth

Volume 14, Number 3
ISSN 1056-4993
ISBN 1-4160-2673-8

The ideas and opinions expressed in *Child and Adolescent Psychiatric Clinics of North America* do not necessarily reflect those of the Publisher. The Publisher does not assume any responsibility for any injury and/or damage to persons or property arising out of or related to any use of the material contained in this periodical. The reader is advised to check the appropriate medical literature and the product information currently provided by the manufacturer of each drug to be administered to verify the dosage, the method and duration of administration, or contraindications. It is the responsibility of the treating physician or other health care professional, relying on independent experience and knowl-edge of the patient, to determine drug dosages and the best treatment for the patient. Mention of any product in this issue should not be construed as endorsement by the contributors, editors, or the Publisher of the product or manufacturers' claims.

Child and Adolescent Psychiatric Clinics of North America (ISSN 1056-4993) is published quarterly by W.B. Saunders Company. Corporate and editorial offices: Elsevier, Inc., 1600 John F. Kennedy Boulevard, Suite 1800, Philadelphia, PA 19103-2899. Accounting and circula-tion offices: 6277 Sea Harbor Drive, Orlando, FL 32887-4800. Periodicals postage paid at Orlando, FL 32862, and additional mailing offices. Subscription prices are $175.00 per year (US individuals), $265.00 per year (US institutions), $200.00 per year (Canadian individu-als), $314.00 per year (Canadian institutions), $220.00 per year (foreign individuals), and $314.00 per year (foreign institutions). Foreign air speed delivery is included in all *Clinics* subscription prices. All prices are subject to change without notice. POSTMASTER: Send address changes to *Child and Adolescent Psychiatric Clinics of North America,* W.B. Saunders Company, Periodicals Fulfillment, Orlando, FL 32887-4800. **Customer Service: 1-800-654-2452 (US). From outside the US, call 1-407-345-4000. E-mail:** hhspcs@harcourt.com.

Child and Adolescent Psychiatric Clinics of North America is covered in *Index Medicus, ISI, SSCI, Research Alert, Social Search, Current Contents,* and *EMBASE/Excerpta Medica.*

Printed in the United States of America.

CONSULTING EDITOR

MELVIN LEWIS, MBBS, FRCPsych, DCH, Professor Emeritus, Senior Research Scientist, Yale Child Study Center, Yale University School of Medicine, New Haven, Connecticut

CONSULTING EDITOR (ACTING)

ANDRÉS MARTIN, MD, MPH, Associate Professor of Child Psychiatry and Psychiatry, Yale Child Study Center, Yale University School of Medicine; and Medical Director, Children's Psychiatric Inpatient Service, Yale-New Haven Children's Hospital, New Haven, Connecticut

GUEST EDITORS

EUGENE V. BERESIN, MD, Director of Child and Adolescent Psychiatry Residency Training, Department of Psychiatry, Massachusetts General/McLean Hospitals; Associate Professor, Department of Psychiatry, Harvard Medical School; and Co-Director, Harvard Medical School Center for Mental Health and Media, Boston, Massachusetts

CHERYL K. OLSON, SD, Co-Director, Harvard Medical School Center for Mental Health and Media, Department of Psychiatry, Massachusetts General Hospital, Waltham; and Clinical Instructor, Department of Psychiatry, Harvard Medical School, Boston, Massachusetts

CONTRIBUTORS

ANNE E. BECKER, MD, PhD, Department of Psychiatry, Massachusetts General Hospital; and Department of Social Medicine, Harvard Medical School, Boston, Massachusetts

EUGENE V. BERESIN, MD, Director of Child and Adolescent Psychiatry Residency Training, Department of Psychiatry, Massachusetts General/McLean Hospitals; Associate Professor, Department of Psychiatry, Harvard Medical School; and Co-Director, Harvard Medical School Center for Mental Health and Media, Boston, Massachusetts

JEFF Q. BOSTIC, MD, EdD, Assistant Clinical Professor of Psychiatry, Harvard Medical School, Boston, Massachusetts

JENNIFER BREMER, MD, Department of Child Psychiatry, University of Chicago, Chicago, Illinois

JEREMY R. BUTLER, MD, Resident in Training, Department of Psychiatry, Columbia University; and the New York State Psychiatric Institute, New York, New York

REBECCA L. COLLINS, PhD, Senior Behavioral Scientist, RAND, Santa Monica, California

RICHARD L. FALZONE, MD, Fellow, Division of Child and Adolescent Psychiatry, Massachusetts General/McLean Hospitals; and Department of Psychiatry, Harvard Medical School, Boston, Massachusetts

WANDA P. FREMONT, MD, Director of Child and Adolescent Psychiatry Training Program; and Assistant Professor, Department of Psychiatry, SUNY Upstate Medical University, Syracuse, New York

JEANNE B. FUNK, PhD, Professor of Psychology; and Director of Clinical Psychology Doctoral Training Program, Department of Psychology, University of Toledo, Toledo, Ohio

HOLLY S. GELFOND, EdD, Research Associate, Harvard Medical School Center for Mental Health and Media, Waltham; and Department of Psychiatry, Massachusetts General Hospital, Boston, Massachusetts

SARAH HALL, BS, Research Assistant, Division of Child and Adolescent Psychiatry, Massachusetts General/McLean Hospitals; and Department of Psychiatry, Harvard Medical School, Boston, Massachusetts

STEVEN E. HYLER, MD, Clinical Professor of Psychiatry, Department of Psychiatry, Columbia University; and the New York State Psychiatric Institute, New York, New York

MICHAEL S. JELLINEK, MD, Professor, Department of Psychiatry, Massachusetts General Hospital, Boston, Massachusetts

LAWRENCE A. KUTNER, PhD, Co-Director, Harvard Medical School Center for Mental Health and Media, Department of Psychiatry, Massachusetts General Hospital, Waltham; and Lecturer on Psychology, Department of Psychiatry, Harvard Medical School, Boston, Massachusetts

ARDIS C. MARTIN, MD, Child and Adolescent Psychiatrist, West Central Mental Health Center, Canon City, Colorado

CHERYL K. OLSON, SD, Co-Director, Harvard Medical School Center for Mental Health and Media, Department of Psychiatry, Massachusetts General Hospital, Waltham; and Clinical Instructor, Department of Psychiatry, Harvard Medical School, Boston, Massachusetts

JENNIFER PATASHNICK, BS, Video Intervention/Prevention Assessment (VIA), Center on Media and Child Health, Division of Adolescent/Young Adult Medicine, Children's Hospital Boston, Boston, Massachusetts

CAROLY PATAKI, MD, Department of Psychiatry, David Geffen School of Medicine, University of California at Los Angeles, Center for Health Sciences, Los Angeles, California

JULIE POLVINEN, BA, Video Intervention/Prevention Assessment (VIA), Center on Media and Child Health, Division of Adolescent/Young Adult Medicine, Children's Hospital Boston, Boston, Massachusetts

MICHAEL RICH, MD, MPH, Video Intervention/Prevention Assessment (VIA), Center on Media and Child Health, Division of Adolescent/Young Adult Medicine, Children's Hospital Boston, Harvard Medical School, Boston, Massachusetts

DOROTHY E. SALONIUS-PASTERNAK, PhD, Research Associate, Harvard Medical School Center for Mental Health and Media, Waltham; and Department of Psychiatry, Massachusetts General Hospital, Boston, Massachusetts

STEVEN SCHLOZMAN, MD, Harvard Medical School, Boston, Massachusetts

SUZANNE R. SUNDAY, PhD, Department of Psychiatry, North Shore University Hospital, Manhasset, New York

KIMBERLY M. THOMPSON, MS, ScD, Associate Professor of Risk Analysis and Decision Science; and Director, KidsRisk Project, Harvard School of Public Health and Division of Adolescent Medicine, Children's Hospital Boston, Boston, Massachusetts

V. SUSAN VILLANI, MD, Assistant Professor, Department of Psychiatry, Johns Hopkins School of Medicine; and Medical Director of School Programs, Kennedy Krieger Institute, Baltimore, Maryland

CLAIRE V. WISEMAN, PhD, Department of Psychology, Trinity College, Hartford, Connecticut

CONTENTS

conceptual model for describing possible relationships among violent video games, brain function, and desensitization by using empathy and attitudes toward violence as proxy measures of desensitization. More work is needed to understand how specific game content may affect brain activity, how brain development may be affected by heavy play at young ages, and how personality and lifestyle variables may moderate game influence. Given the current state of knowledge, recommendations are made for clinicians to help parents monitor and limit exposure to violent video games and encourage critical thinking about media violence.

This article examines how the Internet has entered children's lives and notes some of its potential positive and negative influences on children. Although the Internet's effects on a given child vary based on each child's characteristics and how the child uses the Internet, adults still must have a fundamental understanding of these general potentials. An awareness of the hazards inherent to children's Internet use is essential for all who work with children so they can apply preventive measures and help keep children safe. Whether a child uses the Internet and how a child uses the Internet significantly impact the Internet's influence on him or her. A child's personality and developmental needs also inevitably modify the Internet's influence on him or her.

Terrorist attacks and their aftermath have had a powerful impact on children and their families. Media and television exposure of terrorist events throughout the world has increased during the past few years. There is increasing concern about the effects of this exposure on children who witness these violent images. To develop a proactive and strategic response to reactions of fear, clinicians, educators, and policy makers must understand the psychologic effects of media coverage of terrorism on children. Previous research has focused on media coverage of criminal violence and war. Recent studies have examined the effect of remote exposure of terrorist attacks and have shown a significant clinical impact on children and families.

The mass media have become a powerful force throughout the world and strongly influence how people see themselves and others. This is particularly true for adolescents. This article discusses how the media affect body image and self-esteem and why the media seem to have such strong effects on adolescents. The differences in responses to the media in adolescents of different ethnic, racial, and cultural backgrounds are discussed. Although this article focuses primarily on teenage girls, the data for adolescent boys is reviewed as well. Finally, this article discusses possible ways to help adolescents become more active viewers of the media and help prevent the decrease in body esteem that so often occurs during adolescence.

The depiction of alcohol and drug traffic/usage in films has caused concern since the advent of motion pictures and continues to raise concern with the introduction of new media. This article provides a comprehensive review of much of the existing peer-reviewed published literature about the depiction of substances in the media by focusing on the information obtained in content analyses. This article demonstrates the widespread and overwhelming presence of substances in the media viewed by youth and highlights reviews that discuss the potential impacts of these depictions.

In this article, computer and video games are discussed as electronic play. Major perspectives on play and salient developmental issues are presented, along with similarities and differences between electronic play and other types of play. The authors consider possible benefits and risks associated with this type of play, with particular attention paid to cognitive and socioemotional development. Recommendations for clinicians in their work with children, adolescents, and parents are discussed, as are future directions for research.

II. Clinical Implications and Uses of Mass Media

This article examines the portrayals and myths of child and adolescent psychiatry relevant to the current practitioner. Although behavioral and emotional problems abound onscreen, the formal diagnosis of youth mental illness is uneven and rare. Common myths of brainwashing, incarceration, parent blame, parent supplantation, violence, and evil are explored, with current commercial examples of each. The impact of these portrayals on young patients, peers, parents, and the public at large are examined through the prevalence of different stereotypes across different genres more likely viewed by different ages. Positive and negative depictions of illness and treatment are identified for education and awareness, and the authors provide advice for using Hollywood films successfully as a helpful intervention in the mental health treatment of children and adolescents.

Families and children are in the midst of a media revolution. Television, Internet access, instant messaging, cell phones, and interactive video games are delivering more information for more hours than ever in history. Exposure is occurring at younger and younger ages, often without parental oversight or interpretation. The impact on children is just beginning to be studied. Does media exposure prepare children for the world in which they live or deprive them of critical developmental opportunities? Does the steady display of violence contribute to violent behavior? This article presents a developmental context, discusses the research conducted to date, reviews the recommendations of major organizations, and tries to take a balanced perspective in the midst of a rising tide of media, technology, commercialism, and controversy.

Clinicians and parents share a responsibility to educate themselves in how young people communicate with each other and how it impacts on communication with the adults in their lives. The greater fluency that clinicians have with the world of youth, the easier it is to begin a meaningful dialogue with young people. Such a dialogue always has been the purview of clinicians interested in the developmental trajectory of their young patients. The enormity of media exposure and the changes that characterize current media formats make such a dialogue important and challenging. From watching video clips to listening to music, this assessment affords clinicians a snapshot into the milieu of the modern young world. The dialogue is "virtually" always well worth the effort.

The pediatric illness experience is a complex subject that requires a multidimensional, flexible, and patient-centered approach. Video Intervention/Prevention Assessment (VIA), with its diverse source data and multidisciplinary analytical frameworks, generates findings that can be examined from any number of perspectives simply by asking different questions. As an exploration of human experience, VIA can be applied to various medical and psychiatric conditions. It has been used to investigate the experiences of children and adolescents who live with asthma, obesity, spina bifida, and diabetes mellitus. VIA currently is being applied to a longitudinal examination of the transition to adulthood by pediatric patients with spina bifida, cystic fibrosis, sickle cell disease, and HIV.

Increasing the cultural competence of child and adolescent psychiatrists through the use of film, literature, and music can improve their ability to understand what African Americans experience and the impact these experiences have on mental health. It also may help clinicians recognize their own underlying biases. This understanding, in turn, could improve their ability to address effectively in treatment the issues pertinent to the African-American community and help eliminate the well-documented disparities in the health care quality and health status of minorities.

Videotaping and digital editing (desktop video) provide a therapist with compelling material that can be used for therapy with patients, for teaching and professional presentation, and for therapist development. Despite these advantages, many clinicians are reluctant to record their work for reasons that include self-consciousness on the part of the therapist or patient, concerns about negative effects of videotaping on the session, concerns about confidentiality and legal liability, and lack of familiarity with the process of videotaping and the equipment involved. Understanding the benefits, concerns, and basic process involved in video recording and editing should reduce clinician apprehension and encourage more widespread use of this powerful clinical medium.

Psychiatrists have mixed feelings about working with the mass media. There are many reasons to respond to reporters or proactively reach out to the media, including reducing stigma and other barriers to seeking and complying with treatment, and counteracting media misinformation and distortion. This article addresses ways to increase positive outcomes when psychiatrists respond to calls from reporters, make proactive efforts to influence behaviors or policies, or take advantage of breaking news to educate reporters and the public. The article also reviews examples of planned media campaigns.

FORTHCOMING ISSUES

RECENT ISSUES

THE CLINICS ARE NOW AVAILABLE ONLINE!

Access your subscription at:
http://www.theclinics.com

Child Adolesc Psychiatric Clin N Am
14 (2005) xv–xvi

CHILD AND
ADOLESCENT
PSYCHIATRIC CLINICS
OF NORTH AMERICA

Foreword

Virtually Useful

Mass media are one of the great social equalizers of our time. What may once have been distant and exotic territory has through technology become proximal and familiar. Instant communications across the globe provide daily reminders of this remarkable power: e-mail has effectively shrunk the world and all but eliminated borders and distance. But mass media have been more than a purely democratizing force: they have revealed (when not inflicted) major chasms across countries and individuals. An ever-expanding array of vehicles for electronic communications has highlighted the existence of a world of haves and have nots. And such differences have often been most palpable across the age divide: indeed, when it comes to the media, we stand little chance of keeping up with our own children. So what then? Stick to snail mail instead? Adhere to adultspeak while our patients Instant Message away? Advise against the unfamiliar—those violent video games, raunchy song lyrics, and virtual music studio softwares that allow the untrained, undisciplined musician to fashion an opera with a few keystrokes? Are we but threatened luddites at heart?

Fear not. In this truly pioneer issue, Gene Beresin and Cheryl Olson have delivered more than relief to such generational anxieties: they have contextualized the ubiquity of the mass media within the lives of our youth and given us a framework to approach a topic that through sheer volume and ongoing metamorphoses is all but overwhelming. Moreover, they have done so through contributions that effectively shed light on a topic where heat so often is the norm. Given that mass media and controversy feed off of each other, such editorial balance and clarity is no easy feat.

Media technologies have developed at a much more rapid pace than our ability to understand their impact on developing youths. This issue of the *Clinics* affords us an opportunity to take stock, to make an inventory of sorts. There are real risks of course, and these should not be minimized: the trivialization of sexuality and violence, the impact of advertising targeted at preschoolers who go on to become lifelong "branded" devotees to questionably nutritious products and sedentary lifestyles, the bombardment with unattainable body ideals, the predator on the other side of the internet's anonymity. But the opportunities can be even richer, especially for clinicians working with children. The media-savvy

1056-4993/05/$ – see front matter © 2005 Elsevier Inc. All rights reserved.
doi:10.1016/j.chc.2005.05.001
childpsych.theclinics.com

and -literate clinician will have a new range of ways to connect to and better understand patients. Children in turn may put their own talents and creativity to use in the transitional domain of the virtual. And emerging evidence suggests that video games and the Internet may in fact increase fluid intelligence and certain cognitive abilities. Who knows?: the monotony of *unitasking* may be more dangerous than its feared multiple. Mass media is here to stay, and we should be mindful of its rich yet unwieldy potential.

The purview of our field has greatly expanded, going much further than the consulting room, the hospital, or the school setting. Child psychiatrists need not only be familiar and informed consumers of the media: they may at times be called upon to inform, to shape, to help harness it. Each instance we may come across to reach a wide audience should serve as a reminder of our social contract, and provide an opportunity to responsibly advance the cause for children's mental health. This volume provides necessary guidance to that end. We are indebted to its editors and authors for helping us to proceed as our role has expanded,

> and one man in his time plays many parts.

—William Shakespeare, *As You Like It*

Andrés Martin, MD, MPH
Consulting Editor (Acting, so to speak)
Yale Child Study Center
Yale University School of Medicine
230 South Frontage Road
New Haven, CT 06520-7900, USA
E-mail address: andres.martin@yale.edu

ELSEVIER
SAUNDERS

Child Adolesc Psychiatric Clin N Am
14 (2005) xvii–xix

CHILD AND
ADOLESCENT
PSYCHIATRIC CLINICS
OF NORTH AMERICA

Preface

Child Psychiatry and the Media

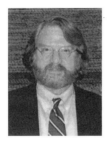 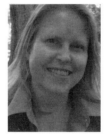

Eugene V. Beresin, MD Cheryl K. Olson, SD
Guest Editors

For the typical American child, mass media are ubiquitous. As of 2004, children in grades 3 to 12 spent over 6 hours a day using some form of media, particularly electronic media such as television, DVDs/videotapes, music, and video games. Although the total amount of media time seems to be stable, more children are multitasking—they are involved with two or more media about a quarter of the time [1].

Many parents, teachers, clinicians, and policymakers have expressed concern about the potential harmful effects of media on youth. Multiple articles in professional journals and the lay press have drawn sometimes dramatic conclusions about media effects. Unfortunately, these are often based on inadequate or poor data, or simply on opinion. This issue of the *Child and Adolescent Psychiatric Clinics of North America* is designed to present a careful, balanced view of the effects of media on youth. In addition to reviewing risks, we have attempted to discern how media may be used in the service of children's health.

Part I of this issue addresses the effects of mass media on children's mental health and health behaviors. Much research on mass media has focused on the effects of (or ways to reduce) the amount of mass media exposure. In recent years, there has been increasing focus on the nature and effects of specific

doi:10.1016/j.chc.2005.03.002   *childpsych.theclinics.com*

media content. Collins presents new research on how sexual content in television programs influences adolescents' behavior. Funk looks at concerns about emotional effects of violent content in video games. Thompson reviews research on the depiction of mood-altering substances (legal and illegal) in mass media, while Wiseman, Sunday, and Becker explore how depictions of unattainable physical perfection can affect children's body image and self-esteem.

Parents are often particularly concerned about the effects of newer media such as interactive games (as addressed by Funk) and the Internet, in part because these media are more difficult for parents to monitor. Bremer looks at how our children are growing up differently due to the influence of the Internet. As parents and clinicians try to grasp the nature and effects of advancing technology, our children are busy incorporating electronic media into their daily lives. Gelfond and Salonius-Pasternak review our understanding of the nature and function of children's play, and how interactive electronic media may be integrated into normal developmental processes. Rounding out Part I of the issue, Fremont, Pataki, and Beresin take us beyond concerns about entertainment programming to the often overlooked effects of exposure to frightening news content—how this can influence children's view of the world as a safe or dangerous place, or even become a traumatic stimulus.

In Part II, we shift our focus to the clinical implications and uses of mass media. Butler and Hyler draw our attention to mass media images of mental illness and psychiatrists and the profound effects these may have on patient and family expectations of treatment and even treatment outcomes.

There are ways that clinicians can influence the use of media to make it a benign or even positive force. Villani, Olson, and Jellinek's article on media literacy provides information that clinicians can use to help parents limit harm and promote constructive uses of mass media. There are also specific ways that clinicians can take advantage of media. Pataki, Bostic, and Schlozman explain how clinicians can ascertain the positive and negative influences of media on a given child's social, cognitive, and emotional development via a "functional media assessment." Rich, Polvinen, and Patashnick describe their method of guiding children coping with chronic medical illness to create their own videotape narratives. These stories can help us understand how chronic illness affects a child's daily life and allow children and clinicians to collaborate better in managing disease and its emotional sequelae. Martin provides detailed insights into the use of film, music, and other media to improve our understanding of other cultures (particularly African American culture), allowing us to recognize assumptions and biases that can interfere with treatment. Falzone, Hall, and Beresin walk us through potential uses of video technology to improve therapeutic skills and help families gain insight into behavior. Finally, Olson and Kutner demonstrate ways that informed clinicians can reach out to news media to influence public perceptions of psychiatrists and of mental illness, and reduce barriers to receiving treatment.

Eugene V. Beresin, MD
Department of Psychiatry
Massachusetts General Hospital
Wang 812
15 Parkman Street
Boston, MA 02114, USA
E-mail address: eberesin@partners.org

Cheryl K. Olson, SD
Harvard Medical School Center for Mental Health and Media
Department of Psychiatry
Massachusetts General Hospital
271 Waverley Oaks Road
Suite 204
Waltham, MA 02452, USA
E-mail address: colson@hms.harvard.edu

Reference

[1] Roberts DF, Foeher UG, Rideout V. Generation M: media in the lives of 8–18-year olds. Menlo Park (CA): Kaiser Family Foundation; 2005.

ELSEVIER
SAUNDERS

Child Adolesc Psychiatric Clin N Am
14 (2005) 371–385

CHILD AND
ADOLESCENT
PSYCHIATRIC CLINICS
OF NORTH AMERICA

Sex on Television and Its Impact on American Youth: Background and Results from the RAND Television and Adolescent Sexuality Study

Rebecca L. Collins, PhD

RAND, 1776 Main Street, Santa Monica, CA 90407, USA

A key period of sexual exploration and development occurs during adolescence. During this time, individuals begin to experiment with sex and consider which sexual behaviors are enjoyable, moral, and appropriate for their age group [1]. During this same developmental period, television plays a central role in life. Teenagers spend more than 3 hours per day in front of a television set—more than with any other medium [2]—and they are not mere passive observers of what is shown there. Adolescents use media to form and assert their identities, for example, as members of the counterculture or as "hip [3,4]. Observation of others' actions and beliefs strongly influences human behavior (a process termed "social learning"), and observation mediated via television can have the same effect [5]. Finally, sexual beliefs and behavior are strongly influenced by culture [6], and television is an integral part of culture in the United States. To the extent that the programming watched by youths includes sexual content, television is likely to influence the sexual socialization process.

Television sexual content

Several studies have measured the extent and nature of television sexual content and can speak to this issue. Their results suggest that television not only

TAS data collection and the preparation of this article were supported by a grant from the National Institute of Child Health and Human Development (R01HD38090) to the author.

E-mail address: Collins@rand.org

1056-4993/05/$ – see front matter © 2005 Elsevier Inc. All rights reserved.
doi:10.1016/j.chc.2005.02.005

childpsych.theclinics.com

contributes to sexual socialization but also has the potential to be a central force in the process. Studies conducted in the 1990s indicated that prime time network portrayals of sex averaged ten per hour [7]. There was an average of 3 sexual acts per hour on the fictional network series watched most often by ninth and tenth graders [8] and 8.5 per hour during the family hour [9]. During this same period, prime time rarely featured depictions or even discussions of intercourse but did present intimate discussions of sexual issues like orgasm, high levels of innuendo and jokes about sexuality, and much touching, hugging, and long kissing [10–14].

In addition to the obvious limitation of their data collection dates, most of these content analyses were limited to 200 shows or fewer and analyzed fairly homogenous content (eg, soap operas, teen programming, prime time or family hour programs). In contrast, recent research by Kunkel et al [15] examined a representative sample of more than 1000 episodes of programming from the 2001–2002 television season. The work includes programs from 11 of the most frequently viewed channels, which represent all segments of the television industry: the four major networks (ABC, CBS, Fox, NBC), an independent broadcast station that aired syndicated programming and was affiliated with the WB (a less established network, popular among teens), UPN, three basic cable channels (Lifetime, TNT, and USA Network), and one premium cable channel (HBO). One week of programming was collected and coded for each channel; daily news and sports were excluded but news magazines such as "20/20" were not.

According to Kunkel et al, sexual content currently appears in 64% of all television programs. Programs that contain sexual content average 4.4 scenes per hour with sexually related material. Talk about sex is found more frequently (61% of all programs) than overt portrayals of sexual behavior (32% of programs). Roughly one in every seven programs (14%) includes a portrayal in which sexual intercourse is depicted (typically under blankets or otherwise partially obscured from sight) or is strongly implied with devices such as "fade to black" and a follow-up morning-after scene [15].

The sexual content rarely includes reference to sexual responsibilities, such as pregnancy and sexually transmitted disease prevention. By some estimates, a single mention of these topics is made per 25 instances of sexual activity in prime time [7,16]. Kunkel's more recent work presents a brighter picture, indicating that 15% of all shows with sexual content make reference to risk [15] and that prime time network dramas include reference to the risks of having sex 22% of the times they include sexual content—more than any other genre [15].

In the past, most shows depicted adults, rather than adolescents, taking part in or discussing sex [9]. More recently, popular programs have emerged that involve a relatively young group of characters and include sex in central plot lines or as a major theme. Similar themes are addressed on shows such as "That 70's Show" and "One Tree Hill," which focus almost exclusively on high school and college students' sexual and relationship issues. In 1999, Kunkel et al estimated that 9% of the characters involved in intercourse portrayals were teens. That percentage dropped to 3% in 2001–2002. Portrayals that involve teens and intercourse more often include a message concerning sexual responsibility (approximately 25% of such shows) [15]. Notably, the shift in programming toward younger characters increases the probability that these programs influence sexual activity among adolescents and young adults, because viewers are more likely to identify with same-aged characters and more readily see their behavior as reflecting relevant norms [17]. Trends in the content of such programs may be crucial in understanding sexual socialization.

In summary, sex is a pervasive presence in a medium that plays a central role during the teenage years. Consequently, the contribution of television to adolescent sexual socialization is likely to be strong. Television's preoccupation with sex, paired with the distorted picture of sexual consequences shown there, suggests that its influence is also likely to be largely negative. One way in which television might affect youth adversely is by leading them to have sexual intercourse without considering its effect on their social and emotional lives, thereby becoming sexually active before they are prepared for the experience. A recent national survey indicated that nearly two thirds of teens who have ever had sex wish they had waited longer to do so [18].

Studies of television viewing and sexual initiation

Emerging research supports the idea that television hastens sexual initiation. This work began with two studies of adolescents published a decade ago, which showed that exposure to portrayals of sex on television and viewers' sexual experience were related [19,20]. Peterson et al [20] tested effects of television viewing using a secondary analysis of two waves of the National Survey of Children. Child and parent reports of the number of hours the child spent viewing television on weekdays were used as measures of television exposure. Each child's listings of favorite television programs were categorized according to amount of sexual content to create a measure of exposure to sexual portrayals. Results revealed some positive associations between amount of television viewing and sexual initiation among boys, especially boys who watched television apart from their parents. No associations between sexual content of favorite shows and sexual behavior were significant, although patterns did suggest such effects.

Brown and Newcomer [19] used similar methodology to Peterson et al [20]. The addition of covariates to their predictive equation, including race, parent education, and peer encouragement of sexual activity, renders their results somewhat stronger, however. Brown and Newcomer also used a more sensitive measure of exposure to sexual content and combined participant ratings of the frequency of watching a list of programs with raters' judgments of the amount of sex content in each. They found that higher proportions of sexual content in an adolescent's viewing diet were related to sexual debut. Findings from these two studies were suggestive, but causality could not be inferred because neither study used a truly longitudinal design. Precocious sexual activity may have led to interest in and increased viewing of television with sexual content, rather than the reverse.

More recent research from our laboratory has extended these findings and provided stronger support for the hypothesis that television causes changes in sexual activity [21]. The RAND Television and Adolescent Sexuality (TAS) study involved a national longitudinal survey of 2003 12- to 17-year-old individuals. At baseline and 1-year follow-up, participants reported their television viewing habits and sexual experience and responded to measures of more than 12 factors known to be associated with adolescent intercourse initiation. Television viewing data were combined with data from Kunkel's sexual content analysis (described earlier) to derive measures of exposure to sexual content, depictions of sexual risks or safe behavior, and depictions of sexual behavior (versus talk about sex but no behavior). This design allowed us to test for changes in sexual behavior that followed television exposure, which eliminated the possibility that sex led to changes in viewing, rather than the reverse. The use of indices of content measured with far greater precision than in prior studies also allowed us to better attribute any association to sexual content, rather than some other characteristic of programming. Finally, the statistical control of a dozen factors, such as parents' attitudes toward sex, their monitoring of teens' behavior, and teens' personalities (eg, sensation seeking), reduced the likelihood that such characteristics might explain any association between viewing habits and behavior.

Results indicated that adolescent virgins who viewed more sexual content at baseline were more likely to initiate intercourse over the subsequent year, even after controlling for respondent characteristics that might otherwise explain this relationship. A one standard deviation increase in exposure to sexual content on television was equivalent in its effect on intercourse to an increase in age of 9 months. Looked at another way, the size of the effect was such that youth in the ninetieth percentile of television sex viewing had a predicted probability of intercourse initiation that was approximately double that of youth in the tenth percentile, across all ages studied (Fig. 1). Exposure to television that included only talk about sex was associated with the same probability of intercourse as exposure to television that depicted sexual behavior. The study found no effect of exposure to portrayals of sexual risk or safe sexual behavior in the sample as a whole; however, African-American youth who watched more depictions of sexual risks or safety were less likely to initiate intercourse over the subsequent year.

The TAS study also examined the relationship between exposure to sexual content and subsequent changes in noncoital sexual behavior. Most research on the sexual behavior of adolescents has focused on intercourse; however, rates of intercourse experience have been declining steadily over the past decade, according to the Center for Disease Control and Prevention's Youth Risk Behavior Survey. This school-based survey regularly assesses various health behaviors among high school attendees across the United States. The percentage

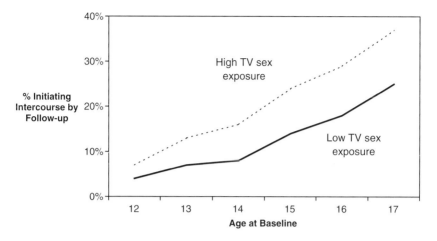

Fig. 1. Predicted probabilities of intercourse initiation among virgins exposed to high versus low levels of TV sexual content.

of youth who reported that they had ever had sexual intercourse in 1991 was 54%, whereas in 2001 the percentage declined to 46% [22]. Although we can only speculate about the reasons for this trend, public health efforts to reduce the rates of pregnancy, HIV, and other sexually transmitted diseases and efforts to increase sexual abstinence may have been involved. Rather than reducing sexual activity per se, however, these interventions may have refocused it, and thereby increased interest in oral sex among youth as an alternative to intercourse. Media reports [23,24] and some emerging research findings [25] suggested that adolescents are increasingly engaged in noncoital sexual behavior, including oral sex, and may be substituting it for coitus.

At baseline and follow-up, TAS assessed adolescents' level of noncoital experience using a measure developed for the study [26]. This measure assumes that noncoital activities are initiated in an ordered sequence by most youths and certain behaviors are more advanced than others. Based on self-reports of experience with various heterosexual activities, youths were classified has having engaged in no noncoital activity or kissing only, "making-out" (kissing for a long time), breast touching, genital touching, or oral sex. These categories were ordered as just described and were made mutually exclusive so that each participant was classified according to the most advanced activity in which he or she had engaged. At follow-up (ages 13–18), 34% of the sample reported experience with oral sex, 14% had reached the stage of genital touching and 9% breast touching, 18% had ever "made-out," and 25% reported no noncoital sexual experience beyond kissing. In comparison to baseline reports when youths were 1 year younger, there had been an average advancement of one noncoital stage, although there was considerable variability in rates of progress among individuals.

Exposure to sexual content strongly predicted which youth progressed to more advanced noncoital activities. After controlling for baseline noncoital stage and multiple covariates, the effect associated with television sexual content was significant and equivalent in magnitude to 17 months of aging. Fig. 2 displays the predicted probabilities of two behaviors—breast and genital touching—generated from the regression results. The probability of initiating breast touching was approximately 50% higher in the high- versus low-exposure group, whereas the probability of initiating genital touching was almost double in the high-exposure group. Results for other noncoital activities fell between these two estimates. Paralleling results for intercourse, exposure to sexual talk versus behavior had similar associations with noncoital advancement, and African Americans were less likely to advance their noncoital activity level with exposure to sexual risk and safety portrayals, whereas change in the noncoital activity level of other races was not related to risk-portrayal exposure.

In summary, results of the RAND TAS to date suggest that television may have a strong influence on the sexual development of teens, at least in regard to the speed with which their sexual behavior advances. These findings are

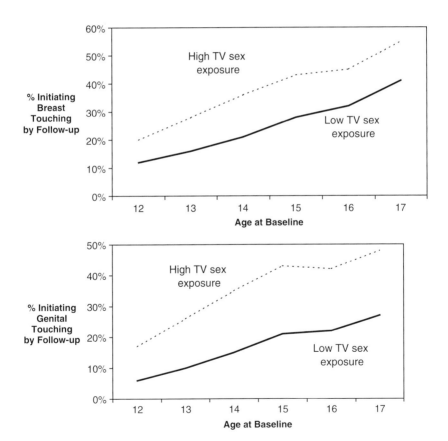

Fig. 2. Predicted probabilities of noncoital advancement among individuals exposed to high versus low levels of TV sexual content.

important, because data indicate that earlier initiation of intercourse increases the probability of sexually transmitted disease infection and pregnancy [27,28] and many sexually active teens wish they had waited longer to have sex [18]. To prevent such outcomes, interventions aimed at reducing or eliminating exposure to television sexual content could be developed. Changes in television diets may be difficult to achieve and maintain, however. Given the centrality of television to teens' lives, they are unlikely to give it up willingly, and their access to television within and outside the home is considerable. The high prevalence of sexual content across most programs and genres means that a "change the channel" approach is also likely to fail. Savvy intervention by clinicians and parents or as part of school curricula can overcome these obstacles by targeting teens' response to television, rather than their exposure to it. To intervene effectively in this way requires information about the process through which television viewing most likely exerts an effect on adolescents' sexual behavior.

Multiple processes may underlie television effects

Social cognitive theory (SCT) [17] argues that television is a source of observational learning and that this form of learning involves several processes. Key among these is a shift in perceived norms. It is hypothesized that people derive their beliefs about what kind of behavior is typical and appropriate by observing the behavior of others, including people portrayed on television. SCT hypothesizes that beliefs about the likely positive or negative outcome of an action, known as "outcome expectancies," are also derived from this observational process. Finally, SCT argues that observational learning involves shifts in self-efficacy. Watching others engage successfully in a behavior helps viewers envision doing the same themselves.

Given the sexual content of television (the rare portrayal of sexual risks and the frequent depiction of sexual behaviors or discussion of sex), SCT predicts that youth who watch more of this content will feel more confident about sex and sexual matters, believe that more of their peers are having sex, and believe that sex seldom has negative consequences. All or any one of these beliefs may be what spurs youths with a heavier diet of sexual fare to have sex sooner than others.

Using the TAS data, Steven Martino, my colleagues, and I recently examined the contribution of SCT processes to the association between sexual content exposure and intercourse initiation in TAS [29]. The analysis used multiple-group structural equation modeling, which allowed us to test and account for any differences that might be present across the different subgroups that participated in TAS. Preliminary analyses revealed no differences by gender but did suggest differences by race/ethnicity (African Americans, Hispanics, non-Hispanic whites/other races). Results of these tests indicated that increased self-efficacy was an important mediator of the effect of television sex exposure on intercourse initiation. Adolescents who more frequently watched people talking about sex and behaving sexually on television were more confident that they could do things associated with being sexually active (eg, obtain condoms, communicate with a potential partner) than were adolescents with less exposure to sex on television. This change was, in turn, associated with a greater probability of subsequent intercourse initiation. The effect held only among African-American and white/other race adolescents. Viewing sexual content on television did not increase self-efficacy among Hispanic youth, and this process could not explain changes in their sexual behavior. Less negative outcome expectancies and shifts in perceived peer sexual behavior occurred across all racial groups and correlated strongly with prior viewing of sexual content. Tests that examined whether these shifts explained the association between television viewing and intercourse initiation in each racial subgroup were somewhat equivocal and reached only marginal levels of statistical significance, but they were based on a statistical test (the Sobel test) widely regarded as conservative [30]. We concluded that shifts toward pro-sex norms and expectancies may account for responses to television sexual content among Hispanic youth, and all three SCT processes (ie, norms, expectancies, and self-efficacy) seem to play a role in the sexual advances demonstrated among television-watching teens from non-Hispanic backgrounds.

Racial and ethnic differences in response to television sexual content

As the findings presented so far have indicated, adolescents with different racial and ethnic backgrounds seem to respond to television sexual content differently. African-American youths differ from whites in their television viewing habits [31,32] and their sexual behavior [33]. Two studies have found that African-American and white adolescents also differ in their reactions to sex-related media content. Walsh-Childers and Brown [34] found that viewing traditionally female-oriented television shows led to acceptance of stereotypes about heterosexual relationships and male dominance among African-American adolescent boys. The male dominance effect also was observed for African-American girls. Little evidence of either effect was obtained for white adolescents of either gender, however. Racial differences also were observed in a study of interpretations of music videos [31]. Whereas African-Americans saw the Madonna video "Papa Don't Preach" as a story about father-daughter issues, whites saw the video's theme as one of teen pregnancy. In earlier work, Greenberg and Atkin [35] presented results that indicated that although African-American and white youths were equally likely to identify with white television characters, African Americans were far more likely than whites to identify with African-American characters, and they viewed characters of both races as more realistic than did whites.

TAS found no racial differences in the behavioral effects of viewing sexual content as a whole. African-American teens were less likely to engage in intercourse if they had seen more portrayals of sexual risk and sexual safety, however, whereas whites and youths of other races showed no effects of exposure to this content. Several factors may have caused this pattern of results. First, although rates of intercourse initiation over the 1-year TAS study period were equivalent across race, more African Americans had had sex at baseline and at follow-up. It may be that risk and responsibility content exerted greater effects on African-American youths because they were more relevant to them (given higher rates of intercourse). Alternatively, it might be that African Americans face disadvantages or barriers to getting sexual risk information from sources other than television and consequently rely on it more heavily.

The finding that Hispanics differed somewhat from other races in the process by which television exposure seemed to influence their behavior suggests a third possibility. This explanation is consistent with the "Papa Don't Preach" work on racial differences in television interpretation: the cultural context provided by race may alter the way in which television portrayals are perceived and processed. Different racial or ethnic groups may pay attention to different aspects of a television scene or may understand and interpret what is happening in a scene differently. Clearly, more empirical research in this area and the development of media theory that addresses the issue of race is needed before these questions can be answered.

Television's potential as a positive force in sexual socialization

Thus far, this article has focused on what many parents and educators would consider to be adverse effects of television on sexual socialization. Television is not an inherently problematic force in adolescent development, however. The medium is not the message, and the effects of viewing sexual content should depend at least in part on the specifics of how sex is portrayed. Television portrayals of people using condoms and birth control, waiting to have sex later in a relationship, or experiencing negative outcomes because they failed to do any of these things should—in theory—deter youth from sex or at least deter them from risky sexual behavior.

Few studies have addressed this issue directly, although research has shown that health messages embedded in entertainment programming can be used to make viewers aware of important sexual health information. For example, an episode of the popular program "ER" that addressed the availability of emergency contraception was associated with increased calls to an HIV/AIDS hotline [36], as were HIV-related plot points contained in a season of the soap opera "The Bold and the Beautiful" [37]. Similarly, when a storyline on the program "ER" addressed the transmission of syphilis among men who have sex with men, an online survey of men who have sex with men showed that individuals who had seen the storyline reported greater intent to be screened for syphilis [36].

None of these studies focused on adolescents. A RAND study that was a spin-off from the TAS did so, however, and tested teens' responses to an episode of what was then the top-rated television sitcom, "Friends" [38]. In the episode, a female character tells her former boyfriend that she is pregnant with his child.

He replies, "But we used a condom!" This fact, and the statement that condoms are "only 95% effective," was repeated several times during the half-hour episode. Nielsen Media Research estimated 1.67 million youth aged 12 to 17 saw the first airing of the episode. Three to 4 weeks after it first appeared, RAND surveyed adolescents enrolled in the TAS who had reported in their baseline surveys that they regularly watch "Friends." Of these youths, at least one in four had seen the episode in question, and 65% of these viewers remembered that it involved a pregnancy resulting from condom failure. Importantly, one in ten teen viewers said that they had talked with an adult about condom effectiveness as a result of seeing the show. Compared with other viewers, teens who talked with an adult were more likely to say that they learned about condoms from the episode.

The study did not find any overall change in viewers' beliefs about how well condoms work to prevent pregnancy compared with what they had said in the TAS survey 6 months earlier. Instead, some teens saw condoms as less effective at preventing pregnancy, others saw them as more effective after viewing the program, and each change occurred equally often. This is not surprising given the information presented, which indicated that appealing characters with whom youths identify use condoms (and think they work) and that condom failure is an unlikely event but it can happen. Different lessons could be learned depending on what aspect of this information the teen viewers focused. The study did document directional changes in beliefs for one subgroup of viewers: youths who discussed the show with adults were less likely to reduce their perceptions of condom effectiveness. It seems that adults directed youth toward the interpretation that most of the time condoms do work.

The "Friends" study indicates that sexual risk information included in entertainment programming reaches youth, is remembered by them, and has the potential to change beliefs and catalyze educational conversations with adults. The question is whether it can have a positive influence on adolescent sexual behavior. Here the evidence is mixed. The reader may recall the results of the main TAS study, which indicated that only the behavior of African-American youths was affected by exposure to sexual risk and responsibility depictions. These teens were less likely to initiate sexual intercourse over the subsequent year when they had viewed relatively more portrayals of the risks of sexual intercourse or more often saw characters behaving in a sexually responsible manner. This effect did not generalize to other racial/ethnic groups, however. It may be that there was simply not enough such material included in the television season studied by TAS to detect an effect in other racial/ethnic groups. The measure of risk and responsibility that was used in TAS did not require that the risk information be central to the television scene in which it occurred (as was required for the other sexual content measures in that study). This was because sexual risk information was so seldom the focus of any scene that TAS could not measure such exposure reliably. An effect of sexual risk might be found in other racial groups when the exposure "dosage" is more substantial or more sensitively measured. We cannot currently conclude that television portrayals of sexual risk have a positive (ie, deterrent) influence on the sexual behavior of most teens.

Another potentially positive effect of television sexual content is the increased sexual self-efficacy observed by Martino et al [29] described earlier. This study found that adolescents who watched relatively more sex on television were more confident that they could do things associated with being sexually active. Brown and Pardun [39] observed a similar relationship between adolescent girls' sexual self-confidence and their exposure to sexual media. At first, this might not seem to be good news; parents might prefer that their children not develop such confidence, at least until they are older. However, Martino and colleagues' measure of sexual self-efficacy assessed adolescents' confidence in their ability to obtain condoms, use condoms consistently, and communicate with a potential partner, which are elements of a more specific construct: safe-sex self-efficacy. Martino et al found that sexual content influenced this more specific self-perception. Importantly, safe-sex self-efficacy has been shown to be instrumental in reducing the risk of unwanted outcomes as a result of having sex [40,41]. These data suggest there is an unexpected benefit of youth exposure to television sexual portrayals, even when those portrayals fail to depict risk. The sexual self-confidence they engender may help youth to resist partners who want to have sex without a condom. It is important to keep in mind, however, that Martino et al also found a link between safe-sex self-efficacy and early intercourse initiation. More confident youth may be having safer sex, but they also seem to be having it sooner.

Recommendations

The findings by Martino et al raise an important issue regarding the goals of intervention in the sexual socialization process. The public and personal health perspective on this topic focuses on increasing avoidance of sexual activity that might lead to pregnancy or sexually transmitted disease infection. Reducing the amount of sexual talk and behavior on television or the amount of time that adolescents are exposed to this content is likely to delay appreciably the age of initiating coital and noncoital sexual activities and indirectly decrease sexual risk (because early intercourse is usually riskier). Some recent analyses of the TAS data set indicate that it also may be possible to reduce exposure to sex on television by implementing household rules regarding television viewing (eg, what to watch, how much to watch) and keeping televisions out of adolescents' bedrooms, where viewing is unsupervised [42]. These simple steps may help delay the onset of sexual activity and indirectly reduce health-related risks.

Health goals also can be met directly by reducing only unprotected intercourse. Increasing the percentage of portrayals of sexual risk and safety on television, relative to other sexual content, should do this, and it might inhibit early sexual activity. A second option is to increase portrayals of characters whose inappropriate sexual comments and activities meet with disapproval or who botch attempts at sexual flirtation. Exposure to such portrayals is likely to increase negative outcome expectancies regarding such behaviors and is unlikely to increase sexual self-efficacy (and thus intercourse initiation). Portraying more of these kinds of events, particularly with teen characters, would be realistic and have much dramatic and comedic potential.

This approach presents some challenges, however, and is not directly useful to parents and others who work with adolescents but have little control over television writers and producers. Moreover, engineering television content so that it depicts negative outcomes of sex more often than positive outcomes brings the risk of teaching youth that sex is about disease, awkwardness, or heartbreak. The broad, long-term goal of sexual socialization, whether from a values or health perspective, is not to prevent sex but to promote healthy sexuality—satisfying sexual relationships that occur at a point when people and relationships are ready.

Some researchers have argued that shielding youth from sexual media may cause harm [43]. Learning about sex and sexuality is a natural and important part of human development. Youth seek out sexual content on television as they begin to develop sexually [42,44]. Brown and colleagues [44] argue that television and other mass media serve as a kind of "sexual super peer" for girls who seek information about sex, especially girls who mature earlier than their peers and for this reason have limited social sources of sexual information. Brown rightfully cautions that television is typically not appropriate to this task, however, because its content is so often distorted. Nonetheless, with some care and effort, parents and clinicians might exploit adolescents' use of television as an educational resource. Parents who watch television with their children have the opportunity to discuss their own beliefs about sex and relationships as these topics arise in programs. As the "Friends" study indicated, discussing television can be an easy way for parents and teens to broach the topic of sex. Parents can choose whether to counter or reinforce any message that is conveyed by the portrayal in question. Viewing shows with their children also would help parents identify any programs that they want to designate as off-limits in the future. Psychiatrists and other counseling professionals also might use television as a tool, using current television plot lines or characters as openings for a discussion of sex or for communicating sex-related information in a manner to which adolescents can relate. The question "Did you see what happened on 'Friends' last week?" may engage attention more effectively than a direct broaching of the topic of unplanned pregnancy.

A nascent field moves forward

Although we recently have learned a fair amount about the role of television in the sexual socialization of America's youth, every one of the areas of research reviewed in this article requires more study. The evidence so far strongly suggests that television sexual content, at a general level, hastens the initiation of various adolescent sexual behaviors. This effect, like all initial scientific findings, must be replicated in other samples by other investigators apart from the RAND TAS, however. Much more must be done before we have established boundaries on the effects of television sexual content. The National Institute of Child Health and Human Development funded several research projects that examined the influence of sexual media on youth, in addition to TAS, and work on these studies is currently underway across the United States. These projects explore some of the same issues as TAS but also test effects of other media, such as music and the Internet. They also examine additional causal pathways between media exposure and behavior. For example, the television-influenced development of gender stereotypes may lead to sex and sexual risk taking among youth [45].

RAND also will be conducting additional work as TAS continues. In addition to further exploring the influence of race on responses to television sexual content, we will be looking at how sexual content on television influences the development of psychologically and socially healthy relationships. Researchers have noted that most sexual activity on television occurs between unmarried couples [46,47]. Other studies indicate that college students who watch more hours of soap operas estimate that the divorce rate is higher and unwed parenthood more common than do students who watch fewer soap operas [48]. These findings have important implications for the kinds of sexual partnerships and intimate relationships likely to be formed by young viewers, and TAS will explore this issue and examine how television portrayals of sex affect young lives more broadly than just hastening sexual initiation. We will look at sexual partnership formation and the psychological consequences of sexual partnerships and activities.

Summary

Television and its effects can be a polarizing topic among lay people, with some people viewing it as a wholly problematic entity and others seeing it as benign entertainment. Media effects research suggests that the truth lies somewhere between these positions and that television effects depend strongly on the specifics of the content, the viewer, and the viewing context. Given current television content and the tendency for many youth to watch television without their parents present [2], there is reason for concern regarding possible effects on sexual development.

Acknowledgments

The contributions of Dale Kunkel, Vicky Rideout at The Henry J. Kaiser Family Foundation, and the RAND TAS research group were invaluable to the work described, as were the support and cooperation of the teen participants and their parents.

References

[1] LeVay S, Valente S. Human sexuality. Sunderland (MA): Sinauer Associates, Inc.; 2003.

[2] Kaiser Family Foundation. Teens, sex and TV survey. Menlo Park (CA): The Henry J. Kaiser Family Foundation; 2002.

[3] Steele JR. Teenage sexuality and media practice: factoring in the influences of family, friends, and school. J Sex Res 1999;36:331–41.

[4] Roe K. The school and music in adolescent socialization. In: Lull J, editor. Popular music and communication. Newbury Park (CA): Sage; 1987.

[5] Bandura A. Self-efficacy: toward a unifying theory of behavior change. Psychol Rev 1977;84: 191–215.

[6] Delameter J. The social control of sexuality. Annu Rev Sociol 1981;7:263–90.

[7] Lowry D, Shidler J. Prime time TV portrayals of sex, "safe sex" and AIDS: a longitudinal analysis. Journal Q 1993;70:628–37.

[8] Greenberg BS, Brown JD, Buerkel-Rothfuss N. Media, sex, and the adolescent. Cresskill (NJ): Hampton Press; 1993.

[9] Kunkel D, Cope KM, Colvin C. Sexual messages in "family hour" TV: content and context. Menlo Park (CA): The Henry J. Kaiser Family Foundation; 1996.

[10] Franzblau S, Sprafkin JN, Rubinstein EA. Sex on TV: a content analysis. J Commun 1977;27(2): 164–70.

[11] Greenberg BS. Content trends in media sex. In: Zillman D, Jennings B, Huston A, editors. Media, children, and the family: social scientific, pschodynamic, and clinical perspectives. Hillsdale (NJ): Lawrence Erlbaum Associates; 1994. p. 165–82.

[12] Sapolsky B. Sexual acts and references on prime-time TV: a two-year look. Southern Speech Communication Journal 1982;47:212–26.

[13] Sapolsky BS, Tabarlet JO. Sex in primetime TV: 1979 vs. 1989. Journal of Broadcasting and Electronic Media 1991;35:505–16.

[14] Sprafkin JN, Silverman LT. Update: physically intimate and sexual behavior on prime-time television, 1978–79. J Commun 1981;31:34–40.

[15] Kunkel D, Eyal K, Biely E, et al. Sex on TV3: a biennial report to the Kaiser Family Foundation. Menlo Park (CA): The Henry J. Kaiser Family Foundation; 2003.

[16] Lowry D, Towles D. Soap opera portrayals of sex, contraception, and sexually transmitted diseases. J Commun 1988;39:76–83.

[17] Bandura A. Social foundations of thought and action: a social cognitive theory. Englewood Cliffs (NJ): Prentice Hall; 1986.

[18] The National Campaign to Prevent Teen Pregnancy. With one voice 2002: America's adults and teens sound off about teen pregnancy. Washington (DC): The National Campaign to Prevent Teen Pregnancy; 2002.

[19] Brown JD, Newcomer SF. Television viewing and adolescents' sexual behavior. J Homosex 1991;21:77–91.

[20] Peterson JL, Moore KA, Furstenberg Jr FF. Television viewing and early initiation of sexual intercourse: is there a link? J Homosex 1991;21:93–118.

[21] Collins R, Elliott M, Kanouse D, et al. Watching sex on TV predicts adolescent initiation of sexual behavior. Pediatrics 2004;114(3):e280–9.

[22] Centers for Disease Control and Prevention. Trends in sexual risk behaviors in high school students: United States, 1991–2001. MMWR Morb Mortal Wkly Rep 2002;51:856–9.

[23] Lewin T. Teen-agers alter sexual practices, thinking risks will be avoided. New York Times. April 5, 1997;section 1:8.

[24] Stepp LS. Parents are alarmed by an unsettling new fad in middle schools: oral sex. Washington Post. July 8, 1999;A1.

[25] Gates GJ, Sonenstein FL. Heterosexual genital sexual activity among adolescent males: 1988 and 1995. Fam Plann Perspect 2000;32:295–7, 304.

[26] Kanouse D, Collins R, Elliott M, et al. Noncoital and coital sexual behaviors of adolescents

in the US. Presented at the Annual Meeting of the Population Association of America. Minneapolis (MN), May 1–3, 2003.

[27] Institute of Medicine. The best intentions: unintended pregnancy and the well-being of children and families. Washington (DC): National Academy Press; 1995.

[28] Singh S, Darroch JE. Trends in sexual activity among adolescent American women: 1982–1995. Fam Plann Perspect 1999;31:212–9.

[29] Martino S, Collins R, Kanouse D, et al. Social cognitive processes mediating the relationship between exposure to sex on television and adolescents' sexual behavior. J Pers Soc Psychol, in press.

[30] MacKinnon D, Lockwood C, Hoffman J, et al. A comparison of methods to test the significance of the mediation and intervening variable effects. Psychol Methods 2002;7:83–104.

[31] Brown J, Schulze L. The effects of race, gender, and fandom on audience interpretations of Madonna's music videos. J Commun 1990;40:88–102.

[32] Comstock G, Chaffee S, Katzman N, et al. Television and human behavior. New York: Columbia University Press; 1978.

[33] Smith EA, Udry JR. Coital and non-coital sexual behaviors of white and black adolescents. Am J Public Health 1985;75:1200–3.

[34] Walsh-Childers K, Brown J. Adolescents' acceptance of sex-role stereotypes and television viewing. In: Greenberg BS, Brown JD, Buerkel-Rothfus NL, editors. Media, sex and the adolescent. Kreskill (NJ): Hampton Press, Inc.; 1993. p. 117–35.

[35] Greenberg B, Atkin C. Learning about minorities from television: a research agenda. In: Mitchell-Kernan GBC, editor. Television and the socialization of the minority child. New York: Academic Press; 1982. p. 215–43.

[36] Kaiser Family Foundation. Documenting the power of entertainment television: the impact of a brief health message in one of TV's most popular dramas. Menlo Park (CA): The Henry J. Kaiser Family Foundation; 1997.

[37] Kennedy M, O'Leary A, Beck V, et al. Increases in calls to the CDC national STD and AIDS hotline following AIDS-related episodes in a soap opera. J Commun 2004;54:287–301.

[38] Collins R, Elliott M, Berry S, et al. Entertainment television as a healthy sex-educator: the impact of condom-efficacy information in an episode of Friends. Pediatrics 2003;112:1115–21.

[39] Brown JD, Pardun CJ. Little in common: racial and gender differences in adolescents' television diets. Journal of Broadcasting & Electronic Media 2004;48(2):266–78.

[40] Jemmott JBD, Jemmott LS, Fong GT. Reductions in HIV risk-associated sexual behaviors among black male adolescents: effects of an AIDS prevention intervention. Am J Public Health 1992;82:372–7 [Published erratum appears in Am J Public Health 1992;82(5):684.]

[41] NIMH Multisite HIV Prevention Trial Group. A test of factors mediating the relationship between unwanted sexual activity during childhood and risky sexual practices among women enrolled in the NIMH Multisite HIV Prevention Trial. Womens Health 2001;33:163–80.

[42] Kim J, Collins R, Kanouse D, et al. Sexual readiness, household policies, and other predictors of adolescents' exposure to sexual content in mainstream entertainment television. Media & Psychology, in press.

[43] Levine J. Harmful to minors: the perils of protecting children from sex. Minneapolis (MN): University of Minnesota Press; 2002.

[44] Brown J, Halpern C, L'Engle K. Mass media as sexual super peer? J Adolesc Health, in press.

[45] Ward L. Does television exposure affect emerging adults' attitudes and assumptions about sexual relationships? Correlational and experimental confirmation. J Youth Adolesc 2002;31:1–15.

[46] Fernandez-Collado C, Greenberg B, Korzenny F, et al. Sexual intimacy and drug use in TV series. J Commun 1978;28:30–7.

[47] Greenberg B, Graef D, Fernandez-Collado C, et al. Sexual intimacy on commercial TV during prime time. Journal Q 1980;57:211–5.

[48] Buerkel-Rothfuss N, Mayes S. Soap opera viewing: the cultivation effect. J Commun 1981;31:108–15.

ELSEVIER
SAUNDERS

Child Adolesc Psychiatric Clin N Am
14 (2005) 387–404

CHILD AND
ADOLESCENT
PSYCHIATRIC CLINICS
OF NORTH AMERICA

Children's Exposure to Violent Video Games and Desensitization to Violence

Jeanne B. Funk, PhD

Department of Psychology, University of Toledo, MS 948, 2801 West Bancroft, Toledo,
OH 43606-3390, USA

Concern about the impact of media violence on children and adolescents is shared by the six signatories to the Joint Statement on the Impact of Entertainment Violence on Children: the American Academy of Pediatrics, the American Academy of Child and Adolescent Psychiatry, the American Medical Association, the American Psychological Association, the American Academy of Family Physicians, and the American Psychiatric Association [1]. Although a less well-researched medium at this point, violent video and computer games (referred to simply as video games) may have particular impact because of their actively engaging, content-generating nature [2,3]. Recent content analyses suggested that up to 90% of all video games contain some sort of violent content, with at least half of these games including the potential for serious harm toward game characters [4]. Such violent video games have become especially popular, even with relatively young children. In a recent survey of first through third graders, 53% of the children's favorite games had violent content, as rated by the children themselves (Jeanne Funk, PhD, Margaret Chan, unpublished data, 2004). In another recent survey of middle school volunteers, students listed and rated up to three favorite games using a list of six categories and descriptors developed with the help of children and adolescents [5] and used in several previous studies. In that study, 99% of boys and 84% of girls categorized at least one of their current preferred video games as having violent content [6]. The inescapable conclusion is that across childhood and adolescence and across gender, violent video games enjoy considerable popularity.

E-mail address: jeanne.funk@utoledo.edu

Given this widespread popularity, concern has been raised about the impact of repeated video game play. Desensitization to violence frequently is cited as being an outcome of exposure to media violence and a condition that contributes to increased aggression, because desensitization prevents the initiation of moral reasoning processes that normally inhibit aggression. This article presents convergent data from neuroscience and behavioral science to examine potential relationships between playing violent video games and desensitization to violence.

Desensitization

Although not yet well studied, desensitization is one of the key mechanisms proposed to explain potential negative impact from playing violent video games (N.L. Carnagey, B.J. Bushman, C. Anderson, unpublished data) [3]. In clinical psychiatry and psychology, desensitization is a well-studied phenomenon, particularly with respect to treatment. For example, desensitization via diminished arousal or systematic habituation of neurophysiologic responses is a well-established and manipulable phenomenon. In behavior therapies the goal is to reduce or eliminate certain responses through graded and supervised exposure to stimuli that are initially anxiety provoking [7]. Helping a patient become desensitized to subconscious cognitive and emotional reactions is one of the key goals of newer trauma-focused therapies, such as eye movement desensitization [8].

Occurring as an unconscious process over time, desensitization to violence can be defined as the reduction or eradication of cognitive and emotional and, as a result behavioral, responses to a violent stimulus [9,10]. Cognitive desensitization is apparent when beliefs about violence are altered. Once believing violence to be uncommon and appalling, persons who experience cognitive desensitization view it as mundane and without particular negative valence. Emotional desensitization is apparent when negative emotional reactions no longer occur to previously disturbing stimuli. For example, in one large sample study of middle school children, researchers found no correlation between greater exposure to community violence and increased distress [11]. Cognitive and emotional desensitization may result in part from diminished negative physiologic arousal.

The behavioral outcome of desensitization to violence may be a failure to intervene to stop violence or the active commission of a violent act. Regarding the possible role of violent video games in desensitization to violence, it has been reported that the US Army frequently uses such games to desensitize soldiers during training [12]. In actual combat situations that involve military aircraft and tanks, there is typically no direct, personal visual identification of targets. Instead, icons tracked on computerized displays that bear an uncanny resemblance to training video games lock on targets automatically. Whether by design or by chance, military training on enhanced video game systems may cause cognitive and emotional desensitization that obscures the moral implications of activating weapons from military vehicles or aircraft. Such potential desensitizing material is not limited to the military. Using actual news clips and satellite pictures, Kuma/ War is a controversial online game that gives players the opportunity to re-enact actual recent battles from the current war in Iraq and Afghanistan, with newer battles being released every few weeks in parallel with actual combat developments. This game has been criticized as exploiting the death of American soldiers. One critic stated: "Have we become so desensitized to images of violence and war that we can no longer take them seriously? Are we willing to watch real deaths turned into our own entertainment" [13]?

Desensitization in context

It is important to understand how desensitization is related to the other processes derived from social cognitive and information-processing traditions to explain how exposure to violent media may have negative impact in the short and long term. Although not as widely tested as for some other media, especially television, these processes can be applied to understanding the potential impact of exposure to violent video games [14,15]. The mechanisms are listed and simplified descriptions are provided in Table 1. As an example of how these processes may be applicable in playing video games, consider the following scenario: While playing a violent video game, a child or adolescent observes and imitates game-specific actions, such as hypervigilance to possible threats and automatic aggressive responses to avoid destruction. This could lead, out of the person's awareness, to the development of aggressive scripts, with scripts being representations of situation-specific behavioral guidelines. These aggressive scripts may be automatized through the repetition required to succeed in playing violent video games, which makes them readily accessible in other situations, even situations that do not involve video game play. If aggressive scripts are primed by a previously neutral cue, then the individual could misperceive a benign situation as one requiring an aggressive response. If an individual has been desensitized to violence through repeated exposure to violent video game play, he or she will lack the capacity to inhibit an aggressive response. For example, a child or adolescent may misjudge an innocent nudge in a school hallway as being intentional and respond with aggression.

In addition to considering these primary mechanisms, it is important to bear in mind potential moderators of the impact of video game and other media violence because it is obvious that individuals are not affected equally by such exposure. Key individual differences include age, gender, characteristic level of aggressiveness (trait aggression), and intelligence. Psychosocial moderators may include cultural environment, socioeconomic status, and family values and control of child's exposure to media violence. Depending on the nature and interactions of each of these variables, individuals may be more or less affected by

Table 1
Mechanisms to explain the impact of violent media

Mechanism	Description	Timespan of impact of violent media
Observational learning	After observing the behavior of others, these behaviors are integrated into the individual's behavioral repertoire	Both short and long term
Imitation	Learned behaviors are taken from the repertoire and exhibited	Short term
Schema development	Knowledge structures about the typical organization of daily experience develop as a way to manage information efficiently	Long term
Script development	Specific types of schemas for events develop to guide behavioral reactions	
Priming	Violent media activate aggressive schemas	Short term
Automatization of aggressive schemas	Repetitive priming of aggressive schemas makes them chronically accessible	
Arousal	Physiologic arousal occurs in response to a particular stimuli; aggressive stimuli cause aggressive arousal	Short term
Excitation transfer	Misattribution of the source of aggressive arousal; could lead to aggression	Short term
Cognitive desensitization	Belief that violence is common and mundane decreases likelihood that moral evaluation will inhibit aggression	Long term
Emotional desensitization	Numbing of emotional response to violent actions or experiences decreases likelihood that moral evaluation will inhibit aggression	Long term

For a comprehensive discussion of these theoretical mechanisms, see Refs. [14,15].

media violence. Two articles have provided a review of the limited research on moderators of exposure to video game violence [2,16].

Desensitization and moral evaluation

In the behavioral realm, measuring correlates of desensitization to violence may improve our ability to study this phenomenon. For example, as may occur in the US Army's use of video games in training, it is proposed that desensitization to violence impacts moral evaluation, a process that is triggered when the situation requires that ethical beliefs guide behavioral choice [17]. Once this process is initiated, higher-order emotions, such as empathy, and knowledge structures, such as attitudes relevant to the situation, are activated. Desensitization to the cues necessary to initiate moral evaluation processes allows behavioral selection without consideration of moral implications. Moral evaluation is a complex process with many triggering and maintaining features. Empathy and attitudes toward violence are two of the critical measurable components of moral evaluation through which desensitization to violence can be examined.

Empathy

Empathy, defined as the capacity to understand and, to some extent, experience the feelings of another, is considered to be critical for the development and use of moral behavior. The experience of empathy results from the activation and interaction of perceptual, cognitive, and emotional processes [18]. There is considerable interest in understanding the neuroanatomy of empathy, and researchers observe that networks of interconnected neurons must be activated for empathic responding to occur [19]. It is worth noting, however, that damage to the prefrontal cortex in childhood is associated with a lack of empathy in adulthood [20].

Behaviors consistent with empathy have been found in children as young as 20 months [21], although some researchers believe that these early manifestations are significantly different from the sophisticated and cognitively mediated processes that develop within the next few years [22]. Although based on inborn potential, the development of mature empathy requires opportunities to view empathic models, interact with others, and experience feedback about one's behavioral choices [23]. The development of self-awareness and self-regulatory behaviors also is necessary for mature empathic responding [24,25].

Hoffman [26] emphasized the role of inductive discipline by parents in the development of moral behavior in relation to empathic responding. Inductive discipline requires children to imagine how they would feel in a victim's situation and encourages the development of scripts for moral behavior. Subsequently, in a conflict situation, these empathy-based scripts automatically are triggered and guide behavioral choice. Considerable experimental evidence exists that empathy inhibits aggressive behavior and that lower empathy is a factor in increased aggression [27–30]. For example, in one questionnaire study, aggressive elementary school children showed less empathy than their nonaggressive peers in that they cared less about the damaging consequences of aggression by themselves on others than did their nonaggressive peers [31]. Examining adolescents' empathy in relation to exposure to community violence, researchers found that exposure to community violence combined with low empathy predicted actual aggressive behavior [32].

Returning to the potential relationship between playing violent video games and empathy, it has been noted that success at these games requires the choice of violent actions that are often presented as normal, acceptable, and fun while concealing realistic consequences [33,34]. In violent video games, victims are frequently dehumanized, a strategy that is commonly used in real-life situations to minimize the activation of moral reasoning [29]. For example, in the popular game "Grand Theft Auto: Vice City," players are rewarded for soliciting and then killing prostitutes. The most recent release of the series, "Grand Theft Auto: San Andreas," features home invasion and robbery as primary rewarded activities. Although unproven as yet, on a theoretical basis, the increasing realism of video games may increase the likelihood of some sort of generalization outside the game situation [14]. In the absence of mitigating factors, playing violent video games could decrease an individual's capacity for empathy, which could contribute to desensitization to violence.

Attitudes toward violence

Attitudes are a type of knowledge structure that result from complex and selective evaluation processes that are based on an individual's experience with, associated cognitions about, and affective reactions to a situation or object [35]. Classical conditioning processes that pair neutral attitude objects with liked or disliked stimuli and reinforcement-based operant conditioning contribute to attitude development [36]. Attitudes may be formed out of awareness, as in the effect of advertising, or with purpose and conscious effort, as in the case of the deliberations of a jury. Experimental evidence exists that powerful attitudes can be developed even in young children. For example, preschoolers differentially evaluate their own group versus another group based on various characteristics, including relatively central ones (eg, race) or more transient ones (eg, the color of t-shirts) [37]. Similar findings are reported in a comparable study of elementary school children [38]. Established attitudes may interfere with accurate perception in new situations, and can exert a direct, cognitively unmediated impact on judgment and behavior.

The development of attitudes toward violence is influenced by many factors, including exposure to violence in real life and in the media and interactions with family and peers [10,39]. Surveys of more than 4000 first- through sixth-grade children living in urban neighborhoods identified a relationship between exposure to community violence and attitudes and beliefs supporting aggression and increases in aggressive behavior [40]. Children who experience abuse have been found to develop biased attitudes, in particular an increased tendency to attribute hostile intent to others [41], and individuals who experienced violence as children are more likely to engage in family violence in later life [42]. It is worth noting, however, that the relationship between early experiences of family violence and later violent behavior has been shown to be moderated by empathy [43]. In a survey of seventh- through ninth-grade students, a positive relationship between being the target of peer aggression and more positive attitudes about aggression was identified [44]. A significant positive relationship was found between pro-violence attitudes and self-reported aggression toward peers.

Pro-violence attitudes play an important role in the translation of negative cognitions and affect into behavior [39,44]. Several studies have demonstrated that pro-violence attitudes in children and adolescents are associated with aggressive behavior [45–48]. Researchers surveyed 473 inner-city middle school students to determine their exposure to community violence and their level of distress and aggression [11]. There were no significant relationships between violence exposure and distress, although higher exposure was related to more aggression in girls. The researchers suggested that children with chronic violence exposure become desensitized to violence and develop the attitude that it is normative. Violent video games also promote the development of the attitude that violence is acceptable, commonplace, and enjoyable.

Surveys relating video game playing and desensitization to violence

Several surveys have investigated potential relationships between playing violent video games and aspects of moral evaluation. In one study, a negative relationship was found between simple frequency of video game use and questionnaire-measured empathy in Japanese fourth- through sixth-grade students [49]. In a survey of 15- to 19-year-old individuals, relationships between game preference, self-esteem, and empathy were examined [50]. Although no significant relationships were found with self-esteem, adolescents whose favorite game was violent had lower empathy scores on the "fantasy empathy" subscale of the Interpersonal Reactivity Index. Sixth-grade students were surveyed to examine relationships between a preference for violent video games, attitudes toward violence, and empathy [51]. It was anticipated that a stronger preference for violent games would be associated with lower empathy and stronger pro-violence attitudes. Relationships were in the expected direction, although marginally significant, with small effect sizes. Perhaps more important, children with a high preference for violent games and high time commitment to playing the games demonstrated the lowest empathy. In a survey of fourth- and fifth-grade students, long-term exposure to violent video games was associated with lower empathy and stronger pro-violence attitudes [3]. In this study, long-term exposure was calculated by multiplying the percentage of favorite games that were violent (as listed and categorized by the participant) by the time spent per week playing video games. This procedure is similar to procedures used by other researchers in categorizing exposure to media violence. In another study, no difference was found in immediate empathic or aggressive responding after 5- to 12-year-old children played a violent or nonviolent video game. A long-term preference for violent video games was associated with lower empathy, however [52]. It must be acknowledged that surveys cannot address the direction of the relationship between lower empathy, stronger pro-violence attitudes, and exposure to violent video games. Although further research is needed to address this question, current results are consistent with the hypothesis that long-term exposure to violent video games may encourage lower empathy and stronger pro-violence attitudes that contribute to and reflect desensitization to violence.

Behavioral evidence for media-moderated desensitization to violence

Behavioral evidence for desensitization to violence as a result of exposure to media violence is limited to a handful of studies, including only one study of video game exposure. In one classic media violence study, children who first viewed a film with aggression took significantly longer to seek adult assistance when faced with an altercation between younger children than children who did not see the film [53]. These findings were replicated more recently using contemporary video materials [54], which provided further evidence that viewing violence can increases one's tolerance for violent behavior. Using a similar paradigm, researchers recently demonstrated that playing a violent video game slowed adults' response time to help a presumed violence victim, relative to individuals who played a nonviolent game (N.L. Carnagey, B.J. Bushman, C. Anderson, unpublished data). In that study, a long-term preference for playing violent video games also was associated with being less helpful to a presumed victim of violence.

Neurophysiologic foundations of desensitization

Based on our current knowledge of brain mechanisms, it is reasonable to hypothesize ways in which desensitization could result from continuous exposure to violent video games from a neurophysiologic perspective. Perry and Pollard [55] suggested that overexposure to technology may deprive children of experiences that promote the development of the caring potentials of their brain. In other words, heavy time commitment to playing video games could prevent children and adolescents from engaging in the social interactions necessary to allow the expression of their genetic potential to develop the neural systems that regulate socioemotional behavior. If this were to occur, brain areas that regulate moral and other social judgments could fail to develop fully. This would not technically be desensitization but rather a failure to develop the processes of moral reasoning that guide behavioral choice.

Apart from sheer time commitment, playing video games with violent content may result in desensitization as a result of repeated exposure to violence presented as necessary, fun, and without negative consequences. An individual's conceptual base for human experience evolves based on a continuous process that involves sensation, processing, and storing life experiences. As time goes on, new input is matched against previously stored representations of situation-specific activity, which are termed "scripts." For some individuals, repeated exposure to violent video games could result in the development of automatized scripts in which aggressive or violent behavior is chronically accessible to behavioral expression. The process of moral reasoning simply would be irrelevant.

Neurodevelopment is a continuous, dynamic process that is sequential and use-dependent [55,56]. When presented with a repetitive, structured, patterned experience, permanent changes in brain reactivity typically occur [56]. If the process of moral reasoning is chronically subverted, then disuse-related extinction of the emotional reactivity substrate of moral reasoning may result. In that case, there would be no arousal of a distress response to violence, which is essentially the definition of desensitization.

Measuring neurophysiologic correlates of emotion and behavior

The development of safer neuroimaging techniques has accelerated interest in establishing neurophysiologic correlates of behavior, particularly aggression and violence. For example, results of one study suggested that the brain activation patterns of aggressive adolescents are different from those of nonaggressive adolescents [57]. In seeking the roots of aggression, some researchers are focusing on the amygdala because of its well-established role in processing emotion. For example, using functional MRI (fMRI) scanning and displays of facial emotion, researchers have demonstrated that the amygdala plays a central role in processing emotion but that this response is moderated by the task relevance of the emotional content of the stimulus [58]. Other fMRI work suggests that although the amygdala is activated by emotional stimuli, moral judgments associated with emotionally evocative stimuli are specific to subregions of the orbitofrontal cortex [59].

Many researchers are examining malfunctions in the prefrontal cortex and associated basal ganglia and limbic systems to explain why brain circuits that typically inhibit aggressive impulses are not effective [60]. In one recent fMRI study, imagining aggression resulted in a shutdown of frontal lobe activity [61]. In a real-life situation, this would be expected to prevent the activation of processes of moral reasoning that would typically inhibit aggression. Grafman [62] proposed that what he terms "structured event complexes" control social behavior. This term parallels what authors in other literature term "scripts." Behavioral and imaging studies suggest that the prefrontal cortex is important for storing and accessing scripts [63,64]. Through studies that used behavioral and imaging data, Wood et al [64] differentially localized social and nonsocial (group versus individual) structured event complexes or scripts in the prefrontal cortex. A review of cases with acquired cerebral damage indicates that disruptions to prefrontal regions cause profound and diverse disturbances in interpersonal relationships [20]. In particular, patients with acquired cerebral lesions scored significantly lower on a measure of empathy than the normal comparison group, and patients with orbitofrontal lesions had the lowest empathy scores when compared with patients with lesions in other areas of the frontal lobe [65].

Video game playing and brain function

Although still limited, imaging studies are beginning to address how playing video games may affect brain function. Two initial reports received considerable media attention but do not seem to have been published in an academic medium. In one study, brain activation patterns while playing a computer-based game were compared with patterns recorded while adolescents were doing arithmetic [66]. Doing arithmetic stimulated the frontal lobe, but playing computer games did not, which raised concern according to the researcher that the frontal lobe could be underdeveloped in frequent game players. That conclusion was considered premature by many experts, however, and the study could not be located in a peer-reviewed publication. Japanese researcher Akio Mori coined the term "video game brain" [67] after finding that more play among 6- to 29-year-old individuals was associated with a lack of beta brainwave activity and more irritability and concentration problems. Mori also speculated that frequent video game playing could lead to underuse and underdevelopment of the frontal region of the brain, which potentially could alter emotional processing. That report was widely criticized because the researcher did not reveal the exact placement of electroencephalographic electrodes or the analytical methods used to interpret the traces in any peer-reviewed venue [66].

Other researchers have presented their findings under traditional peer-reviewed conditions. Results of an fMRI study were presented at the Eighty-eighth Scientific Assembly and Annual Meeting of the Radiological Society of North America [57]. Brain activation patterns were evaluated in response to viewing scenes from violent and nonviolent video games in 19 adolescents with and 19 adolescents without disruptive behavior disorders. Aggressive adolescents had less activation in the frontal lobes and less overall activation than comparison adolescents while viewing scenes from the violent video game. Comparison group adolescents with high past violent media exposure had different activation patterns than control subjects with low violent media exposure. The researchers speculated that past exposure to violent media may change how the brain responds to a current stimulus.

A symposium on the effects of playing video games on brain activity was held in Tokyo at the Thirty-fourth Annual Conference of the International Simulation and Gaming Association in August, 2003. One group of researchers reported on the use of near infrared spectroscopy to examine brain activity in the dorsal prefrontal cortex in three experiments with six adult participants [68]. In the first experiment, four types of games were played for 5 minutes each, including a "first person shooter" game. There was evidence of deactivation of the prefrontal cortex during all types of video game play. In the second experiment, participants simply observed visual stimuli from the video games and two other images (natural scenery and a mosaic). There was significantly more prefrontal deactivation while watching the video game images, possibly because participants were imagining game play. In the third experiment, participants simply tapped a button on a game controller at regular intervals, which resulted in an increase in activation of the prefrontal cortex.

In another study presented at the symposium, researchers examined the relationship between long-term video game playing and functions of the prefrontal cortex [69]. Twelve undergraduates were selected based on their experience playing video games and were divided into two groups: "experts" and "novices." They were given a reading test and spatial working memory tests related to the functions of the prefrontal cortex. There were no negative relationships between long-term play and test performance in this small sample. Expert players were faster than novices on spatial tasks. The researchers proposed that playing video games might improve reaction time even for prefrontal tasks. Cognitive abilities of six high-usage and six low-usage video game players were compared in a study that examined possible relationships between long-term video game play and basic cognitive abilities as measured by the Japanese version of the Wechsler Adult Intelligence Scale-Revised. Positive and negative findings were associated with long-term game playing, with negative relationships found for basic verbal and performance abilities and positive relationships identified for faster reaction times [70].

Symposium organizers concluded that more work is needed, including longitudinal research, to understand how specific game content may affect brain activity, how brain development may be affected by heavy play at young ages, whether prefrontal deactivation occurs during other activities of daily living, and how personality and lifestyle variables may moderate game influence [71]. Research to answer some of these questions is currently underway at the Annenberg School for Communication. For example, one group of researchers is using fMRI technology to examine activation of the anterior cingulate cortex during game play [72]. The anterior cingulate cortex is believed to be involved in linking emotional and cognitive information processing and could play a crucial role in how the cognitive tasks involved in playing a violent video game are transformed into emotional changes found in previous research, such as increased hostility. The activation of the anterior cingulate cortex is higher if the user experiences the game as real or has a feeling of "being there," compared with users who approach the game as pure fiction. Potentially, if players are instructed to approach the game as fiction rather than real, there would be less anterior cingulate cortex activation and less transfer.

Summary and implications

This article presented converging data from behavioral science and neuroscience to examine how playing violent video games may contribute to desensitization to violence. In the behavioral realm, there is limited evidence of immediate desensitization after playing a violent video game. Examining correlates of desensitization, relationships have been reported between lower empathy, stronger pro-violence attitudes, and long-term exposure to violent video games. Neuroimaging studies suggest that a short period of playing video games results in deactivation of the prefrontal area of the cortex, which potentially impacts this area's ability to act as gatekeeper for higher cognitive functions. Research on acquired cerebral damage suggests that the prefrontal cortex may be especially important in empathic processing and the regulation of empathic behaviors. Specifically, researchers speculate that orbitofrontal lesions may inhibit the emotional aspects of empathic processing [20]. Future research on the long-term effects of video game play should pay special attention to the relationship between deactivation of the prefrontal cortex and empathy.

From their review of recent literature, Shuren and Grafman [73] concluded that neural networks, including various regions of the orbitoprefrontal cortex, perform functions that are critical for reasoning processes. These networks allow an individual to identify potential responses and their likely outcomes and recognize the behavioral relevance of response options. Disruptions in the development of the prefrontal cortex may lead to disruption in various aspects of reasoning, including moral reasoning. This finding raises the issue of how video game play may differentially impact children at different ages. Currently, only limited information is available about the long-term neurophysiologic effects of the repeated and lengthy game play that is experienced by many individuals. As noted by Perry and Pollard [55], whereas experience in adults alters the organized brain, in children experience organizes the developing brain. It is important to note that currently the chain of reasoning that links playing video games, brain functioning, and behavior remains hypothetical. It is critical that future research examine the potential long-term relationships between video game event-related changes in brain functioning related to reasoning and the development of reasoning skills in children, especially moral reasoning.

The current attempt to integrate convergent data from different research traditions may not be persuasive for persons who demand unequivocal experimental evidence that exposure to violent video games results in lasting behavioral change [74]. In studies of human behavior, however, randomized, controlled experiments cannot always be held to be the gold standard [75]. Instead, we must seek multiple lines of evidence from different sources—some of which will be correlational—that point in the same direction. Related research already has identified changes in brain functioning and behavior that generalize outside the game-playing situation. For example, game proponents often have claimed that game playing improves visual motor skills, but data that support generalization remain limited. In one supportive study, exposure to action video games (ie, games that require a player's attention to be distributed and rapidly moved around the visual field) led to improvement in aspects of visual attention that generalized to other tasks [76]. Video games also have been used to effect behavioral change in attention deficit hyperactivity disorder using video game–related biofeedback [77]. Developed by NASA researchers and termed "instrument functionality feedback training," the approach uses instrumental learning and classical conditional principles to reward participants with better control of a video game joystick when faster brainwave signals are amplified. After 40 training sessions, attention deficit hyperactivity disorder symptoms improved significantly as a result of the video game–moderated training and after a standard biofeedback approach, as indicated by parent report. Children and parents reported greater satisfaction with the video game–based treatment, however. Other evidence recently was presented for improvement in self-esteem through video game–based training that relies on classical conditioning and the automatization of thoughts [78]. It seems reasonable to conclude that the intentional change that occurs as a result of playing video games in experimental situations supports the position that unintended consequences from typical play must be studied carefully.

In the leisure area, one of the newest developments is a video game that is controlled directly by a player's brain waves [79]. Called "Mind Balance," the game is a prototype that uses a wireless headset called Cerebus, which uses direct electroencephalography, cerebral data nodes, and Bluetooth wireless technology, to make a direct brain-computer interface. This technology is ultimately expected to benefit people who have limited body movement and provide a means of communication for individuals who otherwise would not have this ability. Rapid developments in devices such as the Cerebus probably will make widespread gaming applications a reality within a few years. The developments increase the urgency in examining whether, when, and how playing video games may cause changes in brain functioning and whether those changes that occur are lasting and problematic.

This article has begun the development of a conceptual model to explain the relationship between video game playing, brain functioning, moral reasoning, and behavior. Much more work is needed, however, to identify and understand the complex relationships among initial physiologic arousal, brain activation, social cognitive processing, behavioral outcome, and the possible moderating effects of individual differences. Currently, professionals with a commitment to children and adolescents should work to increase parental awareness of the potential impact of playing video games. At the very least, playing video games may displace other more developmentally valuable activities, such as outdoor activities with friends, and parents should be encouraged to monitor and limit children's playing time. Parents and professionals should familiarize themselves with the industry's game rating system, including content descriptors. The Entertainment Software Rating Board Website (http://www.esrb.com) is a good source of information on the age-based categories and content descriptors. Although not completely representative of the views of the public [80–82], the ratings do provide some useful information about violent games. Because research suggests that there is potential for negative impact for some children, clinicians should encourage parents to restrict younger children's access to violent video games. For older children and adolescents, parents can use examples from the child's experience or news presentations to help them recognize the difference between the impact and consequences of real-life and video game violence. Some schools have media literacy programs that encourage critical thinking about media presentations [83]. Even a brief parallel parent education program could help parents to continue the effort to encourage critical thinking skills at home [84,85].

In the absence of restraint on the part of game developers, public policy to limit the sale of violent games may be made. Several efforts are underway, with Washington being the first state to attempt to regulate the sale of video games, in this case, games that depict violence against law enforcement officials. In July, 2004, the United States District Court found that games are protected under the First Amendment, overturning the Washington legislation. In California, the state senate passed a bill in August, 2004 that required signage that clearly identifies the existence of a video game rating system and provides information about the ratings. The bill was signed into law by Governor Schwarzenegger in September. In December, 2004, Illinois Governor Blagojevich proposed restrictions that subject retailers to potential jail time and fines of up to $5000 if they sell or rent violent or sexually charged video games to individuals under 18 years of age. Previous attempts (eg, by the city of Indianapolis) to impose penalties for failure to regulate sales of games with violent content have been overturned through claims that video games are an art form that is protected by the First Amendment. Because of the increase in gratuitous sexual violence in video games, some leaders believe that obscenity laws or other laws that prohibit the distribution of "harmful matter" to minors (eg, laws that govern sales of tobacco and alcohol) may be invoked. The gaming industry and the research community must communicate more effectively and routinely about extant and emerging data on the effects of playing video games, especially games with violent content. Increasing the moral context of games to force players to live with the real-world consequences of actions within the game context could limit negative impact on moral reasoning. The US Army has released a free online game to demonstrate aspects of Army life to potential recruits. Although this is a first-person shooter game available free of charge to anyone who claims to be age 13 or older, players must follow specific rules of engagement, which prohibit gratuitous violence. A recently released online multiplayer role-playing game, "World of Warcraft," reportedly has a built-in sensor so that players receive diminishing rewards after 6 hours of continuous play, anticipating that this will limit excess time commitment. Although these developments are encouraging, they are far from typical.

Playing violent video games is only one potential route to desensitization to violence. It is, however, a route that is optional and preventable, unlike most exposure to community violence. Current findings from behavioral science and neuroscience are suggestive, incomplete, and troubling. Caveat emptor.

Acknowledgments

The assistance of Dr. Gregory Meyer in providing comments on a draft of the article is gratefully acknowledged.

References

[1] Congressional Public Health Summit. Joint statement on the impact of entertainment violence on children. Available at: http://www.aap.org/advocacy/releases/jstmtevc.htm. Accessed May 7, 2004.

[2] Anderson CA, Bushman BJ. Effects of violent video games on aggressive behavior, aggressive cognition, aggressive affect, physiological arousal, and prosocial behavior: a meta-analytic review of the scientific literature. Psychol Sci 2001;12:353–9.

[3] Funk JB, Bechtoldt-Baldacci H, Pasold T, et al. Violence exposure in real-life, video games, television, movies, and the Internet: is there desensitization? J Adolesc 2004;27:23–39.

[4] Children Now. Fair play? Violence, gender and race in video games. Los Angeles: Children Now; 2001.

[5] Funk JB, Buchman D. Video game controversies. Pediatr Ann 1995;24:91–4.

[6] Funk JB, Fox C, Chan M, et al. A validation study of the Children's Empathy Questionnaire using Rasch analysis. Poster accepted for presentation at the 2005 Biennial Meeting of the Society for Research in Child Development. Atlanta (GA), April 7, 2005.

[7] Wolpe J. The practice of behavior therapy. 2nd edition. Oxford (United Kingdom): Pergamon; 1973.

[8] Shapiro F. EMDR 12 years after its introduction: past and future research. J Clin Psychol 2002; 58:1–22.

[9] Eron L. Seeing is believing: how viewing violence alters attitudes and aggressive behavior. In: Bohart AC, Stipek DJ, editors. Constructive and destructive behavior: implications for family, school, and society. Washington (DC): American Psychological Association; 2001. p. 49–60.

[10] Rule BK, Ferguson TJ. The effects of media violence on attitudes, emotions, and cognitions. J Soc Issues 1986;42:29–50.

[11] Farrell AD, Bruce SE. Impact of exposure to community violence on violent behavior and emotional distress among urban adolescents. J Clin Child Psychol 1997;26:2–14.

[12] Grossman D. On killing. Boston: Little, Brown; 1995.

[13] De Sa PPV. Iraq war should not be a video game. Available at: http://www.alternet.org/wiretap/ 20204. Accessed April 12, 2005.

[14] Anderson CA, Berkowitz L, Donnerstein E, et al. The influence of media violence on youth. Psychological Science in the Public Interest 2003;4:1–30.

[15] Anderson CA, Huesmann LR. Human aggression: a social-cognitive view. In: Hogg MA, Cooper J, editors. The Sage handbook of social psychology. London: Sage; 2003. p. 296–323.

[16] Gentile D, Anderson CA. Violent video games: the newest media hazard. In: Gentile D, editor. Media violence and children: a complete guide for parents and professionals. Westport (CT): Praeger; 2003. p. 131–52.

[17] Guerra N, Huesmann LR, Hanish L. The role of normative beliefs in children's social behavior. In: Eisenberg N, editor. Review of personality and social psychology. Thousand Oaks (CA): Sage; 1995. p. 140–58.

[18] Preston SD, de Waal FBM. Empathy: its ultimate and proximate bases. Behav Brain Sci 2002; 25:1–72.

[19] Atkinson AP. Emotion-specific clues to the neural substrate of empathy. Behav Brain Sci 2002; 25:22–3.

[20] Eslinger PJ. Neurological and neuropsychological bases of empathy. Eur Neurol 1998;39: 193–9.

[21] Zahn-Waxler C, Radke-Yarrow M, Wagner E, et al. Development of concern for others. Dev Psychol 1992;28:126–36.

[22] Brownell CA, Zerwas S, Balaram G. Peers, cooperative play, and the development of empathy in children. Behav Brain Sci 2002;25:28–9.

[23] Feshbach N. Empathy: the formative years. Implications for clinical practice. In: Bohart AC, Greenberg LS, editors. Empathy reconsidered. Washington (DC): American Psychological Association; 1997. p. 333–59.

[24] Gallup GG, Platek SM. Cognitive empathy presupposes self-awareness: evidence from phylogeny, ontogeny, neuropsychology, and mental illness. Behav Brain Sci 2002;25:36–7.

[25] Vreek GJ, van der Mark IL. Empathy, an integrated model. New Ideas in Psychology 2003;21: 177–207.

[26] Hoffman ML. Varieties of empathy-based guilt. In: Bybee J, editor. Guilt and children. San Diego (CA): Academic Press; 1998. p. 91–112.

[27] Bjorkqvist K, Osterman K, Kaukiainen A. Social intelligence-empathy = aggression? Aggress Violent Behav 2000;5:191–200.

[28] Cohen D, Strayer J. Empathy in conduct-disordered and comparison youth. Dev Psychol 1996; 32:988–98.

[29] Guerra N, Nucci L, Huesmann LR. Moral cognition and childhood aggression. In: Huesmann LR, editor. Aggressive behavior: current perspectives. New York: Plenum; 1994. p. 13–33.

[30] Gauthier Y. Infant mental health as we enter the third millennium: can we prevent aggression? Infant Ment Health J 2003;24:296–308.

[31] Boldizar JP, Perry DG, Perry LC. Outcome values and aggression. Child Dev 1989;60:571–9.

[32] Sams DP, Truscott SD. Empathy, exposure to community violence, and use of violence among urban, at-risk adolescents. Child and Youth Care 2004;33:33–50.

[33] Grossman D, DeGaetano G. Stop teaching our kids to kill. New York: Crown; 1999.

[34] Provenzo EF. Video kids: making sense of Nintendo. Cambridge (MA): Harvard; 1991.

[35] Fazio RH, Olson MA. Attitudes: foundations, functions, and consequences. In: Hogg MA, Cooper J, editors. The Sage handbook of social psychology. London: Sage; 2003. p. 139–60.

[36] Olson MA, Fazio RH. Implicit attitude formation through classical conditioning. Psychol Sci 2001;12:413–7.

[37] Kowalski K. The emergence of ethnic and racial attitudes in preschool-aged children. J Soc Psychol 2003;143:677–90.

[38] Bigler RS, Jones LC, Lobliner DB. Social categorization and the formation of intergroup attitudes in children. Child Dev 1997;68:530–43.

[39] Velicer WF, Huckel LH, Hansen CE. A measurement model for measuring attitudes towards violence. Pers Soc Psychol Bull 1989;15:349–64.

[40] Guerra NG, Huesman LR, Spindler A. Community violence exposure, social cognition, and aggression among urban elementary school children. Child Dev 2003;74:1561–76.

[41] Dodge KA, Bates JE, Pettit GS. Mechanisms in the cycle of violence. Science 1990;250: 1678–83.

[42] Markowitz FE. Attitudes and family violence: linking intergenerational and cultural theories. Journal of Family Values 2001;16:205–18.

[43] Shillinglaw RD. Protective factors among adolescents from violent families: why are some youth exposed to child abuse and/or interparental violence less violent than others? Available at: http://wwwlib.umi.com/dissertations/fullcit/9841770. Accessed April 11, 2005.

[44] Vernberg EM, Jacobs AK, Hershberger SL. Peer victimization and attitudes about violence during early adolescence. J Clin Child Psychol 1999;28:386–95.

[45] Guerra N, Slaby R. Cognitive mediators of aggression in adolescent offenders: II. Intervention. Dev Psychol 1990;26:269–77.

[46] Huesmann LR, Guerra NG. Children's normative beliefs about aggression and aggressive behavior. J Pers Soc Psychol 1997;72:408–19.

[47] Slaby R, Guerra N. Cognitive mediators of aggression in adolescent offenders. I. Assessment. Dev Psychol 1988;24:580–8.

[48] Tolan H, Guerra N, Kendall P. A developmental-ecological perspective on antisocial behavior in children and adolescents: toward a unified risk and intervention framework. J Consult Clin Psychol 1995;63:579–84.

[49] Sakamoto A. Video game use and the development of sociocognitive abilities in children: three surveys of elementary school children. J Appl Soc Psychol 1994;24:21–42.

[50] Barnett MA, Vitaglione GD, Harper KKG, et al. Late adolescents' experiences with and attitudes towards videogames. J Appl Soc Psychol 1997;27:1316–34.

[51] Funk JB, Buchman DD, Schimming JL, et al. Attitudes towards violence, empathy, and violent electronic games. Presented at the Annual Meeting of the American Psychological Association. San Francisco (CA), August 14–18, 1998.

[52] Funk JB, Buchman DD, Jenks J, et al. Playing violent video games, desensitization, and moral evaluation in children. J Appl Dev Psychol 2003;24:413–36.

[53] Drabman RS, Thomas MH. Does media violence increase children's tolerance of real-life aggression? Dev Psychol 1974;10:418–21.

[54] Molitor F, Hirsch KW. Children's toleration of real-life aggression after exposure to media violence: a replication of the Drabman and Thomas studies. Child Study J 1994;24:191–208.

[55] Perry BD, Pollard R. Homeostasis, stress, trauma, and adaptation: a neurodevelopmental view of childhood trauma. Child Adolesc Psychiatr Clin N Am 1998;7:33–51.

[56] Perry BD. Childhood experience and the expression of genetic potential: what childhood neglect tells us about nature and nurture. Brain Mind 2002;3:79–100.

[57] Matthews V, Kronenberger WG, Lowe M, et al. Aggressive youths, violent video games, trigger unusual brain activity. Presented at the 88th Scientific Assembly and Annual Meeting of the Radiological Society of North America. Chicago, December 2, 2002.

[58] Gur RC, Schroeder L, Turner T, et al. Brain activation during facial emotion processing. Neuroimage 2002;16:651–62.

[59] Moll J, de Oliveira-Souza R, Bramati IE, et al. Functional networks in emotional moral and nonmoral social judgments. Neuroimage 2002;16:696–703.

[60] Grafman J. Anger is a wind that blows out the light of the mind (old proverb). Mol Psychiatry 2003;8:131–2.

[61] Pietrini P, Guazzelli M, Basso G, et al. Neural correlates of imaginal aggressive behavior assessed by positron emission tomography in healthy subjects. Am J Psychiatry 2000;157: 1772–81.

[62] Grafman J. Experimental assessment of adult frontal lobe function. In: Miller BL, Cummings JL, editors. The human frontal lobes: functions and disorders. New York: Guilford Press; 1999. p. 321–44.

[63] Sirigu A, Zalla T, Pillon B, et al. Planning and script analysis following prefrontal lobe lesions. In: Grafman J, Holyoak KJ, Boller F, editors. Structure and function of the human prefrontal cortex. New York: New York Academy of Sciences; 1995. p. 277–88.

[64] Wood JN, Romero SG, Makale M, et al. Category-specific representations of social and nonsocial knowledge in the human prefrontal cortex. J Cogn Neurosci 2003;15:236–48.

[65] Grattan LM, Eslinger P. Higher cognition and social behavior: changes in cognitive flexibility and empathy after cerebral lesions. Neuropsychology 1989;3:175–85.

[66] NewScientist.com. Video game "brain damage" claim criticized. Available at: http://www. newscientist.com/news/news.jsp?id=ns99992538. Accessed May 7, 2004.

[67] News CNET.com. Video games hurt brain development. Available at: http://news.com.com/ 2100-1040-271849.html?legacy=cnet. Accessed May 7, 2004.

[68] Matsuda G, Hiraki K. Prefrontal cortex deactivation during video game play. In: Shiratori R, Arai K, Kato F, editors. Gaming, simulation and society: research scope and perspective. Tokyo: Springer-Verlag; 2005. p. 101–9.

[69] Tanaka M, Hirasawa K, Suzuki K, et al. The relationship between long-term playing of video games and functions of the prefrontal cortex. Presented at the 34th Annual Conference of the International Simulation and Gaming Association. Tokyo, August 29, 2003.

[70] Suzuki K, Hirasawa K, Tanaka M, et al. Relationship between long-term use of video games and cognitive abilities. Presented at the 34th Annual Conference of the International Simulation and Gaming Association. Tokyo, August 29, 2003.

[71] Suzuki K, Tanaka M, Matsuda G, The effects of playing video games on brain activity. Presented at the 34th Annual Conference of the International Simulation and Gaming Association. Tokyo, August 29, 2003.

[72] Weber R, Ritterfield U. Does playing violent computer games produce specific brain activity? Available at: http://ascweb.usc.edu/asc.php?pageID=337. Accessed April 12, 2005.

[73] Shuren JE, Grafman J. The neurology of reasoning. Arch Neurol 2002;59:916–9.

[74] Freedman JL. Media violence and its effect on aggression: assessing the scientific evidence. Toronto: University of Toronto Press; 2002.

[75] McCall RB, Green BL. Beyond the methodological gold standards of behavioral research: considerations for practice and policy. Soc Policy Rep 2004;18:1–19.

[76] Green CS, Bavelier D. Action video game modifies visual selective attention. Nature 2003;29: 534–7.

[77] Paisson OS, Pope AT. Stress counterresponse training of pilots via instrument functionality feedback. In: Proceedings of the 1999 Association for Applied Psychophysiology and Biofeedback Meeting. Vancouver (Canada), April 10, 1999.

[78] Baccus JR, Baldwin MW, Packer DJ. Increasing implicit self-esteem through classical conditioning. Psychol Sci 2004;15:498–502.

[79] Twist J. Brain waves control video games. Available at: http://newsvote.bbc.co.uk/mpapps/ pagetools/print/news.bbc.co.uk/2/hi/technology/3485918.stm. Accessed May 7, 2004.

[80] Funk JB, Flores G, Buchman DD, et al. Rating electronic games: violence is in the eye of the beholder. Youth Soc 1999;30:283–312.

[81] Walsh DA, Gentile DA. A validity test of movie, television, and video game ratings. Pediatrics 2001;107:1302–8.

[82] Bushman BJ, Cantor J. Media ratings for violence and sex: implications for policymakers and parents. Am Psychol 2003;58:130–41.

[83] Brown GA. Media literacy and critical television viewing in education. In: Singer DG, Singer JL, editors. Handbook of children and the media. Thousand Oaks (CA): Sage; 2001. p. 681–97.

[84] Cantor J, Wilson B. Media and violence: intervention strategies for reducing aggression. Media Psychology 2003;5:363–403.

[85] Dennis EE. Out of sight and out of mind. Am Behav Sci 2004;48:202–11.

ELSEVIER
SAUNDERS

Child Adolesc Psychiatric Clin N Am
14 (2005) 405–428

CHILD AND
ADOLESCENT
PSYCHIATRIC CLINICS
OF NORTH AMERICA

The Internet and Children: Advantages and Disadvantages

Jennifer Bremer, MD

Department of Child Psychiatry, University of Chicago, 5841 South Maryland Avenue, MC 3077, Chicago, IL 60637, USA

Modern children and adolescents are the first to grow up with the Internet as part of their daily lives. Much like radio in the 1920s or television in the 1950s, the Internet rapidly has become an integral part of life and currently is present in homes, schools, libraries, businesses, and coffee shops for work and play.

Children are at the forefront of this technologic frontier, with 30 million children going online annually. Children and adolescents use the Internet more than any other age group, with 65% of children aged 10 to 13 and 75% of young adolescents aged 14 to 17 using the Internet. This number has been growing [1–3].

It seems that "Across the world there is a passionate love affair between children and computers…they seem to know that in a deep way it [computer technology] already belongs to them. They know they can master it more easily and more naturally than their parents. They know they are the computer generation," as observed by Seymour Papert, a renowned expert in the field of computers and artificial intelligence [4].

What is the impact of this technologic sea change on children? A comprehensive review of this multifaceted subject is beyond the scope of this article and reaches across numerous disciplines, from information technology to communications to educational technology to social psychology, among others. An awareness of a basic overview of this subject has become essential for any professional who works with children, because the Internet has become an intimate part of children's lives.

This article examines how the Internet has entered children's lives and notes some of its potential positive and negative influences on children. Although the Internet's effects on a given child vary based on each child's characteristics and

E-mail address: jbremer@ameritech.net

how the child uses the Internet, adults still must have a fundamental under-standing of these general potentials. In particular, an awareness of the hazards inherent to children's Internet use is essential for all who work with children so they can apply preventive measures and help keep children safe.

This article refers to some of the diverse opinions voiced in this field and relevant surveys and a few early studies. Surveys clearly are limited by being cross-sectional and not explaining causation. Does the Internet affect people and their behaviors, or do characteristics of persons surveyed influence their Inter-net use? Empirical evidence is needed to clarify the Internet's impact on children, but it is still relatively sparse.

This article emphasizes the importance of a given child's specific experience of the Internet, which is important to keep in mind because often there seems to be a tendency to generalize this technologic advance as either all bad or all good for all children. "'The Computer' is not a single monolithic entity" [5] but includes an extraordinary range of components. One author on the subject viv-idly stated that "There is no such thing as a…online subculture; it's more like an ecosystem of subcultures, some frivolous, others serious. The cutting edge of scientific discourse is migrating to virtual communities… You can use virtual communities to find a date, sell a lawnmower, publish a novel, conduct a meeting" [6]. For this reason, not only whether a child chooses to use the Internet but also how he or she chooses to use the Internet must have a significant impact on how the Internet influences him or her. A child's personality and develop-mental needs also must modify the Internet's influence on him or her.

Although general messages apply to all children, specifics do matter. As in other realms of a child's life, adults must stay actively aware of an individual child's experience to best offer input and guidance. The online environment inevitably will evolve over time, and consequently this article primarily offers an introduction. Only ongoing engagement with children online keeps adults up to date.

Overview of children's online options

The Internet offers children a tremendous array of communication and enter-tainment choices. Parents report that children largely use the Internet for school research, whereas other online activities tend to include electronic mail (e-mail), chat rooms, Web-based games, Web surfing, and listening to music. Commu-nication with friends and family is a primary use of the Internet. Children's e-mail use increases over time. E-mail, like letters or "snail mail," allows written com-munication, and when the recipient is online simultaneously, it also can be interactive, like chatting, via instant messaging. By using typed messages sent back and forth between computer mailboxes, even when others are not available, e-mail allows a child to communicate with a busy family member or friend in a distant location, and the receiver can respond when time permits. Even wireless phones can "text message," which offers the equivalent of pocket e-mail—no computer necessary. Passing notes has achieved a new technologic level.

Children also "talk" online with others in chat rooms, which are virtual spaces in which children can chat, as the name implies. Communication with strangers online also occurs in other locales, including support groups, newsgroups (which represent an exchange of messages that people post about a particular subject), and multi-user domains (which are forums with a superimposed structure that users join by creating a character that interacts with the characters others have introduced that traverse a virtual terrain). Data suggest that more adolescents frequently go online to take advantage of opportunities to meet new people than do adults. According to information from the Youth Internet Safety Survey [7], 55% of youths communicated online with people whom they did not know in the real world. Chat rooms often have a focus that can range widely from pets to hobbies to sports. Some rooms are designed for specific age groups (eg, teens), and some even include "monitors" who require suitable language and subjects and "lock out" individuals who are inappropriate. Children easily can pose as adults, however, and enter chat rooms that focus on content that is inappropriate for children. Likewise, adults can misrepresent themselves online and pose in chat rooms; online predators may pose as children to lure children into in-person meetings, as discussed in a later section on Internet predators.

Without much experience using written language, without the benefit of facial expressions or body language, and without the formalities of letters to help communicate affect or attitude, children's online communications readily can lead to miscommunications and misunderstandings. Children widely use a couple of techniques to help overcome this. They can use capitals for emphasis and the "smiley face" or "emoticon" to help express emotion online. The following emoticons are used commonly:

:-) Basic smiley, which communicates humor
;-) Winky smiley, which communicates sarcasm or flirting
:-(Frowning smiley, which communicates upset
:- Indifferent smiley, which communicates indifference
:-o Open-mouthed emoticon, which means "oops"[1]

The ease with which e-mails can be forwarded to many others adds further novelty and further potential complications to online communications [8]. A confidential communication sent to and intended for a specific recipient easily can be forwarded widely to others. A child's online secret revelations can be passed on readily.

Computer games are another favorite use of the computer, and many games can be obtained for free online. Even a quick Internet search can identify a wealth of entertaining, educational games. The US government sponsors a child Internet portal—FirstGov for Kids (http://www.kids.gov)—that offers a collection of government-monitored and -approved children's websites. Games also

---

[1] *Data from* Quinion M. Only joking. Available at: http://www.worldwidewords.org. Accessed July 30, 2004.

can be found via more well-known portals such as America Online or "AOL." Adults must be aware, however, that violent and inappropriate computer games are easily accessed at many portals.

Children also go online for schoolwork, which is not surprising, because information gathering is a top use of the Internet [9]. Parents report that they think schoolwork is their children's most frequent online activity [10]. Wonderful resources are available, including research opportunities and specific sites to help with homework. Children just as easily can research inappropriate subjects, however, which is another online hazard discussed later in the article.

The reach of the Internet

The global Internet

Although US Internet use is the focus of this article, it is crucial to understand that Internet access is not only sweeping across the United States but also across the world, especially in Westernized nations. The Internet's extraordinary reach has been underlined by recent terrorist communications online, which showed that the Internet even reaches persons hiding in remote locations and committing unspeakable crimes. The UCLA Center for Communications Policy originated the World Internet Project, which works with international associates worldwide, and they found that the Internet was used to some extent in all countries studied. The percent of the population using the Internet ranged from a high of 71% in the United States to a low of 18% in Hungary (Box 1). South Korea had the largest

---

Box 1. Percentages of Internet users in countries

Britain 59.2
Germany 45.9
Hungary 17.5
Italy 31.2
Japan 50.4
South Korea 60.9
Macao 32.9
Singapore 40.8
Spain 36.4
Sweden 66.1
Taiwan 24.2
United States 71.1

Data from Cole JI, Suman M, Schramm P, et al. The UCLA Internet report: surveying the digital future year 3. Los Angeles (CA): UCLA Center for Communication Policy; 2003.

percentage of its population—56%—online 10 hours or more per week, whereas 41% of the United States population was found to be online to that degree [11].

Although the Internet worldwide tends to remain more accessible to the middle and upper classes, it is reaching across socioeconomic groups. In more than half of the countries studied, 20% or more of the population in the lowest twenty-fifth percentile of income used the Internet. In several countries this number was much higher; approximately half of the poorest income quartile used the Internet in Sweden, South Korea, and the United States [11].

The Internet at home

Most children who go online can do so at home; 62% of families with children in the US reported Internet access in a recent measure [3]. More than 80% of the children who used the Internet in 2002 did so at home [11]. Even young children are online at home, including 7% of 3- to 5-year-old children and 25% of 6- to 11-year-old children. A greater percentage of older children connect to the Internet from home, including approximately 48% of children between the ages of 12 and 17 years [12].

In a home with a computer, the likelihood of having an Internet connection differs according to the parents' experience with the Internet outside the home [10]. Whereas the likelihood of having the home computer connected to the Internet does not differ significantly according to many demographic variables, educational status and age do have an impact [10]. The least educated and oldest individuals in the United States are less likely to have home Internet access [9]. College educational status increases rates of Internet access 35% to 40% compared with persons without a high school diploma. Older Americans tend to have less Internet access and use the Internet less than the rest of the population [9]; they are, however, increasingly online.

Other variables that play a role include race/ethnicity and income. The rates of home Internet access include 55% of white non-Hispanics, 68% of Asians and Pacific Islanders, 32% of Hispanics, 31% of African Americans [13]. Higher income families report more access, with 92.4% of households with an income of $150,000 or more having online computers compared to 29.4% of households with an income of $15,000 to $19,000 [14]. Indirectly, income may have additional impacts by affecting the quality of the computer and the speed of the Internet connection purchased.

The Internet at school

Despite differences in home access, most children can access the Internet in any case in school or in libraries across the United States, where computer and Internet access has grown dramatically. Although 57% of school-aged children access the Internet at home and school, an additional 23% access it at school only, and only 10% have no access [12]. The numbers underline the vast change in school technology. The number of computers in US schools rose from

250,000 in 1983 to 8.6 million in 1998. Whereas only half of US schools had any computers in 1983, by 1998 all schools and half of all classrooms contained one or more computers. Whereas schools averaged 40 students per computer in 1985, they currently average 4 children per computer [15].

Internet access in public schools likewise has risen dramatically, with Internet access growing from 50% in 1995 to 99% by 2001 [15]. The percentage of schools' instructional rooms that contained Internet access likewise increased, rising from 3% in 1994 to 87% by 2001 [15]. Children's access to these online computers also has increased. The student-to-online-computer ratio dropped from 12 students per online computer in 1998 to 5 students per online computer in 2001. Even in impoverished schools, where access lags, the ratio also decreased, dropping from 9 students per online computer in 2000 to 7 students per online computer in 2001. These Internet connections are increasingly high speed. Whereas in 1996, 74% of public schools with Internet access had dial-up connections, by 2001, 55% had T1/DS1 lines (continuous and high-speed Internet connections) and only 5% still used dial-up [15].

Children's online access has grown because they are increasingly permitted access to these school computers outside of school hours, with 51% of public schools offering this opportunity [15]. With such availability, it is important to note that most schools report using monitors and various technologies to protect children online from inappropriate interactions and subjects. Most schools also require a contract signed by a parent or child regarding appropriate Internet use [15]. It is hard to imagine that monitoring across schools after hours achieves uniform vigilance, however, and teachers and parents may wish to keep an eye on this.

Although the impacts of these developments are hotly debated, children not only can but also increasingly must use the Internet at school as it becomes integrated into schoolwork. Most teachers currently incorporate the Internet into classroom instruction or curriculum [16,17].

The Internet in libraries

Even if a child somehow avoids the Internet's incursion into homes and schools, he or she can access the Internet readily in public libraries nationwide, with 92% of libraries offering public Internet access [18]. It is important to note that most of these readily accessible online computers have no filtering mechanisms according to a recent report [19]. Children in this setting can access the unfiltered, uncensored Internet for free, a fact that presents potential hazards. This circumstance may change as laws require such filtering be implemented, as discussed later.

The wireless Internet

More recent technologic advances increase the Internet's reach even further because the Internet is portable. Although only 17% of Americans have tried the wireless Internet and 6% use wireless connections on a given day, these numbers are expected to increase [20]. Such growth is anticipated with the industry's expansion and because 28% of American adults and 41% of Internet users are already prepared to use the wireless Internet because they already use a computer or wireless phone capable of wireless Internet connections. In other words, more than 56 million Americans already are "wireless ready" [20].

The Internet's impact on children

As the expansive scope of the Internet's presence in children's worlds becomes clear, the need to understand how this sweeping technologic change affects children also becomes apparent. Although questions and theories abound and this subject is vigorously debated, there is surprisingly little empirical evidence on this specific subject.

Cognitive and academic impacts

Although comprehensive answers lag, questions are numerous concerning how the Internet affects cognitive and academic development, including: How does the Internet affect how children think and understand? Does it affect different aspects of cognitive development in different ways, such as information processing, language development, and memory? How does the Internet affect the process of learning? Do the vast opinions and information online inhibit or nourish critical thinking and creativity? How does the Internet affect children's school functioning and academic achievement? Does more time online mean less time reading or writing? Does the Internet's wealth of resources nourish children's love of learning?

Most parents see the Internet as having a positive influence on academics, with 84% seeing the Internet as helpful with homework and 81% saying the Internet is a place for children to learn. Indeed, parents describe doing homework as their children's most common use of the Internet [10]. Sixty-eight percent of parents even see children without Internet access as being at a real disadvantage [10]. Most parents who plan to buy personal computers in the near future cite their children's education as a significant motivation [11].

The US government apparently concurs with this positive view of the Internet's role in education. They are spending $4 billion each year to increase Internet-connected computers in classrooms, with a sum of $50 to $80 billion as the projected price for connecting every US classroom to the Internet [21]. A report to the US Congress on the subject underlines the government's enthusiasm, declaring that "the Internet has become a...critical tool for our children's success" [2]. This perspective may stem from the value widely placed on computer skills. In a survey that asked the public what skills are important for graduating students, "computer skills and media technology" ranked third, whereas skills that ranked lower included "values," "good citizenship," "curiosity and love of learning," "knowledge of history and geography," and "knowledge of classic works" (eg, Shakespeare) [21]. Despite this enthusiasm and the Internet's increasing integration into education, little empirical evidence illustrates its benefits for academic achievement or cognitive development.

Even the efficacy of other elements of computer learning is still debated [22,23]. Some researchers in relevant fields strongly object to the emphasis on computers in schooling. "The brutal truth, despite all the hype to the contrary, is that children without computers and with a good education are far more likely to succeed than children walled in by technological fads," writes Dr. Jane Healy, an educational psychologist and author on the subject [21]. Similarly, in 1997, Dr. Samuel Sava, Executive Director of the National Association of Elementary School Principals, underscored US children's poor results in mathematics and science in the face of increasing computer availability and emphasized that computers alone are not adequate to help produce well-educated students [24]. There is concern that computers sometimes may play the role of suboptimal babysitters rather than educational tools to be used to complement classroom work. Some researchers even advocate a discontinuation of further computer introduction into elementary school classrooms [25]. Studies conducted on relevant subjects have widely divergent findings, perhaps partially because of methodologic issues [26]. Several studies have failed to show benefits from computer use for academic achievement or cognitive development, however [25–31].

One study even showed that developmentally inappropriate use of the computer in classrooms could have negative impacts. The study compared three classrooms of 4-year-old children using computer programs 3 hours per week compared to a classroom without computer time and found that children who used "drill and practice" computer software showed a relative decline in creativity compared to the other classes [32].

Conversely, other studies have suggested that although poor computer use should be avoided, thoughtful use of the computer in education can be a boon for children. "Misuse of technology by some and overzealous promotion by others are not valid reasons for...speciously framing the computer as the lightening rod for a broad range of criticism" [33]. Extensive reviews have shown that computer use in education can offer a range of benefits for children [34,35]. Studies have shown that computer use can impact positively children's alphabet recognition, language, early mathematical knowledge, cognitive development, and learning [26,36–43].

Independent computer use, when not part of a school or after-school program, also may support learning. In a recent study of rural, low-income families, 53% of preschool-aged children had a home computer and 29% played with it daily while 44% played with it at least weekly. Of children without home computers, 49% had access to a computer elsewhere and 10% used it daily while 33% played with it at least weekly. The researchers found a significant association between after-school computer accessibility and children's performance on school readiness and cognitive tests after controlling for developmental and socioeconomic factors [26].

Positive cognitive and academic impacts of computer use in an after-school computer club setting are also apparent. Researchers created and studied an after-school computer club, the Fifth Dimension. It offered a range of cognitive and academic benefits, including benefits in computer literacy, following directions, solving mathematics word problems, problem solving, grammar games, reading achievement, and mathematics achievement [44–49]. This club was such a success that it has been replicated many times.

Although these studies are intriguing when considering computer use in general, they offer little to expand our understanding of the impact of children's Internet use in particular. More specific answers may be forthcoming in the near future, however, when large studies are completed. In 2003, the government awarded $15 million in 3-year grants to multiple institutions for pursuit of scientific evaluations in related subjects. The US Secretary of Education, Rod Paige, noted in a US Department of Education press release on November 10, 2003, "We don't want the mere acquisition of advanced education technologies to be the end game—we want it to be the starting point to apply proven strategies to develop more effective teaching and boost student achievement."

Social impacts of the Internet

Strong social networks lead to happier, healthier individuals who are better buffered against hard times [50,51]. Although as an entertainment and communication tool the Internet seems likely to affect these all-important social networks, individuals in the field debate whether the Internet is a benefit or a detriment to community involvement and interpersonal relationships [52]. Relevant questions include "Will the time which children spend online lead them to decrease the time they spend nourishing real world social connections, which will subsequently suffer?" "Will children use the Internet to increasingly nurture existing relationships and build new ones?" "What impacts will new relationships have that are created online and only exist in the virtual world?"

Discussing the Internet's impact on social networks in such a general way, however, necessarily seems overly simplistic and reductionistic. The differing types of Internet use must impact social worlds in differing ways. For example, the impact of the Internet on a child who is chatting with school chums or distant family online must differ dramatically from the impact of the Internet on a child who is downloading games, music, or pornography.

Generalizations ignore what a specific child brings to the equation and the role this plays. How the Internet impacts a child's social connections depends partially on the nature of the child. Some children, especially children with anxious tendencies, may enjoy the anonymity online that permits them to discuss topics and practice social skills in a less stressful setting than in person in the real world. A child has a low stress opportunity to try out various communication approaches. Children can "lurk" passively in chat rooms, which allows them to observe and study social exchanges without the stress of participating. With its anonymity, the Internet may provide a less anxiety-provoking milieu for experimentation with relationships so typical of adolescents [53,54]. The Internet even could be safer for some of the rebellious interactions that can be a part of adolescence. The lack of physical proximity may offer a degree of safety to adolescents who are flirting online or chatting with others who are unsavory characters, assuming that in-person meetings are strictly avoided.

Conversely, the Internet may have negative impacts on social interactions and social systems [52,55,56]. The Internet could lead nervous children to avoid facing fears, a central component to treatment of most anxiety-related issues. Children may be tempted to socialize online to hide from the tribulations of the real social world [53]. Adolescents may be tempted to withdraw from that life phase's sometimes turbulent relationships and escape into online relationships or online distractions. The Internet could be used as yet another escapist pursuit, similar to television viewing. It could yield negative social impacts, similar to what research has found to result from television viewing [57–59]. As yet another leisure device, the Internet could compound the influence of video games, movies, electronic toys, and television as another diversion drawing children away from real-world learning that is essential to development in so many ways [60].

Social skills and relationships could suffer simply from the increased time invested communicating with online contacts at the expense of time essential to real-world friendships [50]. Sixty percent of parents voiced concerns that Internet use might lead to increasing isolation of a child [10]. A survey of more than 4000 parents by the Stanford Institute for Qualitative Study of Society in 1999 supports this concern. The more time individuals reported spending online, the less time they reported spending with people in the real world. Of individuals online 5 hours a week or more, 8% described a decrease in social activities and approximately 25% reported spending less time with family or friends on the phone or in person. A move from phone use to e-mail could account for some of this shift [9]. An early longitudinal study that gave home Internet access to families without access was conducted by the Carnegie Mellon group in the 1990s. The study found decreased social involvement for participants in their first year online, although this impact dissipated over time and was not replicated in a later study by this group [52]. Of note, there have been deliberations about the meaning of these findings [52,61,62]. The study may have interfered with social connections by bringing a technology into a lower socioeconomic community when the community was not yet online, so subjects necessarily communicated with strangers online [52]. In contrast, currently the Internet is primarily used to communicate with real-world friends and family.

Conversely, the Internet often is seen as a communication tool that should strengthen relationships and help build new ones [6,63,64]. E-mail is the most frequent use of the Internet and is used regularly by most persons, including children [9,12,65,66]. Of surveyed adult Internet users, most describe e-mail as helping them more readily communicate with and strengthen their ties to family and friends [11]. In comparison to non-Internet users, persons who go online may have a greater number of friends or social contacts [11]. Despite worries of the Internet pulling people away from friends and family, one large survey found that most people reported that the time they spend with friends and family has not been changed by Internet use [11,63]. According to parents, children also are spending approximately the same amount of time with friends [11].

Social impacts, however, may suffer in the first year online as the Internet is first introduced into a community. Of adults in their first year online, almost 20% described decreased time with friends and family [11].

Another social impact of the Internet includes the formation of a new genre of relationships, the virtual relationship. Such relationships represent a novel type of interpersonal relationship in which a type of friendship emerges purely online. Adolescents increasingly engage in these. One study found that one fourth of adolescent Internet users between the ages of 10 and 17 had formed online friendships in the previous year, and 14% had even developed online relationships that they viewed as close [7]. In a survey of approximately 1500 10- to 17-year-old Internet users, more than 200 had formed relationships that they described as close with people whom they had met online [64]. Young people do tend to be the primary visitors of chat rooms in which such relationships can form. Although more than one fourth of Internet users do frequent chat rooms, fewer do so after the age of 25 [9].

The meaning of such virtual relationships in comparison to real-world relationships is unclear. It may be that online relationships have similarities to real-world relationships and offer meaningful connections [7,67]. Online interactions may even include more intimate and revealing communications than in-person communications for some individuals [68]. This finding is important because self-disclosure is an important ingredient in the development of close relationships [69].

It is interesting to note that youths who are troubled tend to develop virtual relationships more frequently than youths who are not. In a recent study, youths with more online friendships included girls with more conflict with their parents or who were troubled and boys with less communication with parents or who were troubled [64]. It is not yet known whether these adolescents benefit from the online relationships that could offer them support and advice or whether the relationships are detrimental. Among a range of concerns, troubled adolescents may use online relationships as a ready escape and avoid needed work on real-world problems or relationships.

Some people worry that friendships made online cannot be as supportive as those made in day-to-day life because they lack the proximity that is a powerful element in social connections [70]. Online relationships often lead to real-world social contacts, however [7,67]. One author on the subject noted a "breaking down of the borders between online and offline communities" [71]. Illustrating this phenomenon further, another author described "...Just like people who meet in other locales, those who meet in cyberspace frequently move their relationships into settings beyond the one in which they met originally. They do not appear to draw a sharp boundary between relationships in cyberspace and those in real life...cyberspace is becoming just another place to meet" [67]. It is important to note that this movement to the real world is not safe for children because child predators easily can pose as online friends, as discussed later.

In short, data show that although the Internet may bring an initial challenge to social connections, particularly as it first enters a community, it eventually may strengthen relationships. Adolescents may be especially prone to building new friendships online, something that adults should remain alert to as children may be tempted to move to in-person meetings—meetings that should be avoided given the potential dangers involved.

Physical impacts of the Internet

As the Internet invades our children's days, it is essential to discern any impacts on their physical and mental health. There is widespread concern that the sedentary nature of computer use is contributing to westernized society's growing childhood obesity epidemic. There have been further concerns about additional physical risks emerging that tend to plague adult computer users, including eyestrain, deterioration of vision, back strain, and carpal tunnel syndrome [72].

A recent study found that in the United States more than 15% of children age 6 to 19 years were overweight in 1999 to 2000, more than triple the percentage found in the 1960s [73]. Childhood obesity is associated with a plethora of health risks during childhood, including diabetes, hypertension, and orthopedic problems. It also predisposes children to a lifetime of obesity and the long-term considerable morbidities and mortalities it entails. Inactivity seems to be a prime culprit in this epidemic. The average child sits 5 hours each day at the television, the computer, or homework and spends 76% of the day relatively inactive. Studies have found an association between television viewing and decreased physical activity, physical health, and obesity [74,75]. With time online being similarly stationary and absorbing, associations between obesity and computer use do seem likely. One recent study found such a correlation between hours of computer use and childhood obesity in 9- to 12-year old children [76].

On a less bleak note, it is possible that Internet use may not so much increase as continue the problem, because some data suggest that the time using computers and the Internet to some extent comes from displacing television viewing time [11,77–79]. One study found that 60% of regular Internet users reported decreasing their television viewing time since going online [9]. Almost one third of householders described their children watching less television since beginning to use the Internet [11].

The Internet and mental health

Internet use also may affect children's mental well-being. Although initially coined as a parody [80], the term "Internet addiction disorder" has been widely proclaimed in the lay press. "... in the early '90s ... people who spent more than a few hours a day using the Internet would be laughed at for being addicted. Fast-forward to 2003. By that standard pretty much anyone who uses the Internet in the course of their work day, which is pretty much anyone in a desk-bound job these days, could meet some arbitrary early-1990s standard of addiction," aptly described one lay article, underlining a cultural element to this diagnosis [81].

Although a "Diagnostic and Statistical Manual" (DSM-IV) diagnosis is lacking and experts debate whether compulsive computer use represents a primary problem or a symptom of comorbid diagnoses, Internet use does seem to be associated in some individuals with psychological, interpersonal, and professional impairment [82]. On a practical level, computer use can be seen as problematic when time online becomes irresistible and all consuming and interferes with functioning or well-being. There can be an accompanying inability to reduce online time despite negative consequences.

In a study of 16- to 18-year old teens in India, 18 of 100 seemed "Internet dependent." The dependent teenagers skipped work and sleep to go online and feared that life without the Internet would be dull. Individuals who were "Internet dependent" described more loneliness than those who used the Internet moderately [83]. Surveys also reported that compulsive Internet use can impact negatively on academic work and relationships for college students [84,85].

Studies that examined adults who are Internet dependent highlight the presence of comorbid diagnoses. One study found that adults who "depended" on the Internet were online for nonessential purposes for approximately 39 hours per week versus nondependent Internet users, who were online for 5 hours per week [86]. Many comorbidities have been noted in case series of Internet-addicted individuals, including a lifetime mood disorder in 33%, substance use disorder in 38%, anxiety disorder in 19%, and personality disorder in 52% [87]. One case series determined all subjects to meet criteria for impulse control disorder not otherwise specified, and a handful also met criteria for obsessive-compulsive disorder. Most of the subjects (70%) met criteria for a bipolar spectrum disorder [88].

Whether children who use the Internet obsessively suffer comorbidities is not yet known. No psychological or emotional consequences of moderate Internet use have been shown [89]. It seems likely that the specific applications used, the family situation, and the child's characteristics all play a role. For instance, increasing social connections with e-mail may buoy one child's spirits, downloading inappropriate materials (eg, terrorist violence) may feed another child's anxieties, and yet another child struggling with sadness may receive some support and comfort in mental health sites or friendly chat rooms.

In terms of mood, the Carnegie Mellon study found that during the first year of having the Internet in their homes, adolescents had a lowering of mood and increased feelings of loneliness, which dissipated over time and were not present by the follow-up study 3 years later [52]. Conversely, the Internet may benefit children's mental health directly and by serving as a resource. It is not surprising that because the Internet offers children the opportunities to research subjects of their choosing and because children frequently are the family experts on computers, computer use has been found to benefit young children's self-esteem and increase a positive attitude toward learning [32,41]. Four-year-old children who used a computer 3 hours per week in classrooms were found to have an increase in self-esteem when compared with 4-year-old children in a classroom without computer access [32].

The Internet also may play a role in children's mental health by serving as an easily available, private means through which children can seek information and guidance concerning mental health issues. The quality of such resources may be less than ideal, however. A self-report survey of adolescents in 1999 found that 18% had used the Internet to seek help for emotional difficulties; however, only 14% of them found that the Internet offered much help, whereas approximately 20% were dissatisfied with the resources they found [90]. Their dissatisfaction is not surprising because the quality of online information and resources is erratic. Information online often fails to go through the editorial or review process that written publications undergo, and studies have found concerning inaccuracies on medical websites [91–93]. Misinformation could mislead a child and even be unsafe. For example, a multitude of websites object to use of psychotropic agents and advise avoidance of these, which could lead a depressed child toward noncompliance and worsening symptoms.

Exacerbating this problem is the fact that children may be prone to believe what they read, and their parents might not know to correct this tendency when it comes to the Internet. In most of the countries studied in the UCLA World Internet Project, more than half of Internet users describe "most or all" information found online as accurate. Users in South Korea describe the greatest trust in online information, with 70% seeing information found online as generally reliable. In the United States, more than half of people do see information online as mostly reliable and accurate [11].

Dangers online

A primary drawback to children's entrance into the online world is the danger inherent in Internet use. Fortunately, parents are increasingly aware of such perils, with almost three fourths of parents voicing concern that their children may give out personal information on the Internet, for example [94]. Dangers range from exposure to inappropriate information to purchasing inappropriate items to the serious—although fortunately infrequent—hazard of children falling prey to child predators who connect with them online.

Access to information

One hazard for children online is ready access to a range of inappropriate information. An article in *Time* magazine vividly describes that the Internet "bring all the world—in all its glorious, anarchic, beautiful, hateful variety—into your home. We'd all prefer that the porn, the neo-Nazis, the violent misogynists and all the other floating trash of a cacophonous society not wash up in our living room. But...they do..." [95].

Survey results underline the finding that 44% of American adolescents had seen sexual websites, 25% had seen hate group sites, 14% had seen sites with bomb-building instructions, and 12% had seen sites that gave information on gun purchasing [95]. Further inappropriate websites include pro–eating disorder websites, "safe" drug use websites (eg, http://www.dancessafe.org, http://www.lycaeum.org, http://www.erowid.org, which are websites that discuss drug use as if it can be done safely), and websites that promote self-injury, suicide, or violence [95,96]. These sites are numerous. For example, there are more pro-anorexia and pro-bulimia websites than professional and recovery sites [97].

The danger of such websites has been made devastatingly clear when children have acted based on such information. Middle school–aged children used online information to learn how to build a pipe bomb, which they then planted in a school locker. Fortunately, the school was evacuated and the bomb squad successfully detonated it [98]. One of the students responsible for the Columbine massacre in 1999 had detailed bomb-making instructions posted on his website.

Inappropriate websites are difficult to avoid viewing. E-mail boxes fill with spam directing individuals online to pornographic sites. Internet spam is an unsolicited e-mail sent to many e-mail boxes at once, much like junk mail. Advertisements for pornographic sites appear in pop-up boxes on computer screens, also much like junk mail. Not surprising to anyone plagued by such pop-up boxes online, one fourth of children who use the Internet described unwanted exposure to pornographic images in the year before being surveyed [99].

Our government has grappled with how to protect free speech online while increasing appropriateness of content for children. Unfortunately, in 2004 the US Supreme court, concerned about freedom of speech, ruled against the Child Online Protection Act, a law that required age verification procedures for admittance to pornographic sites, which would have decreased child viewing of pornography. It would have allowed for fines for persons who made pornographic material readily accessible to children. Conversely, in 2003, the US Supreme Court favored protection of children. The Supreme Court reversed a lower court ruling and supported the Children's Internet Protection Act, which mandates that schools and libraries that receive discounted telecommunications, Internet access, or internal connections services implement an Internet safety policy and Internet blocks or filters to protect children from obscene or pornographic content.

Purchasing

Online shopping merits brief mention because children, like adults, readily can access stores worldwide. This convenience has been embraced by the public, with US shoppers spending more than $50 billion shopping online in 2003, according to the US Commerce Department, a rate that was up 26% from the year before. Like adults, any child with a credit card number can access the stores of the world online.

As in so many other ways, by offering such extensive availability, the Internet brings a wealth of options and some hazards. A child readily can purchase

inappropriate material—from medications to bomb-making materials to cigarettes. Vendors may implement age verification systems, but these are used in-
frequently. In a recent study, adolescents were able to purchase cigarettes easily
via credit card or money order online [100]. Computer filtering devices could
help but are not used widely. One study found that if filtering devices were used,
the purchase of cigarettes by minors could be blocked [101].

Cyberpredators

Although children falling prey to child predators online is relatively infrequent, it does happen and adults must be aware of predators' existence to help
keep children safe. Child predators may enter chat rooms under various personae
to contact children, have sexual communication with children, and lure children
into real-world meetings [102]. Unawares, children may be "socialize[ing] with
the deviants of society" [98]. The Federal Bureau of Investigation (FBI) and
Justice Department have reported that Internet communications are becoming
a powerful resource for sexual predators to contact children [103].

A significant number of children are sexually solicited online. In 1999, the
Crimes Against Children Research Center, funded by the National Center for
Missing and Exploited Children, surveyed 1501 children and found that 20% of
children who use the Internet and were between the ages of 10 and 17 had
received an online sexual solicitation in the prior year [104]. Similarly, 25% of
children described unsafe online experiences just a few years later in a smaller
survey [1,105]. Individuals at higher risk of such solicitations in the study by
the National Center for Missing and Exploited Children included girls, older
children, troubled children, chat room users, frequent Internet users, and persons
who communicated with strangers online. One in 33 children who used the
Internet received an aggressive solicitation, such as a solicitor who asked to meet
in person, called on the telephone, or sent them regular mail, money, or presents.
One in 17 children was threatened or harassed [104].

Of solicited children, 23% described feeling upset by the incident, 20% described feeling embarrassed, and 20% reported experiencing some subsequent
stress. Individuals who became more upset included younger children, children
who received aggressive solicitations (including attempts at real-world contact),
and children who were solicited on a computer outside of their home [104,106].

Of children approached sexually, only approximately one fourth of the children ever told a parent about it. Only a few children reported it to any type of
authority [106], which may have been contributed to by unawareness concerning to whom it should be reported. Only 17% of children and 11% of parents
could name authorities to report to, such as the FBI, CyberTipline, or the Internet
service provider [104].

Such contacts are of further concern if one considers that children have been
found to have a lower threshold than adults for giving out personal identifying
information online [94]. Of the 17% of youths who described developing close
online relationships in the prior year, 70% had offline contact by mail or tele-

phone with the online friend, and 28% had face-to-face meetings. Overall, 7% of youths who go online have real-world meetings with individuals whom they have met online [7].

Despite the frequency of such disturbing online occurrences, only approximately one third of families with home Internet access use filtering or blocking software [10,65]. An array of technologic resources is available to increase a child's security online, although all of these resources are imperfect. Several companies sell software that blocks children from sites with unsuitable content, and several online services offer ways to stop access to unsuitable material online. Some services allow parents to block children from various services completely, such as the World Wide Web or chat rooms. Other services license technology from software makers to allow persons on their service to bar chosen Internet sites.

Available programs of varying effectiveness include InterGo, CyberSnoop, Rated PG, and Surf Watch [2]. A summary of some filtering effectiveness testing conducted on these programs is available in Appendix 3 of the Children's Internet Protection Act report to US Congress (http://www.ntia.doc.gov/ntiahome/ntiageneral/cipa2003/CIPAreport_08142003.htm#_ftn3). Of note, some programs, including Norton Internet Security software, prevent the exchange of personal information through the Internet, which could help keep a child unidentified to a predator.

Because technology is not foolproof, there is no technologic "silver bullet" to keep children safe online [2]. As an example, one study of popular filtering programs found that they failed to block 25% of inappropriate material but blocked 21% of nonobjectionable websites [107]. Good protection must include rules about Internet use, a child's education about Internet safety, and close monitoring of computer use by adults. Several resources are available that further describe such recommended safety measures (Box 2).

Most recommendations emphasize the importance of adults educating children about how to respond to sexual solicitations or inappropriate content online, how never to communicate identifying information online, and how never to agree to meet anyone from the online world in the real world. Recommendations also include parents limiting children's Internet access to their own home or locations with reliable adult supervision. Some parents confine children's Internet access to public areas in which parents can keep an eye on computer use. "A mother or dad ought to pay just as much attention to their child when they're on the Internet as if they're in a playground, or walking in the mall," President George W. Bush aptly noted in discussing federal efforts to promote children's Internet safety [1].

The international world is embracing the issue of Internet safety. February 6, 2004 was the first "Safer Internet Day" promoted by the Safer Internet Awareness Campaign sponsored by SafeBorders, the European Commission's Safer Internet Program. Involved countries included Australia, Germany, Greece, Italy, Luxembourg, Norway, Spain, The Netherlands, and the United Kingdom. The day aimed to increase awareness of Internet safety issues [108].

Box 2. Online resources for families concerning safety measures

- The "Parent's guide to child safety," available at http://www. missingkids.com, which is from the Department of Justice, the Department of Education, the FBI, and the National Center for Missing and Exploited Children. It offers measures that parents can take to increase safety. It is available in Spanish and English.
- The Department of Justice children's website also describes a safety steps for children. It is available at http://www. cybercrime.gov/rules/rules.htm.
- To report child pornography or online enticement of children, parents can log on to http://www.cybertipline.com or call the Tipline at 1-800-843-5678.
- Online privacy suggestions are available at http://www.ftc. gov/bcp/conline/edcams/kidzprivacy/index.html.
- The FBI offers "A parent's guide to Internet safety," which is available at http://www.fbi.gov/publications/pguide/pguide.htm.

The US government also has worked to increase online safety through the formation of child-safe locations online. In 2002, the Child Internet Safety Legislation, called the Dot Kids Implementation and Efficiency Act, was implemented. Its aim was to create locales online designated as safe for children. The Dot Kids domain parallels the children's section of the library, creating an appropriate place for children to browse. Every site designated ".kids" is monitored for content and safety, with inappropriate materials and links removed.

The child protection community also is actively hunting Internet predators. From 2000 to 2002, the FBI Innocent Images National Initiative increased prosecutions by more than 50%, and since 1998, the Internet Crimes Against Children Task Forces has investigated more than 3000 cases that resulted in more than 1400 arrests [1]. Awareness of recent major operations may make this dark online world seem more real and motivate all to remain vigilant in keeping children safe. Operation Hamlet recently dismantled an international ring of persons who molested their own children and then traded the images and videos online [109]. Operation Candyman discovered and prosecuted a Yahoo! group that traded child pornography online [1,109,110]. Operation Avalanche dismantled the largest child pornography ring ever, with 300,000 subscribers to child pornography websites [1,111,112].

Summary and recommendations

With the speed of the Internet's evolution, by the time of this publication, its contents inevitably will be somewhat out of date. The basic message will not change, however: adults must stay abreast of the evolving Internet world and actively monitor children's activities, therein helping children reap the wealth of possibilities online and avoid the potential negatives.

Child professionals must be aware of the breadth of the Internet's foray into children's lives so they routinely can incorporate appropriate questions and discussions on the subject. Professionals in the mental health field may play a particularly important role in helping a family assess how the applications that a given child uses online may affect that child. Mental health professionals can offer families guidance in ways to use the Internet to minimize harm and maximize advantages. Child psychiatrists, psychologists, or social workers should include discussions about how a child's psychiatric disorders may affect his or her Internet use and the Internet's impact on the child. An awareness of high-quality mental health websites to which to refer families may be useful. (The American Academy of Child and Adolescent Psychiatry "Facts for Families" website is one example of a useful reference site. It is available at http://www.aacap.org/publications/factsfam/.)

Child professionals also want to consider carefully how they choose to use the Internet professionally. Do they communicate with child patients on e-mail? Does this increase accessibility and alliance? Does e-mail lead a given child to speak less in person? Can a child understand the inherent lack of confidentiality in online communications? Does a family know to call or meet in person if a therapist does not reply—in the case of technologic failure or an inadvertently deleted e-mail? Such relevant discussions clearly should precede e-mail exchange with patients. A written e-mail policy can clarify such issues further.

Preventive measures should be considered actively by all who work with children. Pediatricians who see children for check-ups are in an ideal position of authority to include a routine discussion of online safety measures, much as good pediatricians routinely include a discussion of bicycle helmets or car seats. Librarians also have opportunities to help children make wise and appropriate use of Internet resources. Teachers have the opportunity to discuss this subject on an even more regular basis while also closely monitoring school Internet use. Teachers can use their expertise to help children reap educational riches online by encouraging educational forays into topics of interest and promoting the use of developmentally appropriate software. Teachers also can remind families that Internet use is not inherently an educational pursuit but certainly can be, depending on the applications used.

While we await additional studies to inform our Internet decisions further, it seems that families should make thoughtful and careful Internet decisions based on their own children's personalities and characteristics. Families should clarify these decisions with their own children and with all who spend time supervising their children—from significant others to grandparents to baby-sitters. Even adults who actively choose to keep their children off the computer should know that their children are likely to be exposed to the Internet—with its influx into friends' homes, schools, and libraries—and may wish to prepare them for this.

As in so many new worlds that children routinely enter in the course of development—from their first day at school, to their first play date, to their first bicycle ride, to their first sleepover, to their first camp experience—it is essential for adults to stay actively watchful, involved, and available. When it comes to the Internet, that adult presence can ensure that the Internet offers a child a previously unfathomable tool and opportunity rather than fulfill its other potential as a detriment or danger.

References

[1] The White House. Increasing online safety for America's children [press release, October 23, 2002]. Available at: http://www.whitehouse.gov/news/releases/2002/10/20021023-9.html. Accessed April 20, 2005.

[2] Department of Commerce, National Telecommunications and Information Administration. Report to Congress: Children's Internet Protection Act, Pub. L. 106–554. Study of Technology Protection Measures in Section 1703, August 2003. Available at: http://www.ntia.doc.gov/ ntiahome/ntiageneral/cipa2003/CIPAreport_08142003.htm. Accessed July 30, 2004.

[3] US Department of Commerce, National Telecommunications and Information Administration. A nation online: how Americans are expanding their use of the Internet at 1, 13 (Feb. 2002) and based on the September 2001 US Census Bureau's Current Population Survey. Available at: http://www.ntia.doc.gov/ntiahome/dn/index.html. Accessed July 30, 2004.

[4] Papert S. The connected family: bridging the digital generation gap. Atlanta (GA): Longstreet Press; 1996.

[5] Clements DH, Sarama J. Strip mining for gold: research and policy in educational technology. A response to "fool's gold." Educational Technology Review 2003;11:1.

[6] Rheingold H. The virtual community: homesteading on the electronic frontier. Available at: http://www.rheingold.com/vc/book/intro.html. Accessed July 30, 2004.

[7] Wolak J, Mitchell KJ, Finkelhor D. Close online relationships in a national sample of adolescents. Adolescence 2002;37:441–55.

[8] Bremer J. Learning from e-mail hailstorms. Psychiatr News 2003;38:10.

[9] Nie NH, Erbring L. The internet and society: a preliminary report. Supported by the Stanford institute for the quantitative study of society. Available at: http://www.stanford.edu/group/siqss/ Press_Release/internetStudy.html. Accessed July 30, 2004.

[10] Turow J. The Internet and the family. The view from parents. The view from the press. Available at: http://www.annenbergpublicpolicycenter.org/04_info_society/family/rep27.pdf. Accessed July 30, 2004.

[11] Cole JI, Suman M, Schramm P, et al. The UCLA Internet report: surveying the digital future year 3. Los Angeles (CA): UCLA Center for Communication Policy; 2003. Available at: http:ccp.ucla.edu/pdf/UCLA-Internet-Report-Year-Three.pdf. Accessed May 5, 2005.

[12] Newburger EC. US Department of Commerce, Economics and Statistics Administration, US Census Bureau, 2001. Home computers and Intenet use in the United States. Available at: http:// www.census.gov/prod/2001pubs/p23-207.pdf. Accessed July 30, 2004.

[13] US Department of Commerce, National Telecommunications and Information Administration. A nation online: How Americans are expanding their use of the Internet, February 2002. Available at: http://www.census.gov/prod/2004pubs/03statab/inforcomm.pdf. Accessed May 5, 2005.

[14] US Department of Commerce, National Telecommunications and Information Administration. A nation online, 2004, forthcoming report. Available at: http://www.census.gov/prod/2004pubs/ 04statab/infocomm.pdf. Accessed May 5, 2005.

[15] Kleiner A, Farris E; National Center for Education Statistics. Internet access in US pub-

lic schools and classrooms: 1994–2001. NCES 2002018. Available at: http://nces.ed.gov/pubsearch/pubsinfo.asp?pubid=2002018. Accessed July 30, 2004.

[16] US Census Bureau. Statistical abstract of the United States: home computers and Internet use in the United States. August 2000. Available at: http://www.census.gov/prod/2004pubs/03statab/educ.pdf. Accessed May 5, 2005.

[17] US Department of Education Statistics. Teacher use of computers and the Internet in Public Schools (2000d). NCES 2000-090. Available at: http://nces.ed.gov/programs/quarterly/vol_2/2_2/q3-2.asp. Accessed May 5, 2005.

[18] National Center for Education Statistics. Fast response survey system. Available at: http://nces.ed.gov/surveys/frss/publications/2003010/6.asp. Accessed July 30, 2004.

[19] Berlot JC, McClure CR. Public libraries and the Internet 2000: summary findings and data tables. Available at: http://www.nclis.gov/statsurv/2000plo.pdf. Accessed July 30, 2004.

[20] Horrigan JB. Pew Internet and American Life Project. Available at: http://www.pewinternet.org/pdfs/PIP_Wireless_Ready_Data_0504.pdf. Accessed July 30, 2004.

[21] Healy JM. Failure to connect: how computers affect our children's minds, and what we can do about it. New York: Touchstone; 1998.

[22] Cognition and Technology Group at Vanderbilt. Looking at technology in context: a framework for understanding technology and education research. In: Berliner DC, Calfee RC, editors. Handbook of educational psychology. New York: MacMillan; 1996. p. 807–40.

[23] Mayer RE, Schustack MW, Blanton WE. What do children learn from using computers in an informal, collaborative setting? Educational Technology 1999;39(2):27–31.

[24] Sava SG. Electronic genie. Presented at the National Association of Elementary School Principals State Leaders Conference. Arlington (VA), July 25, 1997.

[25] Cordes C, Miller E. Fool's gold: a critical look at computers in childhood. Available at: http://www.allianceforchildhood.net/projects/computers/computers_reports.htm. Accessed July 30, 2004.

[26] Li X, Atkins M. Early childhood computer experience and cognitive and motor development. Pediatrics 2004;113(6):1715–22.

[27] Clements DH, Gullo DF. Effect of computer programming on young children's cognition. J Educ Psychol 1984;76:1051–8.

[28] Howell RD, Scott PB, Diamond J. The effects of "instant" LOGO computing language on the cognitive development of very young children. Journal of Educational Computing Research 1987;3:249–60.

[29] Lehrer R, Harckham LD, Archer P, et al. Microcomputer-based instruction in special education. Journal of Educational Computing Research 1986;2:337–55.

[30] Goodwin LD, Goodwin WL, Nansel A, et al. Cognitive and affective effects of various types of microcomputer use by preschoolers. Am Educ Res J 1986;23:348–56.

[31] Miller MD, McInerney WD. Effects on achievement of a home/school computer project. Journal of Research on Technology in Education 1995;27:198–210.

[32] Haugland SW. The effect of computer software on preschool children's developmental gains. Journal of Computing in Childhood Education 1992;3:15–30.

[33] Clements DH, Sarama J. Strip mining for gold: research and policy in educational technology. A response to "fool's gold." Educational Technology Review 2003;11:1. Available at: http://www.aace.org/pubs/etr/issue4/clements.cfm. Accessed May 6, 2005.

[34] Kulik CC, Kulik JA. Effectiveness of computer-based instruction: an updated analysis. Comput Human Behav 1991;7:75–94.

[35] Ryan AW. Meta-analysis of achievement effects of microcomputer applications in elementary schools. Educ Adm Q 1991;27:161–84.

[36] Schetz KF. An examination of software used with enhancement for preschool discourse skill improvement. Journal of Educational Computing Research 1994;11(1):51–71.

[37] Williams RA. Preschoolers and the computer. Arithmetic Teacher 1984;31:39–42.

[38] McCollister TS, Burts DC, Wright VL, et al. Effects of computer-assisted instruction and teacher-assisted instruction on arithmetic task achievement scores of kindergarten children. J Educ Res 1986;80:121–5.

[39] Howard JR, Eatson JA, Brinkley VM, et al. Comprehension monitoring, stylistic differences, pre-math knowledge, and transfer: a comprehensive pre-math/spatial development computer-assisted instruction and Logo curriculum designed to test their effects. Journal of Educational Computing Research 1994;11:91–105.

[40] Clements DH. Computers in early childhood mathematics. Contemporary Issues in Early Childhood 2002;3:160–81.

[41] Sivin-Kachala J, Bialo ER. Report on the effectiveness of technology in schools, 1990–1994. Washington (DC): Software Publishers Association; 1994.

[42] Shute R, Miksad J. Computer assisted instruction and cognitive development in preschoolers. Child Study J 1997;27:237–53.

[43] Ainsa T. Effects of computers and training in Head Start curriculum. Journal of Instructional Psychology 1989;16:72–8.

[44] Mayer RE, Blanton B, Duran R, et al. Final report to the Andrew W. Mellon Foundation: the Fifth Dimension Cognitive Evaluation. Available at: http://www.psych.ucsb.edu/~mayer/fifth_dim_website/HTML/res_reports/final_report.html. Accessed July 30, 2004.

[45] Mayer RE. Out-of-school learning: the case of an after-school computer club. Journal of Educational Computing Research 1997;16:333–6.

[46] Schustack MW, Strauss R, Worden PE. Learning about technology in a non-instructional environment. Journal of Educational Computing Research 1997;16:337–52.

[47] Mayer RE, Quilici J, Moreno R, et al. Effects of participation in the Fifth Dimension on far transfer. Journal of Educational Computing Research 1997;16:371–96.

[48] Lavezzo A. Cognitive consequences of participation in a Fifth Dimension after-school computer club. Journal of Educational Computing Research 1997;16:353–69.

[49] Mayer RE, Quilici JH, Moreno R. What is learned in an after-school computer club? Journal of Educational Computing Research 1999;20:215–27.

[50] Cohen S, Wills TA. Stress, social support and the buffering hypothesis. Psychol Bull 1985;98:310–57.

[51] Cohen S, Doyle WJ, Skoner DP, et al. Social ties and susceptibility to the common cold. JAMA 1997;277:1940–4.

[52] Kraut R, Patterson M, Lundmark V, et al. Internet paradox: a social technology that reduces social involvement and psychological well-being? Am Psychol 1998;53(9):1017–31.

[53] Bremer J, Rauch P. Children and computers: risks and benefits. J Am Acad Child Adolesc Psychiatry 1998;37(5):559–60.

[54] Bremer J. Computers in psychiatry today. Acad Psychiatry 2000;24(3):168–72.

[55] Stoll C. Silicon snake oil. New York: Doubleday; 1995.

[56] Kroker A, Weinstein MA. Data trash: the theory of the virtual class. New York: St. Martin's Press; 1994.

[57] Brody GH. Effects of television viewing on family interactions: an observational study. Fam Relat 1990;29:216–20.

[58] Jackson-Beeck M, Robinson JP. Television nonviewers: an endangered species? J Consum Res 1981;7(4):356–9.

[59] Neuman SB. Literacy in the television age: the myth of the TV effect. Norwood (NJ): Ablex; 1991.

[60] McKibben B. The age of missing information. New York: Plume; 1993.

[61] Newcomer JM. Deconstructing the Internet paradox. Available at: http://www.acm.org/ubiquity/views/j_newcomer_1.html. Accessed July 30, 2004.

[62] LaRose R, Eastin MS, Gregg J. Reformulating the Internet paradox: social cognitive explanations of Internet use and depression. Available at: http://www.behavior.net/JOB/v1n1/paradox.html. Accessed July 30, 2004.

[63] Katz JE, Aspden P. A nation of strangers? Commun ACM 1997;40(12):81–6.

[64] Wolak J, Mitchell KJ, Finkelhor D. Escaping or connecting? Characteristics of youth who form close online relationships. J Adolesc 2003;26(1):105–19.

[65] Pew Research Center, Pew Internet and American Life Project. The Internet and education:

findings of the Pew Internet and American Life Project. Available at: http://www.pewinternet. org/reports/toc.asp?Report = 36. Accessed July 30, 2004.

[66] Kraut R, Mukhopadhyay T, Szczypula J, et al. Information and communication: alternative uses of the Internet in households. Information Systems Research 1999;10:287–303.

[67] Parks MR, Floyd K. Making friends in cyberspace. Available at: http://www.ascusc.org/jcmc/vol1/issue4/parks.html. Accessed July 30, 2004.

[68] Joinson AN. Self-disclosure in computer-mediated communication: the role of self-awareness and visual anonymity [unpublished paper]. Institute of Educational Technology. Available at: http://iet.open.ac.uk/pp/a.n.joinson/papers/self-disclosure.pdf. Accessed July 30, 2004.

[69] Derlega VJ, Metts S, Petronio S, et al. Self-disclosure. Newbury Park (CA): Sage Publications; 1993

[70] Wellman B, Wortley S. Different strokes from different folks: community ties and social support. Available at: http://www.chass.utoronto.ca/~wellman/publications/differentstrokes/diffstrokes.pdf. Accessed July 30, 2004.

[71] Hamman RB. Computer networks linking communities: a study of the effects of computer networks linking communities. A study of the effects of computer network use upon pre-existing communities. In: Thiedke U, editor. Virtualle gruppen-characteristika und prolemdimensionen. Available at: http://www.socio.demon.co.uk/mphil/short.html. Accessed July 30, 2004.

[72] US Department of Health and Human Services. NIOSH publications on video display terminals (revised). Cincinnati (OH): Public Health Service; 1991.

[73] The National Center for Health Statistics. Health, United States 2002 with chartbook on trends in the health of Americans. Available at: http://www.cdc.gov/nchs/hus.htm. Accessed July 30, 2004.

[74] Andersen RE, Crespo CJ, Bartlett SJ, et al. Relationship of physical activity and television watching with body weight and level of fatness among children. JAMA 1998;279:938–42.

[75] Sidney S, Sternfeld B, Haskell WL, et al. Television viewing and cardiovascular risk factors in young adults: the CARDIA study. Ann Epidemiol 1998;6(2):154–9.

[76] Arluk SL, et al. Childhood obesity's relationship to time spent in sedentary behavior. Mil Med 2003;168(7):583–6.

[77] Vitalari NP, Venkatesh A, Gronhaug K. Computing in the home: shifts in the time allocation patterns of households. Commun ACM 1985;28(5):512–22.

[78] Danko WD, MacLachlan JM. Research to accelerate the diffusion of a new invention. J Advert Res 1983;23(3):39–43.

[79] Kohut A. The role of technology in American life. Los Angeles (CA): Times Mirror Center for the People and the Press; 1994.

[80] Holmes L. Internet addiction: is it real? Your guide to mental health resources. Available at: http://mentalhealth.about.com/cs/sexaddict/a/interaddict.htm. Accessed July 30, 2004.

[81] Hasseldahl A. Gaming ourselves to death. Available at: http://www.forbes.com. Accessed July 30, 2004.

[82] Griffiths MD. Friendship and social development in children and adolescents: the impact of electronic technology. Educational and Child Psychology 1997;14(3):25–37.

[83] Nalwa K, Anand AP. Internet addiction in students: a cause of concern. Cyberpsychol Behav 2003;6(6):653–6.

[84] Scherer K. College life online: healthy and unhealthy Internet use. Journal of College Life and Development 1997;6(38):655–65.

[85] Morahan-Martin J. Incidence and correlates of pathological Internet use. Presented at the 105th annual meeting of the American Psychological Association. Chicago, August 18, 1997.

[86] Young KS. Internet addiction: the emergence of a new clinical disorder. Cyber Psychology and Behavior 1998;1(3):237–44. Available at: http://www.netaddiction.com/articles/newdisorder.htm. Accessed May 6, 2005.

[87] Black D, Belsare G, Schlosser S. Clinical features, psychiatric co-morbidity, and health related quality of life in persons reporting compulsive computer use behavior. J Clin Psychiatry 1999; 60:839–44.

[88] Shapira NA, Goldsmith TD, Keck Jr PE, et al. Psychiatric features of individuals with problematic Internet use. J Affect Disord 2000;57(1–3):267–72.

[89] Shields MK, Behrman RE. Children and computer technology: analysis and recommendations. Available at: http://www.futureofchildren.org. Accessed July 30, 2004.

[90] Gould MS, Munfakh JLH, Lubell K, et al. Seeking help from the Internet during adolescence. J Am Acad Child Adolesc Psychiatry 2002;41(10):1182–9.

[91] Pandolfini C, Impicciatore P, Bonati M. Parents on the web: risks for quality management of cough in children. Pediatrics 2000;105(1):E1.

[92] McClung HJ, Murray RD, Heitlinger LA. The Internet as a source for current patient information. Pediatrics 1998;101(6):E2.

[93] Impicciatore P, Pandolfini C, Casella N, et al. Reliability of health information for the public on the World Wide Web: systematic survey of advice on managing fever in children at home. BMJ 1997;314(7098):1875–9.

[94] Turow J, Nir L. The Internet and the family 2000. View from parents. View from kids. Philadelphia: Annenberg Public Policy Center; 2000.

[95] Okrent D. Raising kids online: what can parents do? Time 1999;153(18):38–43.

[96] Wax PM. Just a click away: recreational drug Web sites on the Internet. Pediatrics 2002;109(6):E96.

[97] Chesley EB, Alberts JD, Klein JD, et al. Pro or con? Anorexia nervosa and the Internet. J Adolesc Health 2003;32:123–4.

[98] Staudenmeier Jr JJ. Children and computers. J Am Acad Child Adolesc Psychiatry 1999; 38(1):5.

[99] Finkelhor D, Mitchell K, Wolak J. Youth Internet safety survey: Crimes Against Children Research Center. Available at: http://www.ncjrs.org/txtfiles1/ojjdp/fs200104.txt. Accessed July 30, 2004.

[100] Ribisl KM, Williams RS, Kim AE. Internet sales of cigarettes to minors. JAMA 2003;290(10): 1356–9.

[101] Bryant J, Cody M, Murphy S. Online sales: profit without question. Tob Control 2002;11(3): 226–7.

[102] Quayle E, Taylor M. Child seduction and self-representation on the Internet. Cyberpsychol Behav 2001;4(5):597–608.

[103] Federal Trade Commission. Privacy online: a report to Congress. Available at: http://www. ftc.gov/reports/privacy3/toc.htm. Accessed April 20, 2005.

[104] US Department of Justice. Office for Victims of Crimes bulletin: Internet crimes against children. Available at: http://www.ojp.usdoj.gov/ovc/publications/bulletins/internet_2_2001/welcome.html. Accessed July 30, 2004.

[105] Stahl C, Fritz N. Internet safety: adolescents' self-report. J Adolesc Health 2002;31:7–10.

[106] Mitchell KJ, Finkelhor D, Wolak J. Risk factors for and impact of online sexual solicitation of youth. JAMA 2001;285(23):3011–4.

[107] Hunter CD. Internet filter effectiveness: testing over and underinclusive blocking decisions of four popular filters. Soc Sci Comput Rev 2000;18(2):214–22.

[108] Today is Safer Internet for Children Day—but the day's bark needs a bite. Available at: http://www.PublicTechnology.net. Accessed June 27, 2004.

[109] US Customs Service. 45 children rescued, 20 arrests in US customs, Danish police investigation of global child molesting, pornography ring [press release]. US Customs Service; August 9, 2002.

[110] Federal Bureau of Investigation. Operation candyman [press release, March 18, 2002]. Available at: http://www.fbi.gov/pressrel/pressrel02/cm031802.htm. Accessed April 20, 2005.

[111] United States Postal Inspection Service. Multimillion-dollar child pornography enterprise dismantled [press release, 2001]. United States Postal Inspection Service; August 8, 2001.

[112] Eiserer T. Child-porn arrests continue as investigation goes global. The Dallas Morning News. September 11, 2002:21A.

ELSEVIER
SAUNDERS

Child Adolesc Psychiatric Clin N Am
14 (2005) 429–451

CHILD AND
ADOLESCENT
PSYCHIATRIC CLINICS
OF NORTH AMERICA

The Impact of Terrorism on Children and Adolescents: Terror in the Skies, Terror on Television

Wanda P. Fremont, MD[a],*, Caroly Pataki, MD[b],
Eugene V. Beresin, MD[c,d,e]

[a]*Department of Psychiatry, SUNY Upstate Medical University, 750 East Adams Street, Syracuse, NY 13210, USA*
[b]*Department of Psychiatry, David Geffen School of Medicine, University of California at Los Angeles, 12-105 Center for Health Sciences, Box 957035, Los Angeles, CA 90095-7035, USA*
[c]*Division of Child and Adolescent Psychiatry, Department of Psychiatry, Massachusetts General/McLean Hospitals, 15 Parkman Street, Boston, MA 02114, USA*
[d]*Department of Psychiatry, Harvard Medical School, 25 Shattuck Street, Boston, MA 02115, USA*
[e]*Harvard Medical School Center for Mental Health and Media, Massachusetts General Hospital, Boston, MA 02114, USA*

Terrorist attacks and their aftermath have had a powerful impact on children and their families. Recent literature has documented the effects of direct and indirect exposure to terrorism. Media and television exposure of terrorist events throughout the world has increased during the past few years. Images of terrorist attacks in the United States, including Oklahoma City and the World Trade Center, the Middle East, Europe, Africa, South America, Asian countries, and other nations have been broadcast into the homes of families throughout the world. There is increasing concern about the effects of this exposure on children who witness these violent images. Parents, teachers, and health care providers are struggling to help youngsters cope with heightened anxiety and fear. To develop a proactive and strategic response to these reactions, clinicians, educators, and policy makers must understand the psychological effects of media coverage of terrorism on children. Research in the past has focused on media coverage of criminal violence and war. Recent studies have examined

* Corresponding author.
E-mail address: fremontw@upstate.edu (W.P. Fremont).

1056-4993/05/$ – see front matter © 2005 Elsevier Inc. All rights reserved.
doi:10.1016/j.chc.2005.02.001
childpsych.theclinics.com

the effect of remote exposure of terrorist attacks and have shown a significant clinical impact on children and families.

Definition of terrorism

Terrorism is defined by the United States Defense Department as "the calculated use of violence or threat of violence to inculcate fear: intended to coerce or to intimidate governments and societies in the pursuit of goals that are generally political, religious, or ideological" [1]. The goal of terrorism is not only to cause visible disaster but also to inflict psychological fear and intimidation at any time, during periods of peace or conflict. Unlike family or community violence or the trauma resulting from war, terrorist activities are not confined to a specific geographic area or time. Terrorist events occur suddenly without any forewarning and frequently result in severe trauma. The threat persists indefinitely. Terrorism capitalizes on media coverage, whose powerful visual images creates strong emotional responses, including fear, panic, despair, and rage, even in individuals who live far away from the traumatic events.

Childhood reactions to terrorism-induced trauma

Terrorism-induced trauma results in unique stressors and reactions in children. By its very nature, terrorism is likely to cause psychological stress. The unpredictable, indefinite threat of terrorist events, the profound effect on adults and communities, and the effect of extensive terrorist-related media coverage exacerbates underlying anxieties and contributes to a continuous state of stress and anxiety. Research on the impact of terrorism and children covers a range of violent acts that are classified as acts of terrorism, including isolated events in countries not at war and repeated terrorist attacks in areas of political conflict. Studies have examined the effects of direct exposure (eg, physical presence, family or friend, or near-miss experiences) and remote exposure through the media.

Many of the effects of terrorism-induced trauma on children are similar to the effects of manmade and natural disaster trauma. Children vary in their reactions to traumatic events [2,3]. Some children suffer from worries and bad memories that dissipate with time and emotional support. Other children may be more severely traumatized and experience long-term problems. Children's responses include acute stress disorder, posttraumatic stress disorder (PTSD), anxiety, depression, regressive behaviors, separation problems, sleep difficulties, and behavioral problems. Children's emotional reactions may develop immediately after the trauma or may occur later. The DSM-IV-TR recognizes these temporal categories of reaction [4]. Acute stress disorder is the most common psychiatric disorder after a traumatic event. PTSD is a reaction that may occur after a period of time. Children and adolescents who suffer from acute stress disorder or PTSD may re-experience the trauma by having nightmares or recurring flashbacks of the trauma. In young children, repetitive play may occur in which themes or aspects of the trauma are expressed. Their dreams may be frightening but without any recognizable content. Trauma-specific re-enactment may occur. Adolescents and children may feel numb and withdraw from the external world or avoid situations that arouse recollection of the trauma. Symptoms of increased arousal may occur, including hypervigilance, sleep difficulties, irritability, difficulty concentrating, and outbursts of anger.

In addition to acute stress disorder and PTSD, children may develop comorbid disorders, including anxiety disorders (eg, panic disorder, agoraphobia, generalized anxiety disorder, phobias, social phobia, obsessive-compulsive disorder), depression, and substance abuse–related disorders. Children may present with partial or variable symptoms of these disorders [5–7].

Risk and protective factors for children and adolescents

Childhood reactions to trauma and terrorist events depend on several risk and protective factors, including factors related to the history and terrorist event itself and individual, family, and community strengths and vulnerabilities.

History and the event

Children's responses vary in accordance to their level of exposure to the terrorist activities, either directly or indirectly. The degree of exposure to terrorist actions is related to the prevalence of PTSD. The more severe the traumatic event, the greater the risk of developing posttraumatic symptoms [8,9]. Children who experience loss directly are more symptomatic [9–17]. Physical injury or witnessing death and physical injury of others is associated with higher rates of PTSD and comorbid depression and anxiety [12,18,19]. The degree of personal loss (ie, the child's relationship to the victim) also has been correlated with the number of posttraumatic stress symptoms in less exposed children. Knowing an injured or deceased person increases the risk of symptom development [17]. The highest rates of PTSD occur in children who lost a parent [20].

In addition to the level of trauma, the duration of exposure to violence predicts risk for development of psychiatric problems in children [13,16,21–23].

Individual factors and vulnerabilities

Individual factors that affect a child's differential response are related to developmental factors, including a child's age and level of psychological maturity [24–29]. Neurobiologic responses, predisposing risk factors, and effects of resiliency also influence a child's individual response to traumatic exposure.

Developmental considerations

What children understand during and after an exposure to a traumatic event is a function of their developmental level with respect to cognition, emotional and social factors.

Preschool-aged children

Young children between the ages of 3 years and 5 years are likely to express their concerns about safety in terms of separation from parents and other primary caretakers. They rely heavily on cues about danger from caretakers, and at this age, their cognitions indicate that they frequently do not understand the finality of death. Although preschoolers understand less of the actual events, they are more comforted than older children by parental behavior that is reassuring [30]. They may have increased difficulties separating from their parents [31]. Children aged 5 and younger may exhibit regressive behaviors, such as bed wetting, thumb sucking, or fear of the dark [25,32–34]. Additional symptoms may include fear, anxiety, sleep problems, and aggressive behaviors [30].

Elementary school–aged children

Elementary school–aged children (6–11 years) are developmentally prone to polarizing even complex situations into "right" and "wrong" and derive a sense of security from clear-cut rules. As children mature from 6 to 12 years of age, they develop an increasing sense of empathy and altruism. When faced with exposure to a terrorist act, for example, children in this age group may fear for others and recognize death as final, although they only may be able to conceptualize it as remote. Elementary school–aged children are profoundly affected by exposure to a traumatic event, even if they are not involved directly. They may suffer from symptoms of anxiety, PTSD, and depression [35]. Signs of anxiety include school avoidance, somatic complaints (eg, headaches, stomachaches), irrational fears, sleep problems, nightmares, irritability, and angry outbursts [17,36,37]. Symptoms of depression may include sadness, feelings of hopelessness, and withdrawal [38,39]. They may have attention problems, and their school work may suffer.

Adolescents

Among early adolescents, although there is a cognitive awareness of the finality and inevitability of death, there is also a competing sense of immunity to being harmed. A sense of omnipotence may overpower a young teen's judgment regarding the actual danger that is present in his or her environment. At the same time, adolescents remain vulnerable to idealized notions, including, for example, the notion that if they helped the world's leaders to set up a meeting, the world's nations would likely be able to resolve their differences and end the threat of terrorism once and for all. When young teens are exposed to extra-ordinary events such as a terrorist attack, they may feel overly responsible for devising a plan that could protect them and their families from danger. Older adolescents are more able to separate personal fears of danger to themselves from world events that have resulted in harm to others. Adolescent (age 12–18) re-sponses are more similar to adult responses and include intrusive thoughts, hyper-vigilance, emotional numbing, nightmares, sleep disturbances, and avoidance [26,29]. They are at increased risk of having problems with substance abuse, peer problems, and depression [40]. Trauma is often associated with intense feelings of humiliation, self-blame, shame, and guilt, which result from the sense of powerlessness and may lead to a sense of alienation and avoidance [15,37,41,42]. Adolescents may internalize the world as riskier and more dangerous [43].

Neurobiologic consequences of trauma in children and adolescents

Evidence suggests that childhood exposure to traumatic events influences the neurobiologic responses to stress in the developing brain in such a way that it predisposes affected individuals to mood and anxiety symptoms later in life [44]. The finding that individuals who have sustained significant trauma during childhood have an increased risk of mood and anxiety disorders later in life may be related to changes in neurotransmitter systems that are stimulated by stress [45]. One important mediator of the stress response is corticotropin-releasing factor. In the presence of stress, this substance is increased in the brain. It is possible that children who have been exposed to chronic or severe stress have dysregulation of the corticotropin-releasing factor system, which may explain some of the symptomatology of traumatic syndromes, such as increased startle response, and symptoms of anxiety and mood disorder [46].

Predisposing risk factors

Some children are at greater risk of developing symptoms of anxiety and depression. Predisposing risk factors include exposure to past traumatic events during childhood [47,48], childhood conduct problems [49], childhood anxiety [49], and antisocial behavior or a family history of psychiatric disorders [40,50]. All children's sense of safety and potential for personal danger is affected, however. Each child reacts differently depending on sensitivity and temperament and whether he or she tends to internalize or externalize experiences and emo-tions [51,52]. Children may become fearful, distractible, anxious, or depressed. Their play and study may be affected, as can their pattern of sleep or eating.

Resilience among children and adolescents

Many children and adolescents who are exposed to traumatic events do not develop pervasive chronic posttraumatic syndromes. Factors associated with resilience among children and adolescents after exposure to severe traumatic events are related to biologic and psychological characteristics. One hypothesis explains resilience in terms of the variability in emotional reaction and physiologic arousal. There is variation in the psychological interpretation of physiologic arousal [53]. For example, when one encounters a fearful event, there is an initial increase in cortisol level in the brain and increase in heart rate in response to the initial fearful event. Recovery from a traumatic event, in this model, includes being able to respond to the event in a supportive environment without extreme avoidance and in the absence of persistent physiologic arousal. Recovery is the normative path, whereas the development of a perpetual state of fear leads to posttraumatic symptoms. It is likely that early intervention might facilitate the process of recovery in vulnerable individuals [53].

Family factors and vulnerabilities

Children's response to violent events and their ability to cope with these disasters are influenced strongly by their parents' responses to the trauma [54–58]. A positive correlation between children's and parents' symptomatology has been noted [59,60]. The importance of parental involvement in mediating stress reactions in children has been studied in families exposed to terrorist attacks [9]. Parents may underestimate their children's reactions and unintentionally hinder their children's process of mastering the trauma [8,61–63]. Because terrorist incidents affect adults profoundly, parents and teachers may not be able to provide the support and reassurance needed to help avoid potential long-term emotional harm to their children. Increased levels of distress were noted in children whose parents responded to traumatic events with negative emotions. Positive coping responses in children were associated with parents who responded with positive emotional reactions to trauma [9]. Family protective factors that have been shown to buffer stress for children and increase resiliency include a stable, secure, emotional relationship with at least one parent [64], a parental model of constructive coping mechanisms [24,54,59,64,65], and physical proximity of children to parents [38].

Community factors

Responses of community members in populations exposed to terrorism have an important influence on children's coping skills. Children's resiliency to traumatic events is influenced by the degree of social support and positive community influences [66–71]. Community educational, political, and religious support fosters moral development in children [67,68]. The presence of a caring adult who is able to provide emotional support, encourage self-esteem, and promote competence has a moderating influence on acute and long-term mental health outcomes [30,32,72,73]. Community ideology, beliefs, and value systems also contribute to resiliency by giving meaning to dangerous events, allowing children to identify with cultural values, and enabling children and adults to function under extreme conditions [63,65,69,73–77].

Children's responses to media exposure of terrorist events

The increased media coverage of terrorist activities has had a significant impact on children's emotional responses. Research studies have shown consistently that one third or more children watch the news [78–81]. The media plays an important role in providing information to the public, especially during times of disaster. The images portrayed are powerful and intensely emotional. They are often unedited and are repeated frequently. Terrorist organizations depend on media dissemination of their activities to increase responses of fear and panic. For decades, research has examined the influence of violence and aggression on children and adolescents. Recently, with the increase in terrorist bombings and access to media coverage throughout the world, more studies have examined the effects of children's reactions to media coverage of terrorism. Research on the impact of the media on children covers a range of violent acts that are classified as acts of terrorism, including the Oklahoma City bombings (1995), the Scud missile attacks and news coverage during the Persian Gulf War (1991), and the attack on the World Trade Center (September 11, 2001). Although the space shuttle Challenger disaster (1986) was not the result of a terrorist attack, studies of children who witnessed the explosion indirectly by viewing it on television provided valuable information on the effects of indirect trauma. The results of the research on children's responses to media coverage has shown that remote exposure, such as viewing terrorism on television, has a significant clinical impact.

The Challenger disaster

Terr et al [82,83] studied children's responses to the space shuttle Challenger explosion [86]. Children watched the explosion on television and were exposed indirectly to the traumatic event. Terr et al [36] defined distant trauma as "the reaction (memory, thinking, symptoms) to a disastrous event, observed at the time of the event, but from a remote, and safe distance." Children's responses included symptom patterns similar to PTSD. Children's reactions to distant trauma also included trauma-specific fear, fear of being alone, the habit of clinging to others, and event-specific fears. Children who lived on the East Coast were more symptomatic than children who lived on the West Coast. East Coast children had a significant increase in dreaming, drawing and behavioral re-enactment, trauma-specific fears (eg, death and dying, taking risks, explosions, fires, airplanes), and clinging behaviors. Latency age children were more affected than adolescents. Children and adolescents throughout the United States had diminished expectations for the future. Most symptoms diminished within a year; however, for children with initial partial PTSD, symptoms (ie, posttraumatic play for young children and hopeless attitudes about the future for adolescents) often would persist. Further studies have described a spectrum of trauma-related conditions that resulted from remote exposure to violence, including viewing media coverage of disaster events [13,15,17,37,54,84].

Oklahoma City bombing

Pfefferbaum et al [11,85] examined children's reactions to news coverage of the 1995 Oklahoma City bombing. More than 2000 middle school students in Oklahoma City were surveyed 7 weeks after the bombing. Television viewing of the bombing after the explosion was extensive. Children who experienced personal losses were at greater risk of watching significantly more terrorist-related television coverage than children without direct losses [11,12]. This further exacerbated the traumatic experience. The degree of television exposure was related directly to posttraumatic stress symptomatology in children. In children who experienced a direct loss, the impact of viewing television was greater (increased initial arousal and fear); however, many nonbereaved youth experienced symptoms after TV exposure. Children who witnessed the bombing on television reported trauma-related stress for more than 2 years [11]. In addition to broadcast media (ie, television and radio) exposure, print media (ie, newspaper and magazine) exposure also was examined. Print media exposure correlated more strongly with enduring posttraumatic stress than broadcast media [86].

Scud missile attacks and news coverage during the Persian Gulf War

The effects of exposure to terrorism and the importance of parental involvement in mediating stress reactions in children have been studied in families exposed to the Scud missile attacks [9,10,30,32,72]. Bat-Zion and Levy-Shiff [9] noted that parents' responses were a central mediating factor for Israeli children's reactions to Scud missile attacks. Parental negative emotional expressions were associated with increased levels of distress in children, whereas positive emotional manifestations were associated with increased coping efforts. Laor et al [30,32,72] studied the long-term consequences of the Scud missile attacks in Israeli children. Children of mothers with poor psychological functioning showed more stress symptomatology in families who were displaced. The association between children's and mothers' symptoms was stronger among younger children (aged 3 and 4). Unhealthy family interactions exacerbate children's stress, children manifest more symptoms, and their capacity to recover from the critical trauma is jeopardized [32].

Parents' positive emotional responses may have a buffering effect on their children's reactions. Children with adequate family cohesion manifest less stress in reaction to trauma and are better able to recover from the initial impact of the trauma [30,32,72]. Unhealthy family interactions—either disengaged or enmeshed styles [87]—exacerbated children's stress. These children manifested more symptoms, and their capacity to recover from the critical trauma was jeopardized. Conversely, children with adequate family cohesion manifested less stress in reaction to trauma and were better able to recover from the initial impact of the trauma.

World Trade Center (September 11, 2001)

Research on children's reactions to the terrorist attacks of September 11, 2001 corroborates the results of previous research studies. The degree of exposure, proximity to the disaster area, association with parental reactions, experience of distant trauma (including media coverage), and history of pre-existing trauma were associated with increased stress symptoms. Children's reactions included symptoms of posttraumatic stress, depression, panic attacks, anxiety, separation anxiety, and agoraphobia. Children who were exposed to trauma before the attacks were more likely to experience PTSD and other psychiatric problems [35]. Halpern-Felsher and Millstein [43] studied adolescents in California 1 month after the September 11 attack. Adolescents experienced heightened perceptions of vulnerability to death, which extended beyond the terrorist attacks and generalized to unrelated risks. After exposure to the terrorist attacks, even from across the country, adolescents internalized a perception of the world as more risky and dangerous.

Media coverage of the September 11 terrorist attacks was extensive, and repeated coverage of the graphic images of planes striking the World Trade Center caused considerable concern about the added emotional effects of viewing the traumatic events. A national study conducted a few days after September 11, 2001 concluded that children (aged 5–18) watched 3 hours of television news on the day of the attacks. Only 8% of children did not watch any coverage of the event [88]. Parents who reported that their children were upset restricted their children's television viewing. In children whose viewing of television was not restricted, the number of hours of television correlated with the number of stress symptoms. A study commissioned by the New York City board of education 6 months after the World Trade Center attacks noted that 62% of children spent much of their time and 33% of children spent some of their time learning about the September 11 attacks on television. Approximately 75% of children increased the amount of time they spent reading newspapers and magazines, and more than 30% obtained information from the Internet. 10.5% (75,000) of students manifested symptoms of PTSD 6 months after September 11, including children who were not affected directly by the event. Among these children, the prevalence of stress was higher among children who spent more time watching television coverage of the events than children who spent less time. The author notes, however, that these results do not determine a direct causality between television viewing and PTSD rates. Exposure to the images on television may have exacerbated children's stress responses; however, anxious children may have been more likely to seek information from the media than nondistressed children [35].

The indirect exposure of September 11 via television, the Internet, and printed media was examined in a study of elementary school children in the southeast United States. More PTSD symptoms were reported in children who saw reports on the Internet (versus television or printed material), saw images of death or injury, or feared that a loved one might have died in the attacks. There was no measurable benefit to seeing "positive" or "heroic" images. Older children and boys were noted to have greater media exposure and more trauma-specific PTSD symptoms [89].

The correlation between television viewing of the September 11 attacks and an increased sense of insecurity and stress symptoms also was shown in a study of elementary school-aged children in Washington, DC [90].

The effects of television viewing of the September 11 attacks also were examined in adults. Specific disaster-related television images were associated with PTSD and depression among persons who were exposed directly to the disaster [91]. The number of hours of television coverage viewed and an index of the content of that coverage were associated with PTSD symptoms [92].

Palestinian children living in a war zone

The impact of the media on children living in a war zone has been studied in Palestinian children and Kuwaiti children during the Gulf War. Palestinian children who were exposed to traumatic events indirectly by the media had a higher incidence of anticipatory anxiety and cognitive expressions of distress than children who were exposed directly, who in turn manifested more symptoms of PTSD [84].

The effect of extensive terrorist-related media coverage further exacerbates the traumatic experience. Television coverage is a secondary source of exposure to trauma and creates a ripple effect. Large numbers of children not exposed directly to terrorist activities are affected. The unpredictable, indefinite threat of terrorist activities exacerbates underlying anxieties and contributes to a continuous state of stress and anxiety.

Television and the media

The extent of children's exposure to television and the media has increased over the past few decades. Forty-one percent of American households have three or more televisions [93]. Approximately 33% of children aged 2 to 7 years and 56% of children aged 8 to 16 have a television in their rooms [94]. The average time per week that American children aged 2 to 17 spend watching television is 19 hours, 40 minutes [93]. The percentage of television time that children aged

2 to 7 spend watching television alone and unsupervised is 81%. Daycare centers use television during a typical day 70% of the time [95]. The number of hours that the average American child spends in school per year is 900; the average number of hours that a child spends watching television per year is 1023.

A survey of children and the media [80] noted that 65% of children reported watching a television news program, and 44% of children read a newspaper. More than 50% of the children reported feeling angry, sad, or depressed after watching the news.

Children's interpretation of the media: developmental considerations

Children's understanding and interpretation of television and the media are related to their cognitive and psychological developmental level [96–98]. Children are less able than adults to regulate their emotions after watching traumatizing images. Preschool-aged children are most affected by visual images and emotional sounds [99,100]. They are more upset by images of dead bodies or bloodied survivors and crying victims or witnesses than falling buildings or announcer commentaries. They are not able to understand the extent of a tragedy. Preschool-aged children cannot distinguish between live pictures and replays. If events are shown repeatedly, they believe that the catastrophe is occurring repeatedly in real life. They are likely to believe that terrorism is happening at the same time that they are watching the coverage, and they believe that it is occurring in close proximity to their home [96].

Elementary school–aged children (7–12 years) have a better understanding of the event but interpret it concretely [96]. They are more sensitive to injured children or children whose parents were killed. They have difficulty understanding the impact of the terrorist threats and adult responses to these threats. School-aged children are more likely to focus on their own safety and that of their family.

Adolescents are more capable of abstraction than younger children. They are equally affected by visual images; however, they also are concerned about community responses and the impact of threats on the future [81]. Their cognitive advances allow them to ponder the broader issues in terrorism, including complex philosophical and existential issues that involve social justice, politics, and theology. Their personal struggles with identity, meaning, and place in society may be compromised seriously or distorted by the perception of the world and its human interactions as dangerous, untrustworthy, and immoral. This world view may have a negative impact on their sense of hope for the future.

Television and the media: constructive and destructive effects

Media coverage of terrorist events has positive and negative consequences. Although there has been extensive research about children's exposure to the entertainment media, there is far less scientific research about children's exposure to the news, especially exposure to terrorist media coverage.

Positive effects

Several constructive effects of the media have been emphasized [101,102]. The media plays a vital role in disseminating information quickly to local, national, and international regions. Media coverage may facilitate family and community cohesion. It facilitates the dissemination of educational information and may serve as a vehicle for discussion in older children and adolescents. Klingman [101] noted that the media, the Internet, and the telephone serve as extensive support systems. Television stations and the Internet are able to broadcast advice on how to help children cope with stress and anxiety related to disastrous events.

Negative effects

The increased incidence of stress-related symptoms in children exposed to media coverage of terrorist events has been mentioned previously. Repeated media exposure is especially detrimental for young children because of their cognitive immaturity. The ubiquitous presence of televisions and computers may compromise further our youths' ability to integrate their exposure given the amount of material they experience alone without adult supervision and guidance. The effect of the repeated coverage may promote the trauma and increase the duration and intensity of the effects. The media may have a continued negative impact on parents and caregivers, which directly affects the coping abilities of their children. More research is needed to measure the effects of media coverage of terrorist events and determine whether they have detrimental or positive effects on mental health outcomes.

Clinical interventions and treatment

The effectiveness and comparative advantages of specific interventions and treatment modalities for children exposed to terrorism have received scant attention. Only recently have researchers developed rigorously designed studies to examine the effectiveness of treatments in children exposed to non–terrorism-induced trauma (eg, single-incident traumas, natural disasters, sexual abuse, community violence, and war-induced trauma). The results of this research are promising. Children exposed to terrorist activities often manifest similar symptoms to children who have experienced other types of trauma. The results of research on the acute and chronic reactions of children to trauma may have significant implications for intervention strategies and treatment of children exposed to terrorism. No research has addressed the issues of treatment and interventions that are helpful to children who have been traumatized specifically by media coverage of terrorist events. Several recommendations can be inferred from the literature on treatment of trauma, however. A general review of community, school-based, individual, and family interventions and treatments is provided, followed by guidelines and suggestions specifically related to media coverage of terrorist events.

The application of trauma-focused interventions addresses several protective and risk factors that have useful implications for treatment of children exposed to terrorism. They emphasize the importance of parental and community reactions. Providing assistance to parents and caregivers and including them in treatment is considered a crucial component of treatment. Psychoeducation, cognitive restructuring, exposure, and coping skills management are emphasized. The importance of the effects of distant trauma and media coverage is taken into consideration.

Essential intervention strategies for dealing with community-wide acts of terrorism include early community-based intervention, clinical needs assessment to identify children at risk, multimodal, trauma-loss-focused treatment programs, and program evaluation of treatment efficacy [61]. Early community-based interventions focus on safety and protection. Restoration of rest and sleep, emotional support by parents and caregivers in the community, and stress-related symptom reduction are emphasized. Community-wide screening—conducted in schools, primary care settings, or neighborhood centers—identifies children at risk. Although there is no consensus on the most effective method of assessment, numerous structured interviews and self-reports are available [103,104]. Screening identifies children at risk and children in need of acute, trauma-related service. An essential component of the screening process is differentiating normal, developmentally appropriate reactions to trauma from abnormal reactions. Screening information may be used to develop specialized treatment programs based on the unique needs of a child, family, or community. Screening results also serve to provide pretreatment data for evaluating outcome studies of treatment effectiveness. Triage and referral, based on knowledge of psychopathology and risk factors, are essential components of intervention.

Family therapy, adult therapy, group therapy, and school and community interventions have been used to treat traumatized children and families, provide them with coping skills, and address issues related to trauma and loss. No systematized studies have proved their effectiveness [105–108]. Psychoeducational group meetings (ie, parent or community meetings) reduce symptoms of individual, family, and community fear and arousal levels [109]. School-based interventions to treat PTSD symptoms have received empirical support in the literature [110–112]. Several manuals on treatment programs for use after community traumatic events, including acts of terrorism, have been developed and distributed internationally [113–118,127]. These intervention programs and materials include active involvement of children's parents, caregivers, health care providers, community leaders, and educators. They present educational materials on basic safety skills, psychological stress responses, and treatment exercises to address symptoms and behavioral difficulties associated with trauma and loss. The preliminary results of the interventions and manuals developed to aid children after terrorist attacks are promising. Outcome data have not been examined, however, and further research is needed to evaluate their effectiveness.

Children and families who manifest significant psychiatric impairment and dysfunction are in need of more intensive mental health interventions treatment. Cognitive behavioral therapy has been the most rigorously studied treatment for traumatized children [119–127]. Studies by March [127] and Goenjian's [125] suggested that cognitive restructuring (ie, reprocessing the traumatic event and identifying traumatic triggers), relaxation training, anger management training, teaching of proactive coping skills, and grief management are important methods for treating PTSD after disasters. Neither study addressed problems faced by children exposed to chronic trauma, comorbid disasters, past history of trauma exposure, and serious family dysfunction, however.

Minimal data are available on the effectiveness of pharmacotherapy to treat symptoms of PTSD in children. Selective serotonin reuptake inhibitors have been shown to have therapeutic effects on symptoms of depression and anxiety disorders in children [128,129]. Because symptoms of anxiety and depression are common in children after trauma, treatment with selective serotonin reuptake inhibitors has been considered an option.

Certain limitations exist when applying trauma-specific interventions to children who have experienced ongoing violence and the continual threat of terrorism. Crisis intervention alone does not prevent the long-lasting effects of children exposed to terrorism [8,19]. Compounded effects of multiple traumas have not been addressed. The unpredictability of terrorist attacks, indefinite nature of violent threats, lack of specific geographic boundaries, and effects of media coverage result in unique stressors and pose specific challenges for treatment of terrorism-induced trauma in children.

Guidelines for parents, health care providers, and educators: trauma and the media

Helping children and adolescents overcome psychological problems in the aftermath of terrorist events is an important challenge for families and communities. Proactive and preventive methods to help children cope with loss and anxiety may help to facilitate positive posttraumatic adjustment and allow for healthier outcomes in children's growth and development. Because the media plays a major role in informing the public about terrorism and may be a causative agent in symptom formation, it is critical for parents and families to have guidance about the use and misuse of media in traumatic times. What follows are media-related suggestions for health care providers, educators, and parents when dealing with children in the aftermath of terrorist attacks.

Parents, educators, health care providers, politicians, and journalists must increase their awareness about the potentially harmful effects of media exposure on children

Disaster-related television viewing by children should be monitored closely by parents. Children's exposure should be limited. Adults also benefit from limiting their own exposure to reduce their stress reactions so that they and their children are better able to cope. Vulnerable persons who have risk factors, such as young children and persons with previous traumatic experiences, should be especially cautious. When children are permitted to watch television, parents and caregivers are advised to watch the coverage with them. This supervision provides adults with the opportunity to observe children's signs of distress and be available to answer questions and discuss relevant topics. School staff also must be aware of the importance of monitoring media exposure and should consider policies related to viewing coverage of traumatic events.

Adults should find positive ways of understanding and coping with their own responses to terrorist events

Since September 11, 2001, many resources have been made available to help parents cope with the terrorism-related fears and anxieties [130–132]. A constructive use of the media may be helpful in this situation to access information to help parents. Any parent who is overwhelmed by the effects of the disaster should seek help from primary health care providers, educators, mental health agencies, and clergy. If parents are not able to manage their own responses to the trauma, they are not effective in reassuring their children and helping them discuss their concerns, particularly when their children see graphic images on television, hear stories on the news, and read about current events in the newspapers and magazines.

Children cannot be sheltered entirely from knowing about or reacting to a disturbing event

In the modern world, children of all ages are likely to have exposure to media. In the youngest age groups, parents may opt to shelter a child from exposure to frightening and disturbing media images. When possible, young children should be encouraged to express their feelings in words. Answers to their questions should be honest and brief. One should not provide more information than is requested. For children in late elementary school who are exposed to some images in school, programs may be previewed by parents and then watched together as a family. Long after an event, children may watch shows with parents to help them understand terrorism, for example, "Through a child's eyes: September 11, 2001," which is an Emmy Award–winning HBO children's special that deals with young school-age children's responses to the September 11 attacks. Children's fears of not knowing or understanding what has happened may be more disturbing than the truth. It is important for parents to present in-formation to children according to a child's developmental level. Children should be encouraged to express their concerns, and their feelings should be validated. Listening is more important than talking. All questions should be treated with respect, not ignored or dismissed. Responses should be made with calm reassur-ance and empathy. If a child's question causes anxiety or discomfort, the adult should not remain silent, because a child may interpret the silence as a sign of danger. It is permissible to tell a child that his or her question cannot be answered immediately but will receive a response after the adult has time to think about it.

Because older children are exposed to media presentation of acts of terrorism at home and most likely in some form in the classroom, discussing terrorist activities with them—without overwhelming them—and encouraging questions or correcting misperceptions are helpful.

Some children's and adolescent's responses may be confusing

Children's and adolescent's defenses may cover up fears and anxieties. For example, they may make comments such as "We should not be upset, nothing has happened to us." Just as adults should be aware of their own defenses and coping styles, they should be sensitive to children's defenses and ways of coping. This awareness may involve judicious use of media chosen at a child's developmental level. Young children should not watch adult-oriented shows. For example, older elementary school–aged children may tolerate being exposed to news "briefs" in which simple concise statements of the facts are made (eg, reports that occur on major networks between television shows) but may not be ready to watch shows such as "20/20" or news shows that spend 30 minutes with interviews, photos, and more detailed discussion of a devastated building or land.

If a child chooses not to talk about the events, parents should respect that decision

Children may not be ready to share their experiences immediately; they may wait days or weeks. Adults should ensure that children know that they are available to listen and discuss their feelings whenever the children need them. Conversely, some children are interested in listening and watching and are pay-ing attention to the media exposure although they are not ready for discussion. Parents should continue to monitor and guide a child's exposure to media reports that contain frightening information and not assume that a child is unaware, unaffected, or disinterested in an event simply because the child is not ready to talk about it.

Adults need to reassure children that they are safe and will be protected

Media reports can be used to help reassure children and adolescents that many adults are working to maintain a safe and protected environment for them. Parents may choose to offer taped news reports or specific types of media discussion that will help a child to feel secure in the knowledge that adults are taking charge and responding in ways that are protective. Films about resilience, survival, family and community consolidation, and triumph over adversity may play a constructive role by giving children a reasonable sense of hope for the future. Maintaining familiar routines helps children know what to expect and is comforting to them. Reassuring children that they are loved and that they will be cared for gives them a sense of security. They should not be offered false assurance, however. Parents should teach children to manage their fears and anger constructively by showing them how to handle their emotions in healthy ways. They can be made to feel more in control by allowing them to make decisions (eg, what to eat at mealtime, what to wear, what movie to see).

Further recommendations

The continuing frequency of terrorism-related events around the world underscores the urgent need for an effective public health approach for children and families. The media have a responsibility to balance their professional goals of delivering news and preventing potentially untoward effects. It is important for journalists and editors to understand the impact of their reporting on children. Mental health care organizations and providers must be educated and prepared to deal with children who need care in the aftermath of terrorist activities. DuFour (Frederick DuFour, PhD, personal communication) has noted that "terrorism is a community mental health issue" because terrorism is "psychological warfare." Collaboration among community, educational, and mental health care organizations has been initiated and is likely to continue to grow and develop. Further collaboration among these agencies and the media is necessary. Advocacy for program development and funding to help children is needed. Efforts should be focused on increasing community services for children affected by terrorism and encouraging further research on terrorism and its unique impact on children and families. Public policy to limit media coverage is a controversial issue but must be addressed. Mental health care providers and organizations, journalists, educators, spiritual leaders, and community organizations will be better prepared to prevent retraumatizing experiences and help children cope, which will minimize long-term psychological problems and enhance healthier outcomes and growth.

References

[1] United States Department of Defense. Department of Defense combating terrorism program (Department of Defense Directive Number 2000.12). Available at: http://www.defenselink.mil/pubs/downing_rpt/annx_e.html. Accessed February 1, 2002.
[2] Yehuda R, McFarlane AC, Shalev AY. Predicting the development of posttraumatic stress disorder from the acute response to a traumatic event. Biol Psychiatry 1998;44:1305–13.

[3] Smith EM, North CS. Posttraumatic stress disorders in natural disasters and technological accidents. In: Wilson JP, Raphael B, editors. International handbook of traumatic stress syndromes. New York: Plenum Press; 1993. p. 405–19.

[4] American Psychiatric Association. Diagnostic and statistical manual of mental disorders. 4th edition (DSM-1V-TR). Washington (DC): American Psychiatric Association; 2000.

[5] Almqvist K, Broberg AG. Mental health and social adjustment in young refugee children 3½ years after their arrival in Sweden. J Am Acad Child Adolesc Psychiatry 1999;38:723–30.

[6] Ayalon O. Children as hostages. Practitioner 1982;226:1773–81.

[7] Macksoud M, Dyregrov A, Raundalen M. Traumatic war experiences and their effects on children. In: Raphael B, Wilson JP, editors. International handbook of traumatic stress syndromes. New York: Plenum Press; 1993. p. 625–33.

[8] Almqvist K, Brandell-Forsberg M. Refugee children in Sweden: post-traumatic stress disorder in Iranian preschool children exposed to organized violence. Child Abuse Negl 1997;21:351–66.

[9] Bat-Zion N, Levy-Shiff R. Children in war: stress and coping reactions under the threat of Scud missile attacks and the effect of proximity. In: Leavitt L, Fox N, editors. The psychological effects of war and violence on children. Hillsdale (NJ): Lawrence Erlbaum Associates, Inc.; 1993. p. 143–79.

[10] Klingman A, Sagi A, Raviv A. The effect of war on Israeli children. In: Leavitt L, Fox N, editors. The psychological effects of war and violence on children. Hillsdale (NJ): Lawrence Erlbaum Associates, Inc.; 1993. p. 75–92.

[11] Pfefferbaum B, Nixon SJ, Tucker RM, et al. Post traumatic stress responses in bereaved children following the Oklahoma City bombing. J Am Acad Child Adolesc Psychiatry 1999; 39:1372–9.

[12] Pfefferbaum B, Gurwitch R, McDonald N, et al. Posttraumatic stress among young children after the death of a friend or acquaintance in a terrorist bombing. Psychiatr Serv 2000;51: 386–8.

[13] Allwood MA, Bell-Dolan D, Husain SA. Children's trauma and adjustment reactions to violent and nonviolent war experiences. J Am Acad Child Adolesc Psychiatry 2002;41:450–7.

[14] Dyregrov A, Gupta L, Gjestad R, et al. Trauma exposure and psychological reactions to genocide among Rwandan children. J Trauma Stress 2000;13:3–21.

[15] Goenjian AK, Pynoos RS, Steinberg AM, et al. Psychiatric comorbidity in children of the 1988 earthquake in Armenia. J Am Acad Child Adolesc Psychiatry 1995;34:1174–84.

[16] Goldstein RD, Wampler NS, Wise PH. War experiences and distress symptoms of Bosnian children. Pediatrics 1997;100:873–8.

[17] Nader K, Pynoos R, Fairbanks L, et al. Children's reactions one year after a sniper attack at their school. Am J Psychiatry 1990;147:1526–30.

[18] Desivilya H, Gal R, Ayalon O. Long-term effects of trauma in adolescents: comparison between survivors of a terrorist attack and control counterparts. Anxiety, Stress, and Coping 1996; 9:1135–50.

[19] Trappler B, Friedman S. Posttraumatic stress disorders of the Brooklyn Bridge shooting. Am J Psychiatry 1996;153:705–7.

[20] Elbedour S, Baker A, Shalhoub-Kevorkian N, et al. Psychological responses in family members after the Hebron massacre. Depress Anxiety 1999;9:27–31.

[21] Gabarino J, Kosteleny K. The effects of political violence on Palestinian children's behavior problems: a risk accumulation model. Child Dev 1996;67:33–45.

[22] Macksoud M. Assessing war trauma in children: a case study of Lebanese children. J Refug Stud 1992;5:1–15.

[23] Pynoos RS, Nader K. Prevention of psychiatric morbidity in children after disaster. In: Shaffer D, Philips I, Enzer NB, editors. OSAP prevention monograph-2: Prevention of mental disorders, alcohol and other drug use in children and adolescents. DHHS Publication ADM 89–1646. Washington (DC): US Government Printing Office; 1989. p. 535–49.

[24] Hanford HA, Mayes SD, Mattison RE, et al. Child and parent reaction to the Three Mile Island nuclear accident. J Am Acad Child Adolesc Psychiatry 1986;25:346–56.

[25] Osofsky JD. The effects of exposure to violence on young children. Am Psychol 1995;50: 782–8.

[26] Realmuto GM, Masten A, Carole LF, et al. Adolescent survivors of massive childhood trauma in Cambodia: life events and current symptoms. J Trauma Stress 1992;5:589–99.

[27] Terr LC. What happens to early memories of trauma? A study of twenty children under age five at the time of the documented traumatic events. J Am Acad Child Adolesc Psychiatry 1988;27:96–104.

[28] Vogel JM, Vernberg EM. Psychological responses of children to natural and human-made disasters. 1. Children's psychological responses to disasters. J Clin Child Psychol 1993;22: 464–84.

[29] Weisenberg M, Schwartzwald J, Waysman M, et al. Coping of school-age children in the sealed room during the scud missile bombardment and postwar stress reactions. J Consult Clin Psychol 1993;61:462–7.

[30] Laor N, Wolmer L, Mayes L, et al. Israeli preschool children under scuds: a 30-month follow-up. J Am Acad Child Adolesc Psychiatry 1997;36:349–56.

[31] Terr LC. Childhood traumas: an outline and overview. Am J Psychiatry 1991;148:10–20.

[32] Laor N, Wolmer L, Mayes L, et al. Israeli preschoolers under the scud missile attacks. Arch Gen Psychiatry 1996;53:416–23.

[33] Scheeringa MS, Zeanah CH, Drell MJ, et al. Two approaches to the diagnosis of posttraumatic stress disorder in infancy and early childhood. J Am Acad Child Adolesc Psychiatry 1995;34: 191–200.

[34] Davidson J, Smith R. Traumatic experiences in psychiatric outpatients. J Trauma Stress 1990;3:459–75.

[35] Hoven CW, Duarte CS, Lucas CP, et al. Effects of the World Trade Center attack on NYC public school students. Initial report to the New York City board of education. New York: Columbia University Mailman School of Public Health and New York State Psychiatric Institute and Applied Research and Consulting; 2002.

[36] Terr LC, Bloch DA, Michel BA, et al. Children's symptoms in the wake of Challenger: a field study of distant-traumatic effects and an outline of related conditions. Am J Psychiatry 1999;156:1536–44.

[37] Pynoos RS, Frederick C, Nader K, et al. Life threat and posttraumatic stress in school-age children. Arch Gen Psychiatry 1987;44:1057–63.

[38] Garbarino J. The experience of children in Kuwait: occupation, war and liberation. Child, Youth, and Family Services Quarterly 1991;14:2–3.

[39] Terr LC. Psychic trauma in children and adolescents. Psychiatr Clin North Am 1985;8:815–35.

[40] Giaconia RM, Reinherz HZ, Silverman AB, et al. Trauma and posttraumatic stress disorder in a community population of older adolescents. J Am Acad Child Adolesc Psychiatry 1995;34: 1369–80.

[41] Cicchetti D, Toth S, Lynch M. The developmental sequelae of child maltreatment: implications for war-related trauma. In: Leavitt L, Fox N, editors. The psychological effects of war and violence on children. Hillsdale (NJ): Lawrence Erlbaum Associates, Inc.; 1993. p. 41–74.

[42] van der Kolk B, McFarlane A. The black hole of trauma. In: van der Kolk A, McFarlane A, Weisaeth L, editors. Traumatic stress. New York: Guilford Press; 1996. p. 3–23.

[43] Halpern-Felsher BL, Millstein GM. The effects of terrorism on teens' perception of dying: the new world is riskier than ever. J Adolesc Health 2002;30:308–11.

[44] Nemeroff CB. Neurobiological consequences of childhood trauma. J Clin Psychiatry 2004; 65(Suppl 1):18–28.

[45] Nemeroff CB. The preeminent role of early untoward experience on vulnerability of major psychiatric disorders: the nature-nurture controversy revised and soon to be resolved. Mol Psychiatry 1999;4:106–8.

[46] Heim C, Nemeroff CB. Neurobiology of early life stress: clinical studies. Semin Clin Neuropsychiatry 2002;7:147–59.

[47] Breslau N, Chilcoat HD, Kessler RC, et al. Previous exposure to trauma and PTSD effects of subsequent trauma. Am J Psychiatry 1999;156:902–7.

[48] Garrison CZ, Weinrich MW, Hardin SB, et al. Post-traumatic stress disorder in adolescents after a hurricane. Am J Epidemiol 1993;138:522–30.

[49] Breslau N, Davis GC. Traumatic events and posttraumatic stress disorder in an urban population of young adults. Arch Gen Psychiatry 1991;48:216–22.

[50] Breslau N, Davis GC. Posttraumatic stress disorder in an urban population of young adults: risk factors for chronicity. Am J Psychiatry 1992;152:529–35.

[51] Lonigan CJ, Shannon MP, Taylor CM, et al. Children exposed to disaster. II: Risk factors for the development of post-traumatic symptomatology. J Am Acad Child Adolesc Psychiatry 1994;33:94–105.

[52] Tyano S, Iancu I, Solomon Z, et al. Seven-year follow-up of child survivors of a bus-train collision. J Am Acad Child Adolesc Psychiatry 1996;35:365–73.

[53] Yehuda R. Risk and resilience in posttraumatic stress disorder. J Clin Psychiatry 2004;65(Suppl 1):29–36.

[54] Breton J, Valla J, Lambert J. Industrial disaster and mental health of children and their parents. J Am Acad Child Adolesc Psychiatry 1993;32:438–45.

[55] Bromet EJ, Goldgaber D, Carlson G, et al. Children's well-being 11 years after the Chernobyl catastrophe. Arch Gen Psychiatry 2000;57:563–71.

[56] Deblinger E, Steer RA, Lipmann J. Maternal factors associated with sexually abused children's psychosocial adjustment. Child Maltreat 1999;4:13–20.

[57] Korel M, Green BL, Gleser GC. Children's responses to a nuclear waste disaster: PTSD symptoms and outcome prediction. J Am Acad Child Adolesc Psychiatry 1999;38:368–75.

[58] McFarlane AC. Family functioning and overprotection following a natural disaster: the longitudinal effects of posttraumatic morbidity. Aust N Z J Psychiatry 1987;21:210–8.

[59] Bryce J, Walker N, Ghorayeb F, et al. Life experiences, response styles and mental health among mothers and children in Beirut, Lebanon. Soc Sci Med 1989;28:685–95.

[60] McFarlane AC. Posttraumatic phenomena in a longitudinal study of children following a natural disaster. J Am Acad Child Adolesc Psychiatry 1987;26:764–9.

[61] Gurwitch RH, Sitterle KA, Young BH, et al. The aftermath of terrorism. In: La Greca AM, Silverman WK, Vernberg EM, et al, editors. Helping children cope with disasters and terrorism. Washington (DC): American Psychological Association; 2002. p. 327–57.

[62] Rigamer EF. Psychological management of children in a national crisis. J Am Acad Child Adolesc Psychiatry 1986;25:364–9.

[63] Sack WH, Angell RH, Kinzie JD, et al. The psychiatric effects of massive trauma on Cambodian children: II. The home and the school. J Am Acad Child Adolesc Psychiatry 1986;25:377–83.

[64] Losel F, Bliesener T. Resilience in adolescents: a study on the generalizability of protective factors. In: Hurrelmann K, Losel F, editors. Health hazards in adolescence. New York: Walter de Gruyter; 1990. p. 299–320.

[65] Kinzie JD, Sack WH, Angell RH, et al. The psychiatric effects of massive trauma on Cambodian children. I: The children. J Am Acad Child Adolesc Psychiatry 1986;25:370–6.

[66] Fergusson DM, Linskey TL. Physical punishment/maltreatment during childhood and adjustment in young adulthood. Child Abuse Negl 1997;21:617–30.

[67] Gabarino J, Kostelny K. Child maltreatment as a community problem. Child Abuse Negl 1992;16:455–64.

[68] Gabarino J, Dubrow N, Kostelny K, et al. Children in danger. San Francisco (CA): Jossey-Bass; 1992.

[69] Miller KE. The effects of state terrorism and exile on indigenous Guatemalan refugee children: a mental health assessment and an analysis of children's narratives. Child Dev 1996;67:89–106.

[70] Smith P, Perin S, Yule W, et al. War exposure and maternal reactions in the psychological

adjustment of children from Bosnia-Herzegovina. J Child Psychol Psychiatry 2001;42: 395–404.

[71] Udwin O, Boyle S, Yule W, et al. Risk factors for long term psychological effects of a disaster experienced in adolescence: predictors of posttraumatic stress disorder. J Child Psychol Psychiatry 2000;41:969–79.

[72] Laor N, Wolmer L, Cohen D. Mother's functioning and children's symptoms 5 years after a SCUD missile attack. Am J Psychiatry 2001;158:1020–6.

[73] Melville MB, Lykes MB. Guatemalan Indian children and the sociocultural effects of government sponsored terrorism. Soc Sci Med 1992;34:533–48.

[74] Baker A. Effects of political and military traumas on children: the Palestinian case. Clin Psychol Rev 1999;19:935–50.

[75] Punamaki RL. Psychological stress response of Palestinian mothers and their children in conditions of military occupation and political violence. Quarterly Newsletter of the Laboratory of Comparative Human Cognition 1987;9:76–9.

[76] Sack WH, McSharry S, Clarke GN, et al. The Khmer adolescent project: I. Epidemiologic findings in two generations of Cambodian refugees. J Nerv Ment Dis 1994;182:387–95.

[77] Sack WH, Gregory C, Seeley M. Posttraumatic stress disorder across two generations of Cambodian refugees. J Am Acad Child Adolesc Psychiatry 1995;34:1160–6.

[78] Atkin C. Broadcast news programming and the child audience. Journal of Broadcasting 1978;22:47–61.

[79] Drew D, Reeves B. Children and TV news. Journalism Quarterly 1978;57:45–54.

[80] Fairbank, Maslin, Maullin, and Associates. Children now: children and the media. Tuned in or tuned out? America's children speak out on the news media. Available at: http://www.childrennow.org/media/mc94/news.html. Accessed April 19, 2003.

[81] Smith SL, Wilson BJ. Children's comprehension and fear reactions to television news. Media Psychology 2002;4:1–26.

[82] Terr LC, Bloch DA, Michel BA, et al. Children's memories in the wake of Challenger. Am J Psychiatry 1996;153:618–25.

[83] Terr LC, Bloch DA, Michel BA, et al. Children's thinking in the wake of Challenger. Am J Psychiatry 1997;154:744–51.

[84] Thabet AM, Abed Y, Vostanis P. Emotional problems in Palestinian children living in a war zone: a cross-sectional study. Lancet 2002;359:1801–4.

[85] Pfefferbaum B, Nixon SJ, Yivis R, et al. Television exposure in children after a terrorist incident. Psychiatry 2001;64(3):202–11.

[86] Pfefferbaum B, Seale T, Brandt E, et al. Media exposure in children one hundred miles from a terrorist bombing. Ann Clin Psychiatry 2003;15(1):1–8.

[87] Minuchin S. Families and family therapy. Cambridge (MA): Harvard University Press; 1974.

[88] Schuster MA, Stein BD, Jaycox LH, et al. A national survey of stress reactions after the September 11, 2001 terrorist attacks. N Engl J Med 2001;345:1507–12.

[89] Saylor CF, Cowart BL, Lipovsky JA, et al. Media exposure to September 11: elementary school students' experiences and posttraumatic symptoms. Am Behav Sci 2003;46(12):1622–42.

[90] Phillips D, Prince S, Schiebelhut L. Elementary school children's responses 3 months after the September 11 terrorist attacks: a study in Washington, DC. Am J Orthopsychiatry 2004; 74(4):509–28.

[91] Ahern J, Galea S, Resnick H, et al. Television images and psychological symptoms after the September 11 terrorist attacks. Psychiatry 2002;65:289–300.

[92] Schlenger WE, Caddell JM, Ebert L, et al. Psychological reactions to terrorists attacks: findings from the national study of Americans' reactions to September 11. JAMA 2002;288:581–8.

[93] Neilson Media Research. Report on television. Available at: http://www.neilsonmedia.com. Accessed August 30, 2004.

[94] Annenberg Public Policy Center. Media in the home national survey. Available at: http://www.annenbergpublicpolicycenter.org/05_media_developing_child/mediasurvey.htm. Accessed August 30, 2004.

[95] Kaiser Family Foundation. Kids and the media @ the new millennium. Available at: http://www.kff.org/entmedia/1535-index.cfm. Accessed August 30, 2004.

[96] Cantor J, Nathanson AI. Children's fright reactions to television news. J Commun 1996; 46(4):139–52.

[97] Cantor J. Mommy, I'm scared: how TV and movies frighten children and what we can do to protect them. San Diego (CA): Harvest/Harcourt Brace & Co; 1998.

[98] Smith SL, Wilson BJ. Children's reactions to a television news story: the impact of video footage and proximity of the crime. Communic Res 2000;27:641–73.

[99] Cantor J, Mares ML, Oliver MB. Parents' and children's emotional reactions to TV coverage of the Gulf War. In: Greenberg BS, Gantz W, editors. Desert Storm and the mass media. Cresskill (NJ): Hampton Press; 1993. p. 325–40.

[100] Hoffner C, Cantor J. Developmental differences in responses to a television character's appearance and behavior. Dev Psychol 1985;21:1065–74.

[101] Klingman A. Children under the stress of war. In: La Greca AM, Silverman WK, Vernberg EM, et al, editors. Helping children cope with disasters and terrorism. Washington (DC): American Psychological Association; 2002. p. 359–80.

[102] Raviv A. The use of hotline and media interventions in Israel during the Gulf War. In: Leavitt L, Fox N, editors. The psychological effects of war and violence on children. Hillsdale (NJ): Lawrence Erlbaum Associates, Inc.; 1993. p. 319–37.

[103] American Academy of Child and Adolescent Psychiatry. Practice parameters for the assessment and treatment of children with posttraumatic stress disorder. J Am Acad Child Adolesc Psychiatry 1998;37(Suppl 10):4S–26S.

[104] Cohen JA, Berliner L, March JS. Treatment of children and adolescents. In: Foa EB, Keane TM, editors. Effective treatments for PTSD: practice guidelines for the International Society for Traumatic Stress Studies. New York: Guilford Press; 2000. p. 106–38.

[105] Nader K. Treatment methods for childhood trauma. In: Wilson JP, Friedman M, Lindy J, editors. PT treating psychological trauma and PTSD. New York: Guilford Press; 2001. p. 278–334.

[106] Pope L, Campbell M, Kurtz P. Hostage crisis: a school-based interdisciplinary approach to posttraumatic stress disorder. Soc Work Educ 1992;14:227–33.

[107] Prinstein MJ, La Greca AM, Vernberg EM, et al. Children's coping assistance after a natural disaster. J Clin Child Psychol 1996;25:463–75.

[108] Terr LC. Childhood posttraumatic stress disorder. In: Gabbard GO, editor. Treatment of psychiatric disorders. 3rd edition. Washington (DC): American Psychiatric Press; 2001. p. 293–306.

[109] Nader K. Treating traumatic grief in systems. In: Wilson JP, Friedman M, Lindy J, editors. Death and trauma: the traumatology of grieving. New York: Guilford Press; 1997. p. 278–334.

[110] La Greca AM, Silverman WK, Vernberg EM, et al. Symptoms of posttraumatic stress after Hurricane Andrew: a prospective study. J Consult Clin Psychol 1996;64:712–23.

[111] Swenson CC, Saylor CF, Powell MP, et al. Impact of a natural disaster on preschool children: adjustment 14 months after a hurricane. Am J Orthopsychiatry 1996;66:122–30.

[112] Vernberg EM, La Greca AM, Silverman WK, et al. Predictors of child's post-disaster functioning following Hurricane Andrew. J Abnorm Psychol 1996;105:237–48.

[113] American Red Cross. Facing fear: helping young people deal with terrorism and tragic events. Falls Church (VA): American Red Cross; 2001.

[114] Gurwitch RH, Messenbaugh A. Healing after trauma skills: a manual for professionals, teachers, and families working with children after trauma/disaster. Oklahoma City (OK): Children's Medical Research Foundation; 2001.

[115] La Greca AM, Vernberg EM, Silverman WK, et al. Helping children cope with natural disasters: a manual for school personnel. Coral Gables (FL): University of Miami; 1994.

[116] La Greca AM, Sevin SW, Selvin EL. Helping America cope: a guide to help parents and children cope with the September 11th terrorist attacks. Coral Gables (FL): 7-Dippity; 2001.

[117] Storm V, McDermott B, Finlayson D. The bushfire and me. Newtown (Australia): VBD Publications; 1994.

[118] Vernberg EM. Intervention approaches following disasters. In: La Greca AM, Silverman WK, Vernber EM, et al, editors. Helping children cope with disasters and terrorism. Washington (DC): American Psychological Association; 2002. p. 55–72.

[119] Berliner L, Saunders B. Treating fear and anxiety in sexually abused children: results in a two-year follow up study. Child Maltreat 1996;1:294–309.

[120] Celano M, Hazzard A, Webb C, et al. Treatment of traumatogenic beliefs among sexually abused girls and their mothers: an evaluation study. J Abnorm Child Psychol 1996;24:1–17.

[121] Cohen JA, Mannarino AP. A treatment outcome study of sexually abused preschool children: initial findings. J Am Acad Child Adolesc Psychiatry 1996;35:1402–10.

[122] Cohen JA, Marrarino AP. Factors that mediate treatment outcome of sexually abused preschool children: six and 12-month follow-up. J Am Acad Child Adolesc Psychiatry 1998;37:44–51.

[123] Deblinger E, Lippman J, Steer R. Sexually abused children suffering posttraumatic stress symptoms: initial treatment outcome findings. Child Maltreat 1996;1:310–21.

[124] Deblinger E, Steer RA, Lippman J. Two-year follow-up study of cognitive behavioral therapy for sexually abused children suffering post traumatic stress symptoms. Child Abuse Negl 1999;23:1371–8.

[125] Goenjian AK, Karayan I, Pynoos RS, et al. Outcome of psychotherapy among pre-adolescents after the 1988 earthquake in Armenia. Am J Psychiatry 1997;154:536–42.

[126] King NJ, Tonge BJ, Mullen P, et al. Treating sexually abused children with posttraumatic stress symptoms: a randomized clinical trial. J Am Acad Child Adolesc Psychiatry 2000;39:1347–55.

[127] March JS, Amaya-Jackson L, Murray MC, et al. Cognitive-behavioral psychotherapy for children and adolescents with PTSD after a single incident stressor. J Am Acad Child Adolesc Psychiatry 1998;37:585–93.

[128] Emslie GJ, Mayes TL. Mood disorders in children and adolescents: psychopharmacological treatment. Biol Psychiatry 2001;49:1082–90.

[129] RUPP Anxiety Study Group. An eight-week placebo-controlled trial of fluvoxamine for anxiety disorders in children. N Engl J Med 2001;344:1279–85.

[130] National Mental Health Association. Available at: http://www.nmha.org/reassurance/second anniversary/kidscopingtips.ctm. Accessed April 5, 2005.

[131] Centers for Disease Control. Available at: http://www.bt.cdc.gov/masstrauma/copingpub.asp. Accessed April 5, 2005.

[132] American Academy of Child and Adolescent Psychiatry. Available at: http://www.aacap.org/publications/factsfam/87.htm. Accessed April 5, 2005.

ELSEVIER
SAUNDERS

Child Adolesc Psychiatric Clin N Am
14 (2005) 453–471

CHILD AND
ADOLESCENT
PSYCHIATRIC CLINICS
OF NORTH AMERICA

Impact of the Media on Adolescent Body Image

Claire V. Wiseman, PhD[a],*, Suzanne R. Sunday, PhD[b],
Anne E. Becker, MD, PhD[c,d]

[a]Department of Psychology, Trinity College, 300 Summit Street, Hartford, CT 06106, USA
[b]Department of Psychiatry, North Shore University Hospital, 400 Community Drive,
Manhasset, NY 11030, USA
[c]Department of Psychiatry, Massachusetts General Hospital, Harvard Medical School, WAC 816,
15 Parkman Street, Boston, MA 02114, USA
[d]Department of Social Medicine, Harvard Medical School, Boston, MA 02114, USA

The mass media have become a powerful force throughout the world and strongly influence how people see themselves and others. This is particularly true for adolescents. This article discusses how the media affect body image and self-esteem and why the media seem to have such strong effects on adolescents. The authors discuss differences in responses to the media in adolescents of different ethnic, racial, and cultural backgrounds. Although this article focuses primarily on teenage girls, the authors also review the data for adolescent boys. Finally, this article discusses possible ways to help adolescents become more active viewers of the media and help prevent the decrease in body esteem that so often occurs during adolescence.

Media defined

Media is defined as an intervening agency that provides wide reaching communication and has significant influence [1]. This ubiquitous force is multi-

Dr. Sunday is supported in part by grants from the National Institute of Mental Health (RO1 MH602642) and the Substance Abuse and Mental Health Services Administration (U79 SM54251).
Dr. Becker is supported in part by a grant from the National Institute of Mental Health (5K23MH068575-02).
* Corresponding author.
E-mail address: Claire.wiseman@trincoll.edu (C.V. Wiseman).

1056-4993/05/$ – see front matter © 2005 Elsevier Inc. All rights reserved.
doi:10.1016/j.chc.2005.02.008

dimensional and seems to penetrate our minds without our conscious awareness. It seems logical that the media affect our attitudes about ourselves and about the world. The influences can be subtle and affect self-concept, but they also can be relatively direct, because the media often give explicit instructions on achieving the thin ideal that is displayed. Selective editing, casting, and reporting frame the fictional and news stories in ways that shape our response. The seamless and idealized worlds portrayed in print and film media present a generally unrealistic but compelling standard for self-comparison. With chronic viewing and media consumption, this standard generally becomes integrated into our taken-for-granted world. Values promoted through television, which often are directly related to the consumerism that funds it, are incorporated—often unexamined—into quotidian life. Our capacity to critique the images and values is likely undermined by the chronicity and ubiquity of exposure. Admiration, identification, and self-comparison with the models and characters are facilitated in advertisements designed for this purpose. Product sales depend on consumers being made aware of a need or a desire to acquire social acceptability or prestige [2].

Historical changes in the portrayal of women's body size and shape

Media portrayal of adolescent girls and women has shifted considerably in the past decades. Whereas much of this change has been positive in providing templates for independent choices and behavior for girls and women, changes in body size and shape have followed a more disturbing trend. In America, we have seen an increasing trend toward a thin ideal for women [3–5]. In the 1950s, the average American model was within 5% of the size of the average American woman. The gap in body weight between models and the average women has increased dramatically; currently, almost two thirds of Americans are overweight [6] and the average model is 15% to 20% below what would be considered a healthy weight for her height [4]. Beauty icons of the 1950s and 1960s were voluptuous, shapely, and "healthy" looking. Since that time, the trend in women's body image has been tall, slender, and athletic [4,5,7]. Multiple studies have reported a decrease in women's body size and changes in body shape as portrayed in the media from the 1950s to current time. For example, in a frequently cited study, Garner et al [5] concretely demonstrated that beauty standards reflected in *Playboy* centerfolds (for which actual bust, waist, and hip measurements were published) grew progressively tubular over the 1970s and 1980s. A subsequent study that analyzed body shape trends in *Playboy* centerfold models between 1953 and 2001 corroborated this finding [8]. Although it is not clear that this publication represents media depiction of women, additional analysis showed that 70% of centerfold models were underweight (ie, body mass index [weight in kilograms/height in meters squared] less than 18.5 kg/m^2) from 1978 to 1998, which further illustrated the idea that icons of male desire are apparently portrayed as thin in at least some influential media [9]. Similarly, results of a content analysis of the popular women's magazine *Vogue* demonstrated that women's figures depicted in the magazine also became less curvaceous between 1901 and 1993 [10]. Currently, the average American woman is 64 inches tall and weighs 164 pounds. In stark contrast, the average American female model is 71 inches tall and weighs 117 pounds. We see that most fashion models are thinner than 98% of American women [11]. As the female ideal has become thinner and thinner, American women seem to be more dissatisfied with their own bodies [12] and may use more extreme techniques to try to achieve the ever-shrinking media images.

The media and its importance to adolescent girls

Several popular press books have appeared over the last two decades arguing that the media have presented maladaptive and dangerous images of women that have become internalized, particularly by adolescent girls [13–16]. They have argued that we are presented only with pictures of extremely thin women, which strongly affects young women's body image and sense of self.

The media affect adolescents so significantly because they are at a vulnerable point in their lives—they are seeking their own identity [17]. During adolescence, they are turning away from parents as their primary source of information and support and turning to peers. Most of them wish to fit in to whatever they perceive as the "norm" of the society and their peers [18]. Adolescents' thinking becomes less grounded in actual fact and becomes more theoretical and based on deductive reasoning [19]. If teens perceive something to be a desired behavior or image, they may deduce that their acceptance by others depends on the achievement of that goal. Adolescents experience the "imaginary audience" [20]—the belief that people are watching them as if they are on stage all the time. This belief can lead them to feel the need to look a certain way much of the time, and the way they should look often is defined by the media.

In his "Social Comparison Theory," Festinger [21] ventured an explanation for this phenomenon. People in general compare themselves to others to gain information. According to Festinger and others, people prefer to use a form of "upward comparison," which includes comparing themselves to people they perceive to be better than themselves [22]. This provides an excellent explanation for the power that the media hold in our society, especially for teens. As long as adolescents perceive the media as "better than " themselves and use the media for a basis of comparison, then they are likely to conform to the media images. Conformity to group pressure has been demonstrated in numerous studies over the years [23–26]. The combination of the two forces—upward comparison and conformity to group pressure—may explain the influence of the media. Studies on norms within groups have indicated that people conform after they essentially have compared themselves to others [27–29]. Adolescents use upward comparison, and television, movies, and magazines provide numerous figures who fulfill that function [21,22].

Taylor et al [30] examined factors that predicted weight concerns that affected young adolescent girls in a study. For middle school–aged students, the best model accounted for more than half the variance, with the importance peers placed on weight and eating being the strongest predictor (33% of the variance), followed by self-confidence, actual weight, trying to look like women on television or in magazines, and being teased about weight. Body image is an important element in a girl's psychology because it plays a significant role in the development of self-esteem. For girls in contemporary American society, unfortunately self-esteem is linked to appearance, particularly the appearance of their bodies [31].

In a 1997 survey of *Psychology Today* readers [32], viewing thin models resulted in approximately half of the women feeling more negatively about themselves and wanting to lose weight. Additional research has demonstrated that the body image of white adolescent girls became more negative after viewing images of thin, beautiful women [33–37]. For example, Richins [38] found that women who viewed images of beautiful, thin, female models experienced decreased satisfaction with their own physical appearance. Although it is unclear how long this effect persists, these studies demonstrated conclusively that viewing images in the media can have at least a temporary effect on a girl's opinion of her body. This is particularly significant as the body sizes displayed in the media continue to shrink and images are increasingly digitally enhanced. Unfortunately, experience teaches us that the lack of correspondence with reality within the media is not a factor about which girls think when making a comparison. When girls compare themselves with an unrealistic standard, they set themselves up for inevitable failure that, in turn, threatens self-efficacy and self-esteem. A possible explanation for the significant impact that the media have lies in the internalization of the media norms. The media become important and viable as an influence only once the norms are internalized, otherwise the influence is fleeting. In a recent study by Lokken et al [39], internalization of the thin ideal was found to correlate directly with subjects' preferences for fashion magazines. They also found that the internalization of the cultural ideal of thinness predicted two major risk factors for eating disorders: drive for thinness and body dissatisfaction. Several recent studies have investigated the internalization of the media images and ways in which we can target the internalization in prevention programs [40–42]. The goal of these programs is to reduce the amount of internalization and thereby reduce the effectiveness of the media. It is clear that the media send out a message that can be dangerous to young girls in particular by presenting images and ideas that encourage them to be thinner [4,5].

Perceived unfavorable comparison with media standards and ensuing body dissatisfaction has been shown to associate strongly with disordered eating behaviors and a distorted body image. Eating disorders, such as anorexia nervosa and bulimia nervosa, primarily affect girls, especially during adolescence. These disorders result from a multitude of factors [43], although most researchers agree that poor self-esteem plays a significant role in their onset. The progression may be that adolescent girls experience a decrease in their satisfaction with their bodies, which may lead to a decline in self-esteem. In looking for ways to feel better about themselves, teenage girls may look toward remedies suggested by the media; unfortunately, one of the solutions that is offered frequently is weight loss and appearance-based solutions for low self-esteem. These solutions solidify further the link between self-esteem and body image.

Dieting may place some girls on the pathway toward an eating disorder. Dieting behavior is ubiquitous in the United States, with 45% of American women being on a diet on any given day [44]. It is estimated that 35% of dieters end up with some form of pathologic dieting, and of this group, 20% to 25% eventually develop partial- or full-syndrome eating disorders [45]. Most eating disorders—as many as 95%—begin with some form of dieting [43]. Although research has not demonstrated that dieting causes eating disorders, it is clearly one of the strongest risk factors. Forces that encourage adolescents to diet may contribute to the current rates of eating-disordered behavior. Printed media targeted at adolescent girls and young adult women promote not only unrealistically thin beauty standards but also dieting strategies. Dieting then becomes routinized and may be described as culturally normative among populations of adolescent and young adult women.

To the extent to which media promote and validate particular body ideals, they are implicated in perpetuating, if not amplifying, the "social pressure to be thin" that is believed to contribute to environmental risk for eating disorders [4,5,43,46,47]. For vulnerable adolescent girls, visual media often present an idealized picture of slender bodies paired with affluent lifestyles. Women's magazines highlight the "gap" between their readership and the cultural ideal. Products are promoted by suggesting that the magazine and its advertisers can assist women in reshaping their bodies or remaking themselves according to cultural ideals [48]. The pressure to conform to body ideals portrayed in Western media may be especially powerful among populations in which Western products and styles are seen as prestigious [49,50]. Studies that demonstrated increased risk for disordered eating in modernizing, urban, immigrant, and upwardly mobile populations (Eileen Anderson-Fye, EdD, unpublished dissertation, 2002) [51,52] are consistent with this hypothesis. The specific ways in which media may impact on adolescent body image are likely somewhat culturally particular, however (see later discussion).

Observational studies on media consumption and body image can establish neither directionality of effect nor mechanism of effect. Although it seems intuitively obvious that women, especially adolescent girls, would be influenced strongly by the media, relatively few empirical studies have explored the issue. Groesz et al [53] recently conducted a meta-analysis of 25 experimental studies and concluded that women's body image is affected negatively by viewing images of thin models, and the effects are most pronounced among teenage girls and girls with pre-existing body image problems. Unfortunately, half of the studies that were reviewed did not measure body dissatisfaction before and after presenting media images. These studies cannot begin to document the undoubtedly profound influences of chronic exposure to strongly appealing, yet virtually unattainable, body shapes and lifestyles depicted in the media. We can glean some important information from experimental studies that examined the effects of brief exposures, however.

Irving [34] speculated that an increased preference for the thin body ideal would result in increased pathologic eating conditions among young women. Attitudes and behaviors of more than 100 women with varying levels of self-reported bulimic symptoms were recorded after viewing thin, average, or over-weight fashion models. Subjects who viewed the thin models had lower levels of self-esteem than the other two groups. Subjects who viewed the oversized models experienced greater weight satisfaction than subjects who were exposed to the average sized models. Pinhas et al [37] examined self-esteem, body dissatisfaction, and mood of normal women who viewed only images of thin female models in comparison to women who viewed non-human images. Viewing photos of thin models had an immediate negative effect on the body satisfaction and mood of the participants.

Our research group (C.V.W. and S.R.S.) recently completed a study that examined the effects of viewing thin and plus-size professional models on college women's drive for thinness, body satisfaction, and esteem [33]. Viewing super-thin and plus-size models had an inverse effect on drive for thinness compared with baseline responses. Body esteem-appearance and -weight subscales and eating disorder inventory body dissatisfaction scores improved after exposure to plus-size models when they were compared with the group that viewed super-thin models. These findings are especially interesting given the number of thin and plus-size models depicted in magazines read by adolescent girls. From 2000 to 2003, 71% of the pictures in *Cosmopolitan, Glamour, Teen People*, and *Seventeen* magazines depicted thin models and only 1% of the images showing plus-size models [32]. The possible positive effects of viewing plus-size models on the body image of adolescent girls may be entirely moot given the low frequency of these images in magazines targeting teenage girls. It is possible that increasing the number of plus-size models in media advertisements may help inoculate (or "protect") young women against some potential risks to their self- and body-esteem. These and other possible methods to prevent problems with body image and disordered eating are discussed in more detail later.

Ethnic, racial, and cultural differences and the media

The media and ethnic/racial differences in the United States

The impact of the media depends on one's body image, and evidence suggests that body image is not viewed consistently across diverse ethnic and racial populations. African-American women have been reported to have lower levels of drive for thinness [54] and lower body weight dissatisfaction [55] than their white counterparts. When African-American and white college women were compared for eating disorder risk factors and eating disorder symptoms, the correlations were similar for the two groups, but the endorsement of the risk factors and the symptoms was considerably lower for the African-American women [56]. Compared with white teenage girls, black adolescent girls of equivalent weights were more likely to say their friends and family viewed them as thin [57]. There also seems to be a racial difference in the age at which body dissatisfaction peaks. For white teenage girls, the peak has been reported to begin during adolescence and extend into young adulthood [58], whereas body dissatisfaction peaked in early adolescence and then declined for black teens [59]. Unfortunately, these studies did not give details concerning the ethnic composition of their white subjects. Non-Latina white girls also have been reported to have lower levels in overall self-esteem during elementary school and a greater drop in esteem during high school than black girls [60]. Further studies in this area are needed to understand what factors (eg, family, cultural, or social norms in the community for an ideal female body) inoculate African-American adolescent girls from the thin images to which they are exposed.

The differences between young non-Latina white women and young Latina white women seem to be less clear than differences between white and African-American teenage girls. Some studies have found that Latina women had larger ideal body sizes than white women [61]; however, other studies have drawn different conclusions. A qualitative study of college-educated Latina and African-American women found that respondents perceived themselves as subject to the same esthetic body ideals as non-Latina white women. Although these minority women reported experiencing these ideals as relatively more unattainable to them, they also rejected the inherent beauty in them, rejected pressures to reshape their bodies to match this perceived ideal, and instead emphasized a body ethic of self-acceptance and self-nurturing [62].

Acculturative stressors and processes seem to be critical to differences between Latina and white women. For example, Pumariega [63] found higher levels of disordered eating symptoms in Latina teenagers who reported a higher level of integration into American culture. Among women of Mexican origin in the United States, Chamorro and Flores-Ortiz [64] found a significant positive relationship between disordered eating attitudes and higher levels of acculturation. The second-generation Mexican-American women had the highest acculturation levels and the highest levels of pathologic eating attitudes. Not all researchers have reported differences that reflect acculturation, however. Joiner and Kashubeck [65] did not find that acculturation affected body dissatisfaction or perceived body shape preference in their Latina sample. Latinas are culturally heterogeneous, and transnational migration likely has variable impact across these diverse groups. Because Latinas are the fastest growing "minority" group in the United States [66], developing a greater understanding of the changes in Latina body image in diverse contexts of social transition is important in understanding the effects of media on this ethnic group and developing appropriate interventions.

Introduction of the media into media-naïve societies

Although helpful to our understanding of the effects of media images, experimental studies may have limited ability to establish the relation between exposure and outcome in populations that have had chronic media access. The results may not generalize to media-naïve societies. For these reasons, investigation into the effects of media on adolescent body image in media-naïve populations provides critical insights into ways in which media-disseminated images and values exert their impact. Clarification of the effects of media on adolescent body image across diverse social contexts outside of the United States is essential to thoughtful, strategic, and culturally sensitive public health interventions. Media exposure to Western ideas, images, values, and lifestyles is believed to play a key role in the apparently global distribution of eating disorders.

Few opportunities remain to discern the relation between media exposure and its effects in a media-naïve population. Television and other media invariably arrive in the setting of other social change, the effects of which are difficult to separate from those of the media exposure. For example, a remote village accessing television for the first time likely is the result of new access to electricity or disposable income sufficient to purchase electronic equipment. Conversely, ethnographic and qualitative data-based studies often can illuminate ways in which youth respond to media, albeit in the context of other social change.

The introduction of television has had a demonstrable impact on local values or behavior across a wide variety of cultural contexts [67–74]. The introduction of television to Korea was associated with intensification of traditional values among male students [75]. Although television is often maligned for its putative adverse effects on youth risk behaviors and violence [76–81], some have pointed out its potential benefits either in providing young women with positive role models or providing ideas for navigating social change in the context of globalization [50,82–84]. Many experts have recognized the utility of television and other media for promoting pro-social messages in areas in which health information access otherwise may be limited [85–89].

Effects of the media on body image across diverse cultural settings

The ways in which media impact on body image may be similar in important ways across disparate cultural contexts. For example, a study of middle school–aged and adult women in India found that media internalization mediated the effect of body size on body dissatisfaction [90]. This finding is consistent with models that link appearance comparison, media internalization, and body dissatisfaction in Western populations [91,92]. Notwithstanding this interesting finding, media effects likely also differ in important ways across cultural contexts, although few studies have addressed this issue specifically.

There may be reason to believe that adolescent girls and women in modernizing societies may be particularly vulnerable to media effects on body image. This vulnerability may stem from less experience in viewing media critically

[93,94], a perceived material gap between lifestyles of characters portrayed in Western programming and of the far less affluent viewership, and the introduction of ideas and values about self-representation through the body. A study on the effects of television on adolescent schoolgirls in peri-urban Fiji found that prevalence of indicators of disordered eating increased significantly in the setting of recent rapid modernization there. This study on ethnic Fijian adolescent girls presented a unique (and time-limited) opportunity to study the impact of new television exposure on risk for disordered eating and body image disturbance for several key reasons. First, traditional Fijian attitudes toward food, dieting, weight, body esthetic ideals, and reshaping the body relevant to dis-ordered eating and body image are substantially distinct from Western attitudes. Eating disorders were believed to be rare in ethnic Fijians before 1995 [95]. Next, because of relative geographic isolation and Fiji government policies that did not allow broadcast television in Nadroga until 1995, Fijians have had only recent substantial exposure to Western ideas, values, and media imagery. A two-wave cross-sectional design was used to compare ethnic Fijian adolescent schoolgirls before (1995) and after (1998) prolonged regional television exposure with a modified 26-item Eating Attitudes Test (EAT-26), which was supplemented with a semi-structured interview to confirm self-reported symptoms. Narrative data from a subset of 30 purposively sampled respondents with a range of disordered eating attitudes and behaviors and television viewing habits from the exposed sample were collected by semi-structured, open-ended interview and were ana-lyzed for content relating television exposure to body image concerns [94]. Adolescent Fijian girls exposed to television (ie, the 1998 cohort) had a significantly higher prevalence of history of inducing vomiting to lose weight and scores above 20 on the 26-item Eating Attitudes Test than the girls un-exposed to television in their community (the 1995 cohort) [94]. Qualitative data from the television-exposed cohort in 1998 demonstrated a clear shift in esthetic body ideals in Fiji linked to television access. Concomitant with this shift in body ideals, study participants perceived that weight loss would enhance social and economic opportunities [50]. For example, most (77%) schoolgirls sampled reported that television influenced their body image, 40% of respondents indi-cated that they believed losing weight would promote economic opportunities, and 30% used television characters as role models for job access [94].

Although the shift in body ideals was not subtle, the ideas and values in-troduced through Western television programming also may have had substantial impact. For example, the portrayal of American values supporting achievement and competition may have stimulated social comparison and interest in com-petitive social positioning in this indigenous small-scale society. The results of this study suggested that exposure to Western media images and ideas may have contributed specifically to poor body image and disordered eating by promoting (1) comparisons that result in perceived economic and social disadvantage and (2) the notion that efforts to reshape the body will enhance social status [50]. The impact of media exposure in Fiji is undoubtedly tied closely to the social context in which economic changes have increased pressures on youth to find wage-earning jobs. Although it is difficult to generalize the results of this study to other social contexts, the data illustrate the potentially powerful influence of television on body image ideals.

A study of media exposure and body image in girls and women in Papua New Guinea provided noteworthy contrast to the previously mentioned study conducted in Fiji. Although women with greater exposure to television had less desire to match the traditional larger body ideal by comparison with women with less exposure, they did not indicate a desire to pursue a thinner ideal. Compared with women with less frequent viewing, women aged 16 years and older in this study with greater frequency of television and movie viewing actually selected a body size closer to their own as "beautiful." The study investigator acknowledged, however, that the women with less television exposure admired a bigger body size than their own, whereas the women with greater exposure tended to admire a body size similar to or smaller than their own. Women with greater television exposure in this study were more likely to wish to be taller by comparison with other women in Papua New Guinea, which suggested that height—rather than weight—may have been a more salient body dimension in this population (Sarah Wesch, PhD, unpublished dissertation, 2004). Similarly, in Belize, indigenous body ideals that favor a "coca-cola shape" over a specific body size preference seem to have persisted despite widespread availability of Western televised and print media [96].

Other important effects of media on adolescent body image may be indirect. For example, programming may stimulate an interest in behaviors associated with weight control [50] or disordered eating [96]. The association of television viewing with pediatric and adult obesity is nearly ubiquitous across diverse populations [97–104]. Television viewing arguably may contribute to a vicious cycle of overweight, disappointment in comparative appearance, and body disparagement. Additional research will be helpful in exploring the ways that television viewing may mediate overweight and body image among adolescents.

Body image, the media, and adolescent boys

The media also have portrayed men in unrealistic ways. During the 25 years from 1973 to 1997, men who appeared in the centerfolds of *Playgirl* magazine became thinner, but more importantly, they became far more muscular [105]. Even boys' action figures, such as G.I. Joe and Star Wars characters, have become significantly more muscular from the 1960s to the 1990s [106].

Until recently, it was assumed that the media's negative effect of body image and self-esteem occurred only for young women. Within the past 10 years, however, several researchers have examined body image and self-esteem for adolescent boys and found that young men have become increasingly more dissatisfied with their bodies [107,108]. In a 1997 survey of their readers conducted by *Psychology Today*, approximately one third of the men said that viewing muscular male magazine models made them feel insecure [32]. In a recent study by Leit et al [109], college men who viewed pictures of ideal male bodies rated their own bodies more negatively. It seems that the media effects may be similar for adolescent boys as they are for adolescent girls.

The media and prevention of body image problems in adolescents

Because adolescents struggle with challenges to their body image and self-esteem that are partly related to the messages they receive from the media, several researchers have tried to address this problem through educational programs. The portion of these programs that may help to inoculate participants against the negative messages from the media is called "media literacy." In these programs, students are made aware that the images we see in the media are frequently digitally altered and air brushed to enhance the illusion of their perfection, and the statements that are made in advertisements are fictitious. By incorporating such a piece into a school-based program, it is hoped that adolescents will learn to approach the media with a sense of strength through knowledge, thus inoculating them against the negative messages. Students often are asked to participate actively in this component, with such tasks as a homework assignment to view and analyze television commercials and popular magazines so that they hopefully will become active consumers in the future.

It is probably important to present information about the media to students in a positive, empowering manner based on the data concerning smoking prevention programs. Although much of the early school-based smoking prevention work initially focused on the negative health effects of smoking (eg, showing black lung tissue from lung cancer victims and pictures of people smoking often through tracheotomies while dying from lung cancer or emphysema), more recent smoking prevention programs have provided reasons not to smoke. This latter type of smoking prevention program has been found to be more effective in preventing tobacco use among youth [110]. Dalton et al [111] suggested that we will be more successful if we challenge students' positive expectations associated with smoking (eg, decreasing stress and boredom, helping to control weight, making social situations easier) and help them to find alternative means for achieving these positive outcomes.

Media literacy programs may help adolescents—especially adolescent girls—develop more positive body images. Irving et al [112,113] conducted several small studies in which they were able to demonstrate the positive effects of a media literacy program. In one of the studies, high school students who participated in the program were less likely to internalize messages from the media and believed the media was less realistic than nonparticipants [113]. They also reported that two media literacy conditions (externally oriented and cognitively oriented) increased college women's skepticism about advertising.

Despite the theoretical appeal and practical logic of such an approach, few published studies have tackled media literacy as a primary issue. We could find few studies that focused primarily on the impact of media literacy. Of these studies, three examined general effects [114–116], one looked at effects on children's decision making about alcohol [117], and several others investigated whether media literacy had an impact on preventing eating disorders [118–121]. With the premise that teaching youth to deconstruct and critique media images will help to mitigate their powerful and harmful effects, Neumark-Sztainer et al [118] incorporated media literacy training into an eating disorders prevention program. The study did find changes in body-related attitudes initially, but they were not sustained. Similar to many other prevention programs that have included media literacy training as one component [118,122], they did not find changes in disordered eating behaviors after the intervention [118]. McVey and Davis [120] also failed to find an effect of a combined media literacy and life skills program on body image and disordered eating in middle school girls. A controlled study of a ten-lesson prevention program, including one lesson on media literacy given to 9- to 11-year-old boys and girls (386 students received the intervention and 166 were controls), also yielded disappointing results. The investigators concluded that the media literacy portion of the program was largely ineffective and not well received by teachers. They noted that the program as a whole was found to improve knowledge relating to nutrition, weight, and shape among the students and improve attitudes toward overweight people among fifth graders. The researchers suggested that some of the effects may have related to media literacy content throughout the curriculum [121]. Finally, another large controlled study that investigated efficacy of a program designed to promote body satisfaction and prevent disordered eating (incorporating a substantial media literacy component) in a sample of 236 sixth-grade girls failed to demonstrate significant differences between intervention and control groups [120].

Although the limitations in sustained effects on disordered eating behaviors are discouraging, the impact on attitudes in the short term strongly suggests that investigators may be on the right track in targeting media literacy as one of the means of intervening in the harmful effects of media exposure. A controlled study that compared media literacy and self-esteem with controls in 86 eighth-grade students found promising results in a short-term follow-up at 3 months. The students who underwent the media literacy intervention demonstrated significantly lower scores on weight concern compared with the self-esteem intervention and control groups [119].

Our research group (C.V.W. and S.R.S.) also has developed a media literacy program combined with health education: the "Building Better Bodies" program [123,124]. This program helps students recognize the ways in which the media alter our perspective and has been shown to decrease known risk factors for eating disorders. Programs such as these could be used in schools to help protect adolescents from media pressure.

In addition to media literacy programs as a prevention strategy, others have proposed and tested the use of prevention programs that target other risk factors, such as body dissatisfaction and drive for thinness [40–42]. This approach seems reasonable because media effects were strongest in adolescents who were dissatisfied with their bodies before viewing thin models (Eileen Anderson-Fye,

EdD, unpublished dissertation, 2002). Although the concept of these programs seems excellent, the scientific proof is mixed [119,120]. Some prevention studies have reported clear beneficial effects, whereas others have not, and many of the studies on these prevention programs lack scientific rigor [125]. Additional research in this area is needed.

Because we know that the media can have deleterious effects on adolescents, it is strategically appealing to consider potential ways to channel the media's potency to promote positive body image or at least neutralize the negative effects it has been shown to incur on body image. One way the media could be used proactively to mitigate body image disturbance would be to show more realistic images. As was suggested by our research, despite the importance of other factors (eg, family, peers, biology), the media could have a more positive effect on women's body image by showing more images of plus-size models [33].

Summary

It seems clear that media images are likely a factor in the increasing body image dissatisfaction seen in many adolescent girls and some adolescent boys over the past two to three decades. Although these effects are the strongest in Western societies, such as the United States, as societies become more Westernized and are exposed to more Western media images and values, young women in these populations also are showing an increase in body dissatisfaction and drive for thinness.

Because adolescents inevitably compare themselves to persons around them, including persons depicted in media images, we must develop means of neutralizing the impact of media exposure on adolescents. Theoretically, this goal can be pursued at individual, school-based, industry, or public policy levels. Parental awareness of the effects of media on children can provide a springboard for limiting or better selecting programming for adolescent girls. School-based or after-school–based media literacy programs can disseminate information about how media affect teenagers and teach them to view media critically to question and deconstruct the images they view and messages they receive. Clinicians who see adolescents with weight or shape concerns should remain sensitive to the social context that exacerbates these concerns, including exposure to esthetic standards and consumeristic values promoted within the mass media. Many such patients may benefit from a mode of psychotherapy (eg, cognitive behavioral therapy) that can address directly the cognitive distortions perpetuated by television viewing or reading fashion magazines. Clinicians also can address media consumption patterns with patients and their parents and recommend media literacy training when appropriate. Teaching our young people to be sophisticated viewers of the media may attenuate some of the adverse effects of the overly thin images that are portrayed, although further research is essential for clarifying the most effective ways to implement media literacy.

Finally, because of the well-documented negative effects of media on children (including teen risk behaviors, such as substance use, sexual activity, and violence [81,126,127]), we likely will need to intervene at a societal level to influence entertainment industry portrayals of adolescents and embed pro-social messages about the diversity of body sizes and shapes. Despite their theoretical appeal and promise, however, the proposed remedies for the adverse impact of television, which range from family- and school-based interventions (eg, parental supervision and media literacy training), to consumer pressure on the entertainment industry, to social policy (eg, more rigid constraints on programming), appear inadequate in substantively resolving the problem [128–131]. For this reason, additional research that documents the means by which the media exert adverse effects and demonstrates the positive effects of modifications (eg, showing realistic body shapes and sizes) is critical if we are to promote healthy body image development of young women.

References

[1] Morris W, editor. The American heritage dictionary of the English language. New York: American Heritage; 1975. p. 815.

[2] Cambell R, Martin CR, Fabos B. Media and culture: an introduction to mass communication. Boston: Bedford/St Martin; 2004.

[3] Puhl RM, Boland FJ. Predicting female attractiveness: waist-to-hip ratio versus thinness. Psychology Evolution and Gender 2001;3(1):27–46.

[4] Wiseman CV, Gray J, Mosimann J, et al. Cultural expectations of thinness in women: an update. Int J Eat Disord 1992;11:85–9.

[5] Garner DM, Garfinkel PE, Schwartz D, et al. Cultural expectations of thinness in women. Psychol Rep 1980;47:483–91.

[6] Flegal KM, Carroll MD, Ogden CL, et al. Prevalence and trends in obesity among US adults, 1999–2000. JAMA 2002;288:1723–7.

[7] Silverstein B, Perdue L, Peterson B, et al. The role of the mass media in promoting a thin standard of bodily attractiveness for women. Sex Roles 1986;14(9/10):519–33.

[8] Voracek M, Fisher ML. Shapely centrefolds? Temporal change in body measures: trend analysis. BMJ 2002;325(7378):1447–8.

[9] Katzmarzyk PT, David C. Thinness and body shape of Playboy centerfolds from 1978 to 1998. Int J Obes Relat Metab Disord 2001;25(4):590–2.

[10] Barber N. Secular changes in standards of bodily attractiveness in women: tests of a reproductive model. Int J Eat Disord 1998;23(4):449–53.

[11] Levine MP, Smolak L. Media as a context for the development of disordered eating. In: Smolak L, Levine MP, Striegel-Moore R, editors. The developmental psychopathology of eating disorders: implications for research, prevention, and treatment. Hillsdale (NJ): Lawrence Erlbaum Associates, Inc.; 1996. p. 235–57.

[12] Timoko C, Striegel-Moore R, Silberstein L, et al. Femininity/masculinity and disordered eating in women: How are they related? Int J Eat Disord 1987;6(3):701–12.

[13] Blyth M. Spin sisters. New York: St. Martins Press; 2004.

[14] Cortese A. Provocateur. Lanham (MD): Rowman & Littlefield; 1999.

[15] Kilbourne J. Deadly persuasion. New York: The Free Press; 1999.

[16] Wolf N. The beauty myth. New York: William Morrow and Company, Inc.; 1991.

[17] Adams GR, Abraham KG, Markstrom CA. Adolescent development: the essential readings. Malden (MA): Blackwell; 2000.

[18] Berndt T. Developmental changes in conformity to peers and parents. Dev Psychol 1979;15: 608–16.

[19] Piaget J. The construction of reality in the child. New York: Basic Books; 1954.

[20] Elkind D. Child development and education: a Piagetian perspective. New York: Oxford University Press; 1976.

[21] Festinger L. A theory of social comparison processes. Hum Relat 1954;7:117–40.

[22] Wheeler L. Motivation as a determinant of upward comparison. J Exp Soc Psychol 1966; 1(Suppl):27–31.

[23] Asch SE. Opinions and social pressure. Sci Am 1955;193:31–5.

[24] Sherif M. The psychology of social norms. New York: Harper and Row; 1966.

[25] Newcomb TM. Personality and social change. New York: Dryden Press; 1943.

[26] Schachter S. The psychology of affiliation. Stanford: Stanford University Press; 1959.

[27] Prentice DA, Miller DT. Pluralistic ignorance and alcohol use on campus: some consequences of misperceiving a social norm. J Pers Soc Psychol 1993;64:243–54.

[28] Crandall C. Social contagion of binge eating. J Pers Soc Psychol 1988;55:588–98.

[29] Cialdini RB, Kallgren CA, Reno RR. A focus theory of normative conduct: a theoretical refinement and reevaluation of the role of norms in human behavior. Advances in Experimental Social Psychology 1991;24:201–34.

[30] Taylor C, Sharpe T, Shisslak C, et al. Factors associated with weight concerns in adolescent girls. Int J Eat Disord 1998;24:31–42.

[31] Feingold A. Good looking people are not what we think. Psychol Bull 1992;111:304–41.

[32] Garner D. The 1997 body image survey results. Psychol Today 1997;30–44, 75–80, 54.

[33] Wiseman CV, Sunday SR, Cohen AR, et al. Plus-size vs. super-thin: impact of media images. Ravello (Italy): Eating Disorders Research Society; 2003.

[34] Irving LM. Mirror images: effects of the standard of beauty on the self and body-esteem of women exhibiting varying levels of bulimic symptoms. J Soc Clin Psychol 1990;9:230–42.

[35] Levine MP, Smolak L, Hayden H. The relation of sociocultural factors to eating attitudes and behaviors among middle school girls. J Early Adolesc 1994;14:472–91.

[36] Stice E, Shaw H. Adverse effects of the media portrayed thin-ideal on women and linkages to bulimic symptomatology. J Soc Clin Psychol 1994;13:288–308.

[37] Pinhas L, Toner B, Ali A, et al. The effects of the ideal of female beauty on mood and body satisfaction. Int J Eat Disord 1999;25(2):223–6.

[38] Richins M. Social comparison and the idealized images of advertising. J Consum Res 1991; 18:71–83.

[39] Lokken K, Worthy SL, Trautmann J. Examining the links among magazine preference, levels of awareness and internalization of sociocultural appearance standards, and presence of eating-disordered symptoms in college women. Fam Consum Sci Res J 2004;32:361–81.

[40] Stice E, Trost A, Chase A. Healthy weight control and dissonance based eating disorder prevention programs: results from a controlled trial. Int J Eat Disord 2003;33:10–21.

[41] Stice E, Ragan J. A controlled evaluation of an eating disturbance: psychoeducational intervention. Int J Eat Disord 2002;31:159–71.

[42] Stice E, Mazotti L, Weibel D, et al. Dissonance prevention program decreases thin-ideal internalization, body dissatisfaction, dieting, negative affect, and bulimic symptoms: a preliminary experiment. Int J Eat Disord 2000;27:206–17.

[43] Striegel-Moore RH, Silberstein LR, Rodin J. Toward an understanding of risk factors for bulimia. Am Psychol 1986;41:246–63.

[44] Smolak L, Levine MP, Striegel-Moore R, editors. The developmental psychopathology of eating disorders: implications for research, prevention, and treatment. Hillsdale (NJ): Lawrence Erlbaum Associates; 1996.

[45] Shisslak CM, Crago M, Estes LS. The spectrum of eating disturbances. Int J Eat Disord 1995; 18(3):209–19.

[46] Stice E, Ziemba C, Margolis J, et al. The dual pathway model differentiates bulimics, subclinical bulimics, and controls: testing the continuity hypothesis. Behav Ther 1996;27: 531–49.

[47] Becker AE, Hamburg P. Culture, the media, and eating disorders. Harv Rev Psychiatry 1996;4: 163–7.

[48] O'Connor A. Media exposure and eating disorders: current knowledge and implications for prevention. Presented at the Ninth New York International Conference on Eating Disorders. New York, May 4–7, 2000.

[49] Mazzarella W. Shoveling smoke: advertising and globalization in contemporary India. Durham (NC): Duke University Press; 2003.

[50] Becker AE. Television, disordered eating, and young women in Fiji: negotiating body image and identity during rapid social change. Cult Med Psychiatry 2004;28:533–59.

[51] Katzman MA, Hermans KME, van Hoeken D, et al. Not your "typical island woman": anorexia nervosa is reported only in subcultures in Curacao. Cult Med Psychiatry 2004;28(4): 463–92.

[52] Becker AE. Eating disorders and social transition. Primary Psychiatry 2003;10:75–9.

[53] Groesz L, Levine M, Murnen S. The effect of experimental presentation of thin media images on body satisfaction: a meta-analytic review. Int J Eat Disord 2002;31:1–16.

[54] Cash TF, Henry PE. Women's body images: the results of a national survey in the USA. Sex Roles 1995;33:19–28.

[55] Wilfley D, Schreiber G, Pike K, et al. Similarities in eating disturbances among black and white women. Int J Eat Disord 1996;20:377–87.

[56] Atlas J, Smith G, Hohlstein L, et al. Similarities and differences between caucasian and African American college women on eating and dieting expectancies, bulimic symptoms, dietary restraint, and disinhibition. Int J Eat Disord 2002;32:326–34.

[57] Kemper K, Sargent R, Drane J, et al. Black and white females' perceptions of ideal body size and social norms. Obes Res 1994;2:117–26.

[58] Rosen J, Silberg N, Gross J. Eating attitudes test and eating disorder inventory: norms for adolescent girls and boys. J Consult Clin Psychol 1998;56:305–8.

[59] Brown K, McMahon R, Biro F, et al. Changes in self-esteem in black and white girls between the ages of 9 and 14 years: the NHLBI growth and health study. J Adolesc Health 1998;23:7–19.

[60] American Association of University Women. How schools shortchange girls: a study of major findings on girls and education. New York: Marlowe; 1992.

[61] Winkleby M, Gardner C, Taylor C. The influence of gender and socioeconomic factors on Latina/white differences in body mass index. Prev Med 1996;25:203–11.

[62] Rubin LR, Fitts ML, Becker AE. Whatever feels good in my soul: body ethics and aesthetics among African American and Latina women. Cult Med Psychiatry 2003;27:49–75.

[63] Pumariega A. Acculturation and eating attitudes in adolescent girls: a comparative and correlational study. J Am Acad Child Psychiatry 1986;25(2):276–9.

[64] Chamorro R, Flores-Ortiz Y. Acculturation and disordered eating patterns among Mexican American women. Int J Eat Disord 2000;28:125–59.

[65] Joiner GW, Kashubeck S. Acculturation, body image, self-esteem, and eating-disorder symptomatology in adolescent Mexican American women. Psychol Women Q 1996;20:419–35.

[66] United States Census Bureau. Projected population of the United States, by race and Hispanic origin 2000–2050. Available at: http://www.census.gov/ipc/www/usinterimproj/natprojtab01. Accessed August 25, 2004.

[67] Granzberg G. Television and self-concept formation in developing areas. J Cross Cult Psychol 1985;16:313–28.

[68] Miller CJ. The social impacts of televised media among the Yucatec Maya. Hum Organ 1998; 57:307–14.

[69] Tan AS, Tan GK, Tan AS. American TV in the Philippines: a test of cultural impact. Journal Q 1987;64:65–72.

[70] Cheung C-K, Chan C-F. Television viewing and mean world value in Hong Kong's adolescents. Soc Behav Pers 1996;24:351–64.

[71] Wu Y-K. Television and the value systems of Taiwan's adolescents: a cultivation analysis. Diss Abstr Int 1990;50:3783A.

[72] Reis R. The impact of television viewing in the Brazilian Amazon. Hum Organ 1998;57: 300–6.

[73] Varan D. The costs and benefits of television: applying the emerging paradigms of development communication to the Cook Islands experience. Diss Abstr Int 1993;53:3031A.

[74] Charlton T, O'Bey S. Links between television and behaviour: students' perceptions of TV's impact in St Helena, South Atlantic. Support for Learning 1997;12:130–6.

[75] Kang JG, Morgan M. Culture clash: impact of US television in Korea. Journal Q 1988;65: 431–8.

[76] Klein JD, Brown JD, Childers KW, et al. Adolescents' risky behavior and mass media use. Pediatrics 1993;92:24–31.

[77] Villani S. Impact of media on children and adolescents: a 10-year review of the research. J Am Acad Child Adolesc Psychiatry 2001;40(4):392–401.

[78] Wood W, Wong FY. Effects of media violence on viewer's aggression in unconstrained social interaction. Psychol Bull 1991;109:371–83.

[79] Paik H, Comstock G. The effects of television violence on antisocial behavior: a meta-analysis. Comm Res 1994;21:516–46.

[80] American Academy of Pediatrics. Sexuality, contraception, and the media. Pediatrics 1995; 95(2):298–300.

[81] Altman DG, Levine DW, Coeytaux R, et al. Tobacco promotion and susceptibility to tobacco use among adolescents aged 12 through 17 years in a nationally representative sample. Am J Public Health 1996;86:1590–3.

[82] Anderson-Fye EP. Never leave yourself: ethnopsychology as mediator of psychological globalization among Belizean schoolgirls. Ethos 2003;31:59–94.

[83] Varan D. The cultural erosion metaphor and the transcultural impact of media systems. J Comm 1998;48:58–85.

[84] Barker C. Television and the reflexive project of the self: soaps, teenage talk and hybrid identities. Br J Sociol 1997;48(4):611–28.

[85] Capone PL, Lane JC, Kerr CS, et al. Life supporting first aid (LSFA) teaching to Brazilians by television spots. Resuscitation 2000;47:259–65.

[86] Elkamel F. The use of television series in health education. Health Educ Res 1995;10:225–32.

[87] Brown WJ. Prosocial effects of entertainment television in India. Asian J Commun 1990;1: 113–35.

[88] McDivitt JA, Zimicki S, Hornik R, et al. The impact of Healthcom mass media campaign: no timely initiation of breastfeeding in Jordan. Stud Fam Plann 1993;24:295–309.

[89] Jaramillo E. The impact of media-based health education on tuberculosis diagnosis in Cali, Colombia. Health Policy Plan 2001;16:68–73.

[90] Shroff H, Thompson JK. Body image and eating disturbance in India: media and interpersonal influences. Int J Eat Disord 2004;35:198–203.

[91] van den Berg P, Thompson JK, Obremski-Brandon K, et al. The tripartite influence model of body image and eating disturbance: a covariance structure modeling investigation testing the mediational role of appearance comparison. J Psychosom Res 2002;53:1007–20.

[92] Durkin SJ, Paxton SJ. Predictors of vulnerability to reduced body image satisfaction and psychological wellbeing in response to exposure to idealized female media images in adolescent girls. J Psychosom Res 2002;53:995–1005.

[93] Granzberg G. Television as storyteller: the Algonquin Indians of Central Canada. J Comm 1982;32:43–52.

[94] Becker AE, Burwell RA, Gilman SE, et al. Eating behaviours and attitudes following prolonged television exposure among ethnic Fijian adolescent girls. Br J Psychol 2002;180:509–14.

[95] Becker A. Body, self, society: the view from Fiji. Philadelphia: University of Pennsylvania Press; 1995.

[96] Anderson-Fye EP. A Coca-Cola shape: cultural change, body image, and eating disorders in San Andres, Belize. Cult Med Psychiatry 2004;28:561–95.

[97] Hu RB, Li TY, Colditz GA, et al. Television watching and other sedentary behaviors in relation to risk of obesity and type 2 diabetes mellitus in women. JAMA 2003;289:1785–91.

[98] Ma GS, Li YP, Hu XQ, et al. Effect of television viewing on pediatric obesity. Biomed Environ Sci 2002;15:291–7.

[99] Ruangdaraganon N, Kotchabhakdi N, Udomsubpayakul U, et al. The association between television viewing and childhood obesity: a national survey in Thailand. J Med Assoc Thai 2002;85(suppl 4):S1075–80.

[100] Robinson TN. Television viewing and childhood obesity. Pediatr Clin North Am 2001;48: 1017–25.

[101] Crespo CJ, Smit E, Troiano RP, et al. Television watching, energy intake, and obesity in US children: results from the third National Health and Nutrition Examination Survey, 1988–1994. Arch Pediatr Adolesc Med 2001;155:360–5.

[102] Vioque J, Torres A, Quiles J. Time spent watching television, sleep duration and obesity in adults living in Valencia, Spain. Int J Obes Relat Metab Disord 2000;24:1683–8.

[103] Hernandez B, Gortmaker SL, Colditz GA, et al. Association of obesity with physical activity, television programs and other forms of video viewing among children in Mexico City. Int J Obes Relat Metab Disord 1999;23:845–54.

[104] Gortmaker SL, Must A, Sobol AM, et al. Television viewing as a cause of increasing obesity among children in the United States, 1986–1990. Arch Pediatr Adolesc Med 1996;150:356–62.

[105] Leit R, Pope H, Gray J. Cultural expectations of muscularity in men: the evolution of Playgirl centerfolds. Int J Eat Disord 2001;29:90–3.

[106] Pope H, Olivardia R, Gruber A, et al. Evolving ideals of male body image as seen through action toys. Int J Eat Disord 1999;29:65–72.

[107] Cohane G, Pope H. Body image in boys: a review of the literature. Int J Eat Disord 2001;29: 373–9.

[108] Pope H, Phillips K, Olivardia R. The Adonis complex: the secret crisis of male body obsession. New York: The Free Press; 2000.

[109] Leit R, Gray J, Pope H. The media's representation of the ideal male body: a cause for muscle dysmorphia? Int J Eat Disord 2002;31:334–8.

[110] Huang TTK, Unger JB, Rohrbach LA. Exposure to, and perceived usefulness of, school-based tobacco prevention programs: associations with susceptibility to smoking among adolescents. J Adolesc Health 2000;27(4):248–54.

[111] Dalton MA, Sargent JD, Beach ML, et al. Positive and negative outcome expectations of smoking: implications for prevention. Prev Med 1999;29(6):460–5.

[112] Irving LM, Berel SR. Comparison of media-literacy programs to strengthen college women's resistance to media images. Psychol Women Q 2001;25:103–11.

[113] Irving LM, DuPen J, Berel S. A media literacy program for high school females. Eating Disorders: The Journal of Treatment and Prevention 1998;6:119–31.

[114] Irving L. A bolder model of prevention: science, practice and activism. In: Piran N, Levine MP, Steiner-Adair C, editors. Preventing eating disorders. East Sussex (United Kingdom): Brunner-Routledge; 1999. p. 63–84.

[115] Irving LM. Prevention of eating disorders: problems, pitfalls and feminist possibilities. In: Collins LH, Dunlap MR, Chrisler JC, editors. Charting a new course for feminist psychology. Westport (CT): Praeger Publishers/Greenwood Publishing Group; 2002. p. 255–81.

[116] Stormer SM, Thompson JK. The effect of media images and sociocultural beauty ideals on college-age women: a proposed psychoeducational program. Presented at the Meeting of the Association for the Advancement of Behavior Therapy. Washington (DC), November 16–19, 1995.

[117] Austin EW, Johnson KK. Effects of general and alcohol-specific media literacy training on children's decision about alcohol. J Health Commun 1997;2:17–42.

[118] Neumark-Sztainer D, Sherwood NE, Coller T, et al. Primary prevention of disordered eating among preadolescent girls: feasibility and short-term effect of a community-based intervention. J Am Diet Assoc 2000;100:1466–73.

[119] Wade TD, Davidson S, O'Dea JA. A preliminary controlled evaluation of a school-based media literacy program and self-esteem program for reducing eating disorder risk factors. Int J Eat Disord 2003;33(4):371–83.

[120] McVey GL, Davis R. A program to promote positive body image: a 1-year follow-up evaluation. J Early Adolesc 2002;22(1):96–108.

[121] Levine MP, Smolak L, Schermer F. Media analysis and resistance by elementary school children in the primary preventions of eating problems. Eating Disorders: The Journal of Treatment and Prevention 1996;4:310–22.

[122] Austin BS. Prevention research in eating disorders: theory and new directions. Psychol Med 2000;30:1249–62.

[123] Wiseman C, Sunday S, Halmi K. Decreasing eating disorder risk factors in middle school boys and girls:Edi-3 scoring unveils changes. Amsterdam: Eating Disorders Research Society; 2004.

[124] Wiseman CV, Sunday SR, Bortolotti F, et al. Primary prevention of eating disorders through attitude change: a two country comparison. Eating Disorders: The Journal of Treatment and Prevention 2004;12:241–50.

[125] Stice E, Shaw H. Eating disorder prevention programs: a meta-analytic review. Psychol Bull 2004;130:206–27.

[126] Villani S. Impact of media on children and adolescents: a 10-year review of the research. J Am Acad Child Adolesc Psychiatry 2001;40:392–401.

[127] American Academy of Pediatrics. Sexuality, contraception, and the media. Pediatrics 1995; 95(2):298–300.

[128] Feingold M, Johnson GT. Television violence: reactions from physicians, advertisers, and the networks. N Engl J Med 1977;296:24–7.

[129] Sege R, Dietz W. Television viewing and violence in children: the pediatrician as agent for change. Pediatrics 1994;94:600–7.

[130] Charren P, Gelber A, Arnold M. Media, children, and violence: apublic policy perspective. Pediatrics 1994;94:631–7.

[131] Strasburger VC, Donnerstein E. Children, adolescents, and the media: issues and solutions. Pediatrics 1999;103:129–39.

ELSEVIER
SAUNDERS

Child Adolesc Psychiatric Clin N Am
14 (2005) 473–489

CHILD AND
ADOLESCENT
PSYCHIATRIC CLINICS
OF NORTH AMERICA

Addicted Media: Substances on Screen

Kimberly M. Thompson, MS, ScD

*KidsRisk Project, Harvard School of Public Health and Division of Adolescent Medicine,
Children's Hospital Boston, 677 Huntington Avenue, 3rd Floor, Boston, MA 02115, USA*

Concern related to the depiction of alcohol and drug traffic/usage in films dates back decades, with the Hayes Production Code severely restricting their depiction on screen between 1930 and 1967: "The illegal drug traffic must not be portrayed in such a way as to stimulate curiosity concerning the use of, or traffic in, such drugs; nor shall scenes be approved which show the use of illegal drugs, or their effects, in detail... The use of liquor in American life, when not required by the plot or for proper characterization, will not be shown" [1]. The Production Code did not address cigarettes, however, probably because the Code preceded the large growth in popularity of cigarettes and active efforts to market cigarettes using popular media.

In the context of the cultural revolution of the 1960s, however, the Production Code did not mesh with the prevailing societal norms, which in part contributed to its demise. In 1968, the movie industry replaced the Production Code with the current voluntary ratings system that currently exists for movies [2,3]. Although the current movie ratings sometimes indicate depiction of drugs or alcohol as a reason for the rating, they do not systematically provide information about the depiction of substances, and they rarely provide any information about tobacco depiction/use [2–4]. In contrast, the video game rating system includes specific content descriptors for substances but lacks clearly communicated criteria for when the rating board does and does not apply them [5–7]. Current television ratings provide no information about substances, with the content designation "D" indicating dialog [8], not drugs, as many parents incorrectly expect [9].

Parents must rely on nonexistent or imperfect information about the depiction of substances in popular media, and they must expect that their kids will

Dr. Thompson used unrestricted gifts to the KidsRisk Project to cover her effort in writing this article.

E-mail address: kimt@hsph.harvard.edu

experience messages about substances from media and recognize that these
messages may influence their children's perceptions, attitudes, beliefs, and behaviors about substances. This article provides a comprehensive review of much
of the existing peer-reviewed published literature about the depiction of substances in the media and its potential impacts, particularly on children. The article
organizes the body of research by focusing on the information obtained in media
content analyses to synthesize the vast body of research that collectively demonstrates the widespread and overwhelming presence of substances in media viewed
by children and adolescents. The article then highlights reviews that provide
insights about the potential impacts of these depictions. With some current
demand that any movie that contains smoking receive an "R" rating (eg, http://
www.smokefreemovies.ucsf.edu), the discussion of this article highlights the
challenges of creating and encouraging healthy media for children while also
allowing maximum freedom for individuals who are involved with the media.

Methods

To identify media content analyses related to substances, the author conducted
an extensive literature search for published peer-reviewed articles that contained
the words alcohol, drug, tobacco, substance(s), and movie, motion picture,
television, video game, magazine, or media and synthesized them. For purposes
of this effort, "substances" refers to alcohol, tobacco, or illicit drugs but does not
include pharmaceutical products (unless the intent for misuse as a drug is clear),
medicinal herbs, tonics, or ambiguous tonics or brew. Although this article aims
for comprehensive coverage of the existing US peer-reviewed, published literature, it does not exhaustively include every study because of space limitations.

Results

Content analyses

Review of the literature identified hundreds of papers in the peer-reviewed
literature related to substances in media. Notably, several US researchers contributed significantly to our understanding by dedicating a significant portion of
their research to the topic (eg, Drs. Warren Breed, William DeJong, Stanton
Glantz) [11,12,15,16,30–32,40,47–53,59,65–68,77,97]. This study identified
more than 50 original content analyses published in peer-reviewed journals that
reported some information about the depiction of substances in various media.

Print media
Several studies explored the information in newspapers and newsweeklies
[10–13] and women's magazines [14] that documented the depiction of substances in print media targeted at children and adolescents. Several additional

studies characterized substances shown in advertisements in newspapers [15,16] and popular consumer magazines [17], and they explored the features of smoking [18–23] and antismoking [24] print ads. Overall, these studies clearly show significant numbers of depictions of substances in print media targeted at children, adolescents, and young adults.

A recent study that counted and classified types of alcohol advertisements in magazines reported a significantly higher placement rate for beer and liquor ads in magazines with higher numbers of adolescent readers [25] and minority readers [26]. An analysis of alcohol control policy issues found similar coverage in black-oriented compared with mainstream newspapers, with less coverage of economic alcohol policy issues in black-oriented papers, which possibly suggests less salience of these issues in communities served by these papers [27].

Only one study provided insights about the depiction of substances in popular children's literature. The first content analysis to explore the depictions of tobacco in children's picture books reported a decline in the depiction of tobacco over time, dropping from 2.4% of pages in a sample of books published before 1960 to 0.4% in books published after 1980 [28].

Movies

As a medium, movies received considerable attention from researchers, with most of the studies focusing on tobacco use in films. The first analysis that assessed the depiction of illegal drugs, legal drugs, tobacco, and alcohol in the 20 top box-office films released each year between 1977 and 1988 found an increase in the depiction of smoking over time [29]. Using 5-minute intervals of film for analysis, the study also reported increased smoking and illegal drug use in R-rated movies but greater alcohol consumption in non–R-rated movies. A subsequent analysis of top grossing films released between 1960 and 1990 reported that movies did not represent accurately actual US smoking behaviors and found a consistent rate of tobacco use in films over the three decades, with three times as much smoking among elite characters than in the actual population [30]. Subsequent updates of these data suggested an increase in the depiction of tobacco in films released between 1990 and 1996 [31] and then up through 2002 [32]. The authors also extended the results back to 1950, but their insights depended on dropping 3 out of 20 films (15% of their sample) because these films contained "essentially continuous smoking," which suggested that analysis with a larger sample size would reveal whether these films truly represented outliers or the beginning of the era of films that featured tobacco.

Other recent content analyses of tobacco depiction in popular movies showed depiction of alcohol or tobacco in more than half of the animated G-rated feature films [33,34]. Although analyses suggested that the depiction of substances in these films declined significantly over time [33], the number of depictions in current G-rated animated films still remains at a level that may surprise some parents, and all of these depictions represent deliberate additions of substances to the films, because artists must draw them in. A recent study of more than 1200 films rated G, PG, PG-13, and R and released between 1996 and 2003 reported that 95% of films contained some depiction of substances (ie, tobacco, alcohol, or drugs visible on screen regardless of whether they were in use), whereas the Motion Picture Association of America mentioned alcohol or drugs in its rating reason for only 18% of the films and did not mention tobacco use as a rating reason for any of these films [4]. The authors noted that most of the films that depict alcohol or drugs also depict tobacco, and they reported depiction of tobacco in 79% of all the films.

Other studies reported finding more pro-substance than anti-substance (eg, anti-tobacco) events in films [35], more than 85% of popular films depicting tobacco and a strong correlation of character smoking with other risk factors (eg, alcohol use, drug use, illegal activities) [36], and significant gender differences with respect to tobacco use by popular actors [37]. A study of specific brand appearances found brands depicted in 28% of popular films, with no evidence of a decrease in brand depiction after a voluntary ban on tobacco product placement [38,39]. Notably, a study that explored the development of the relationship between the tobacco industry and Hollywood suggested significant financial ties [40] and highlighted specific high-profile actors who received large payments for featuring cigarettes (eg, Sylvester Stallone, who received $500,000 in 1983 for agreeing to use one particular brand of cigarettes in no less than five feature films). A study that explored Hollywood insiders' understanding of tobacco portrayal suggested heterogeneous perspectives and some influence of the actors' off-camera tobacco use on on-camera use [41]. In 1999, a study that reviewed 38 films from 1994 to 1996 found that teens who had smoked at least once—versus teens who had never smoked—identified a significantly higher percentage of actors who smoked on and off screen among their top ten favorite stars, and the authors suggested that this might provide preliminary evidence that films stars smoking in movies might encourage youth smoking [42]. A similar study published in 2001 that included a content analysis of tobacco use by 43 "stars" in all films in which they appeared between 1994 and 1996 found that 65% of the stars used tobacco at least once. The study reported an association between adolescents with favorable attitudes toward smoking and their identification of their favorite stars as ones who smoked in this sample of films [43].

Television

The role of substances depicted on television also raised many questions and led to a large number of content analyses, with most of them focusing on alcohol. One study assessed the depiction of alcohol in the top ten prime-time fictional series programs on television from 1979 to 1980 and reported a range of 3 to 16.5 incidents of alcohol consumption per program hour for the top ten shows, but almost no smoking or illicit drug incidents [44]. A content analysis of 14 daytime soap operas aired over 4 consecutive weeks in 1977 reported 3 alcohol-related events per program, with drinking most frequently depicted in homes [45]. In 1982, a content analysis of a representative week of major network programming and commercials (ie, ABC, CBS, and NBC) from 1975 coded all drinking events, including alcoholic and nonalcoholic beverages, and reported a low overall rate of alcohol consumption but slightly more alcoholic beverages consumed during prime time than nonalcoholic beverages [46].

Breed et al [47–54] performed several studies in the 1980s that assessed drinking and smoking on television. The first study identified several situational comedies that presented marijuana use as harmless and humorous and suggested that these types of depictions, although rare [55], could impact public attitudes toward drug use [47]. An analysis of top television dramas and situation comedies from 1976 to 1977 reported that characters in these programs were more likely to drink alcohol than all other beverages combined and that these shows failed to depict negative consequences associated with drinking too much [48]. Based on a review of television programming between 1950 and 1982, Breed and DeFoe [49] observed an increase in alcohol use and a decrease in tobacco use over these three decades. A study that assessed nearly 5 years of daytime soap opera programming for "All My Children" found realistic depiction of drinking and drinking problems but suggested that because negative consequences occurred only when characters drank to escape reality, the program might encourage the perception that alcohol helps in social facilitation or in managing a crisis [50]. Looking at alcohol depictions from fall 1984 prime-time dramas, one study reported references to alcohol in 90% of the 127 programs viewed, with alcohol shown in 80% and consumed by a character in 60%—at a rate of more than ten consumptions of alcohol per program hour [51]. A study of top-ranked prime-time programs from 1976 to 1986 identified only 74 scenes with problem drinkers out of more than 1400 episodes and characterized a wide range of responses to these problem drinkers by other characters [52]. Using this same sample of programs and focusing specifically on youth, DeFoe and Breed [53] reported that underage characters accounted for less than 2% of televised alcohol consumption and that these depictions generally occurred in the context of criminal activity or with portrayals of gangs. Finally, analysis of a sample of 3 weeks of prime-time fictional programs from 1986 revealed alcohol depicted in 64% and consumed in 50% of episodes, at a rate of more than eight alcohol consumption acts per program hour [54].

Studies by other researchers reported similar findings and provided some additional insights. A 1987 analysis of week-long samples of prime-time and weekend daytime network television dramas shown from 1969 to 1985 reported an increase in alcohol depiction over the time period, with 37% of major characters shown drinking and an association noted between drinking and sexual behavior [56]. A 1988 qualitative analysis of alcohol depictions in 77 prime-time episodes from 1984 suggested that alcohol-related behavior serves as a cue to viewers for character attributes, for example, with preferred alcoholic beverage providing an indication of social class and lifestyle [57].

Content analyses of tobacco depiction on television document the presence of smoking in some prime-time programs. Although no existing content analyses seem to go back to the beginning of television programming, many early programs depicted popular media stars smoking (eg, Lucille Ball, Milton Berle). An analysis of a composite sample of 2 weeks of 1984 prime-time programs reported one act of smoking per hour, with more smoking by lead characters and in dramas compared with situation comedies [58]. A study that analyzed the depiction of tobacco and alcohol advertising shown during 166 sports events televised between 1990 and 1992 (nearly 444 hours of programming) noted viewer exposure to alcohol and tobacco advertising from on-site promotions and sponsorship recognitions and highlighted the near absence of moderation and public service announcements [59]. This study also reported more commercials for alcohol than for any other beverage, with beer commercials dominating [59]. Based on analysis of 3 composite weeks of 1992 prime-time programs on major networks, one study reported 24% of programs depicting tobacco, with most depictions promoting its use (92%) and a higher rate of smoking depicted by characters on television than in the actual population [60].

Recent content analyses provided indications of significant amounts of depictions of substances in current programming. A study of the portrayal of women in television beer commercials that aired from 1991 to 1992 found significantly more camera shots of the chests, buttocks, legs, or crotches of women than men [61]. An analysis that evaluated televised content for the week of September 16 to 22, 1990 reported nearly 40 times as many commercials that promoted drugs and alcohol than networks' news stories, documentaries, and public service announcements about illegal drugs [62]. Analysis of alcohol portrayal in 2 weeks of prime-time programming from major networks from 1994 to 1995 identified alcoholic beverages as the most frequently portrayed food or drink, accounting for a significant percentage of the food and drink consumption by adolescents, although programs typically associated adolescents consuming alcohol with negative personality characteristics [63]. Based on 36 national network news broadcasts from 1977 to 1996, one study reported a shift in the nature of the portrayals of pregnancy and alcohol from white, middle-class women to minority women [64]. A 2002 study that quantified the prevalence of substance use among characters on prime-time TV during 1995 to 1996 reported significantly lower prevalence of substance use by TV characters than exhibited by the US population (ie, 11%, 6.1%, and 0.8% of TV characters who consumed alcohol, tobacco, or illicit drugs, respectively, compared with US population prevalence estimates of 51%, 28.9%, and 6.1%, respectively) [65]. Recent content analyses of television advertising characterized the focus of public service announcements about alcohol-impaired driving [66], the nature of the Massachusetts Tobacco Control Program [67], and the messages about drug users in public service announcements aimed at preventing the spread of HIV/AIDS [68]. The analyses questioned the effectiveness and responsibility of the moderation message in alcohol ads [69] and reported differences in these messages with corporate versus nonprofit sponsorship [70].

Billboards

In addition to reassessing the content of existing media, researchers continue to evaluate the content of new media as they emerge. After placement of restrictions on advertising, several researchers performed content analyses of tobacco advertising on billboards [71–74]. For example, a study of tobacco and alcohol advertising on billboards in Chicago found that billboards in minority neighborhoods showed three times as many tobacco ads and five times as many alcohol ads as billboards in white neighborhoods [71].

Music and music videos

A 1997 content analysis of tobacco and alcohol depiction in music videos aired on four music channels during peak adolescent viewing times in 1994 found more smoking depicted on MTV than on other networks and in rap videos than in other genres [75]. The study also reported that videos that contained sexual content portrayed more alcohol use behaviors and alcohol content and that lead singers smoked twice as much and consumed alcohol three times as much as background performers [75]. Another study provided some historical perspective on illegal drugs in song lyrics and noted a shift in the 1990s, with some artists singing about drug hazards and harms and providing some pro-social messages [76].

Video games

Analyses of video games found relatively few depictions of substances in games rated "E" for "Everyone" [77], but a significant number of games rated "T" for "Teen" (15% of a random sample of 81 games) depicted alcohol, tobacco, or illicit drugs [6]. One study found that most of these depictions did not receive content descriptors for substances from the Entertainment Software Rating Board [6] (only 1 game or 1% received this label), and another study presented specific examples of games that did not receive content descriptors in which players were required to acquire substances to advance in the game [7]. An analysis of tobacco industry marketing documents reported on the aggressive advertising, brand-sponsored activities, and distribution of samples in bars and nightclubs aimed at increasing smoking in the 18- to 24-year-old age group [78].

The Internet

With widespread access to the Internet, researchers appreciate the importance of assessing the depiction of substances on websites [79–88]. A study focused on identifying and characterizing information on hallucinogens identified 81 sites in December, 1998 that provided thousands of pages on obtaining, synthesizing, extracting, identifying, and using hallucinogens, with almost no information from highly reliable (eg, US government agency) sites offering cautionary material [79]. A subsequent study highlighted the significant role of the Internet as an unmonitored, unregulated, and untouched (by the Master Settlement Agreement against tobacco companies) vehicle for delivering pro-tobacco messages and found that consumers could order products directly from approximately half of the 318 pro-tobacco sites reviewed, with only 23% of these sites attempting to verify age and only 11% including health warnings [80]. A similar study that assessed the tobacco content of 30 pro-tobacco websites in April, 1999 reported no restrictions on access to any of these sites, an age-related warning on only one third of the sites, and no sites that allowed the user to purchase cigarettes, although 2 sites sold cigars and 2 sold smoking paraphernalia [81]. The study further reported depictions of cigarettes on 63% and cigars on 17% of the main pages of websites, with 24% of sites showing a brand image, 35% providing a brand name in writing, and nearly 15% of sites showing nudity [81]. A study 2 years later reported that minors successfully purchased cigarettes using a credit card (93.6% of 47 attempts) or money order (89% of 36 attempts) from 55 websites identified by the authors as selling cigarettes online and that none of the vendors or delivery services attempted age verification [82].

Significant non–peer-reviewed analyses

Several key reports that do not appear in a search of the peer-reviewed published articles but frequently appear in references in these articles also documented the extent of the depiction of substances in popular television, movies, music, and music videos [89–92]. These studies allowed for some comparisons of the amount of depictions in the different media [89]. They also provided a wealth of information about the nature of the depictions, for example, documenting the large percentages of alcohol depictions in movies and music that associate alcohol use with wealth and sex [90] and the lack of the depiction of harmful consequences associated with illicit drug use [91,92].

Potential impacts of these depictions

Several prior reviews summarized the decades of strongly suggestive evidence of media depictions of substances that influenced children's perceptions, attitudes, beliefs, and behaviors [93–97]. The reviews collectively suggested that exposure to glamorous or normalized depictions of substances in media increases youth initiation and perception of the acceptability of substance use, although no study definitively answers the question: How would substance usage rates change in the absence of media messages about substances? The clear implication for clinicians is that the media present an important risk factor that should be a topic of discussion during well-child annual examinations.

Several reviews of the impact and effectiveness of counteradvertising emerged in the last decade [98–102]. These reviews, combined with evaluations of media literacy programs [103], suggested that the media can teach kids about avoiding substance use. Measuring the strength of media effects continues to be problematic [104], and assessing the role of media in the broader social context remains the elusive challenge as researchers try to understand the roles of parents [105–107], peers [108], musical preferences [109,110], and sociocultural [111], psychosocial [112], and other factors, such as skepticism [113] or disengagement from school, that associate with youth susceptibility to tobacco promotions [114,115]. Some studies suggested that tobacco marketing may be a stronger influence on youth initiation of smoking than exposure to peer or family smokers or perceived school performance and other sociodemographic factors [116]. Other studies suggested that tobacco advertising and promotion activities can undermine the influence of parents [117], encourage all youth to smoke [118], and even induce nonsusceptible never-smokers to start the process that leads to addiction [119].

We must acknowledge, however, that the multi-billion dollar annual substance advertising budgets clearly work and continue to play a role in influencing perceptions, attitudes, beliefs, and behaviors about substances, as they have for decades [120–127], with two historical analyses demonstrating the impacts of the tobacco industry's early marketing campaigns and targeting of women [126,127]. The money spent on promoting substance use has led to extensive brand recognition, even by young children [18,128–134]. A recent estimate suggested that the nearly $60 million spent in 2000 to advertise cigarette brands popular with youth in magazines led to ads that reached 80% of young people more than 17 times each and noted that the Master Settlement Agreement did not significantly change spending or youth exposure to these ads [135]. All of the literature taken as a whole suggests that we should expect that researchers will continue to observe increased rates of youth substance use initiation with increased exposure to media [136–139].

Summary and discussion

The reality that the media reflect actual practices in society means that they will depict unhealthy behaviors, such as smoking, unless media producers make a point of eliminating them or counteradvertisers succeed in producing the dominant message (which would represent an impressive shift given the lack of any observed public service announcements on tobacco or alcohol in a study of 1989 advertisements in a composite day of programming [140]). The remarkable rise of tobacco use that accompanied the widespread growth and diversification of entertainment media provides a powerful example of the ability of the media to influence perceptions, attitudes, beliefs, and behaviors.

Although many physicians and researchers have continued to call for greater control of media messages about substances targeted at children and adolescents [141–145] and the American Academy of Pediatrics has issued several policy statements [146–148], we have not seen recently the medical community take as strong a position on media depictions of substances as it has on media depictions of violence [149]. The same observation also applies to the government, with recent discussions about the marketing of violent entertainment to children by the Federal Trade Commission [150] similarly focusing exclusively on violence and not considering the impact of marketing of substances in popular entertainment media targeted at children. Clinicians must emphasize the risks of substance use with patients at every opportunity and encourage patients to evaluate media content critically and pay attention to media ratings.

Some recent efforts that have focused on changing the movie ratings eventually could make it easier. For example, some efforts focus on changing the ratings so that they provide an indication of any depiction of tobacco in a film (ie, smoking movies receive an automatic "R" rating) [151]. According to a recent study, that change could imply that in the absence of changes in the behavior of producers, 79% of films could be rated R just for smoking alone [4]. If that same demand were generalized to depiction of all substances, it would imply that more than 95% of films could be rated R for depiction of substances [4]. Although we can reasonably expect that such a change in the rating system could lead some media producers whose products target young audiences to remove tobacco and other substances from some percentage of future productions, the reality of the large body of existing media containing depictions of substances still would present an important issue for parents. Efforts to educate parents about the depiction of substances in media and develop and expand media literacy programs should remain in high demand.

A significant issue that arises in the context of providing rating information about substances comes from the nature of the depictions, with current depictions including a spectrum from minor or background characters to lead characters and from pro-substance to anti-substance depictions. The questions about definitions arise quickly (eg, Which substances count? Do they have to be identified as real substances, or is it enough that they produce effects like real substances? Does the character actually have to use the substance or does presence of the substance itself require parental warning? For tobacco products, must they be lit?) In the context of making progress toward a system that could provide parents with better information to enable them to discriminate between healthy and unhealthy depictions of substances in media, efforts to work toward standardized definitions offer some promise for progress.

One of the difficult questions with which researchers, parents, teachers, and others must grapple arises from the reality of the mixed messages that media provide about substances and the reality of the convergence of media. A review of the body of literature of content analyses of substances in media demonstrates that it does not make sense to talk about individual media in isolation, and efforts to bring all of the media together in a standardized approach (eg, a universal labeling or rating system) offers the most promise for ensuring that all media share the same incentives. Recognizing that all media interact, particularly with the existence of the Internet, the challenge for researchers becomes even larger as they also attempt to understand children's media diets and combine these with information about exposure. Clinicians can begin to understand better the role of media in their patients' lives by asking questions about media use in physical examinations. With diseases and injuries associated with substance use topping the list of the leading causes of death in the United States, clinicians must help patients see the potential short- and long-term effects of substance use and understand the lack of depiction of the real consequences of substance use in the media.

Focusing on the lack of a national strategy to protect children from media messages that promote unhealthy and harmful behaviors while simultaneously protecting individual freedoms to create and choose media should emerge as national priorities for action, not only among clinicians but also in the community. Although further research is needed to understand the role of substance depictions in the media, the existing evidence shows widespread depiction of substance use and raises the question of how to fight this apparent addiction [152–159]. The larger theme that emerges centers on the need to promote media that value youth instead of devalue them [160] and the ability to use media to help children make better choices about the numerous risks that they face [161]. Clinicians must take a leading role in asking patients about their exposure to substances and ask not only about use but also about depictions in their environments, including the media and their attitudes. Clinicians must help to find ways to correct patients' misperceptions of the risks of substance use and ensure that children hear about the potential health consequences of bad choices. Individuals interested in an online guide to the media that may provide a useful resource for distributing to parents can check the guide to media on the KidsRisk website [162].

Acknowledgments

Dr. Thompson thanks Brandy King of the Center on Media and Child Health, Children's Hospital Boston, for assistance with finding some of the papers.

References

[1] Hayes D. The production code of the motion picture industry (1930–1968). Available at: http://prodcode.davidhayes.net/. Accessed August 1, 2004.

[2] Motion Picture Association of America. Movie ratings: how it works. Available at: http://www.mpaa.org/movieratings/about/index.htm. Accessed August 1, 2004.

[3] The Classification and Rating Administration. Available at: http://www.filmratings.com. Accessed March 1, 2004.

[4] Thompson KM, Yokota F. Violence, sex, and profanity in films: correlation of movie ratings and content. Available at: http://www.medscape.com/viewarticle/480900. Accessed August 1, 2004.

[5] Entertainment Software Ratings Board. Available at: http://www.esrb.org. Accessed August 1, 2004.

[6] Haninger K, Thompson KM. Content and ratings of teen-rated video games. JAMA 2004; 291:856–65.

[7] Haninger K, Ryan MS, Thompson KM. Violence in teen-rated video games. Available at: http://www.medscape.com/viewarticle/468087. Accessed August 1, 2004.

[8] The TV Parental Guidelines. Understanding the TV ratings. Available at: http://www.tvguidelines.org/ratings.asp. Accessed August 1, 2004.

[9] Rideout V. Parents, media, and public policy: a Kaiser Family Foundation survey. Available at: http://www.kff.org/entmedia/7156.cfm. Accessed October 1, 2004.

[10] Atkin CK, DeJong W. News coverage of alcohol and other drugs in US college newspapers. J Drug Educ 2000;30(4):453–65.

[11] Balbach ED, Glantz SA. Tobacco information in two grade school newsweeklies: a content analysis. Am J Public Health 1995;85(12):1650–3.

[12] DeJong W. When the tobacco industry controls the news: KKR, RJR Nabisco, and the Weekly Reader Corporation. Tob Control 1996;5(2):142–8.

484 THOMPSON

[13] Lemmens PH, Vaeth PAC, Greenfield TK. Coverage of beverage alcohol issues in the print media of the United States, 1985–1991. Am J Public Health 1999;89:1555–60.

[14] Feit MN. Exposure of adolescent girls to cigar images in women's magazines, 1992–1998. Am J Public Health 2001;91(2):286–8.

[15] DeFoe JR, Breed W. The problem of alcohol advertisements in college newspapers. J Am Coll Health Assoc 1979;27(4):195–9.

[16] Breed W, Wallack L, Grube JW. Alcohol advertising in college newspapers: a 7-year follow-up. J Am Coll Health Assoc 1990;38(6):255–62.

[17] Strickland DE, Finn TA, Lambert MD. A content analysis of beverage alcohol advertising: magazine advertising. J Stud Alcohol 1982;43:655–82.

[18] Lancaster AR, Lancaster KM. Teenage exposure to cigarette advertising in popular consumer magazines: vehicle versus message reach and frequency. Journal of Advertising 2003;32(3): 69–76.

[19] Pucci LG, Siegel M. Features of sales promotion in cigarette magazine advertisements, 1980–1993: an analysis of youth exposure in the United States. Tob Control 1999;8(1):29–36.

[20] Altman DG, Albright CL, Slater MD, et al. How an unhealthy product is sold: cigarette advertising in magazines, 1960–1985. J Commun 1987;37:95–106.

[21] Albright CL, Altman DG, Slater MD, et al. Cigarette advertisements in magazines: evidence for a differential focus on women's and youth magazines. Health Educ Q 1988;15(2):225–33.

[22] Basil MD, Schooler C, Altman DG, et al. How cigarettes are advertised in magazines: special messages for special markets. Health Commun 1999;3:75–91.

[23] Botvin GJ, Goldberg CJ, Botvin EM, et al. Smoking behavior of adolescents exposed to cigarette advertising. Public Health Rep 1993;108(2):217–24.

[24] Beaudoin CE. Exploring antismoking ads: appeals, themes, and consequences. J Health Commun 2002;7(2):123–37.

[25] Garfield CF, Chung PJ, Rathouz PJ. Alcohol advertising in magazines and adolescent readership. JAMA 2003;289:2424–9.

[26] Cui G. Advertising of alcoholic beverages in African-American and women's magazines: implications for health communication. Howard Journal of Communications 2000;11(4): 279–93.

[27] Jones-Webb R, Baranowski S, Fan D, et al. Content analysis of coverage of alcohol control policy issues in black-oriented and mainstream newspapers in the US. J Public Health Policy 1997;18(1):49–66.

[28] Nakahara S, Ichikawa M, Wakai S. Depiction of tobacco use in popular children's picture books. Arch Pediatr Adolesc Med 2004;158(5):498.

[29] Terre L, Drabman RS, Speer P. Health-relevant behaviors in media. J Appl Soc Psychol 1991; 21:1303–19.

[30] Hazan AR, Lipton HL, Glantz SA. Popular films do not reflect current tobacco use. Am J Public Health 1994;84(6):998–1000.

[31] Stockwell TF, Glantz SA. Tobacco use is increasing in popular films. Tob Control 1997;6: 282–4.

[32] Glantz SA, Kacirk KW, McCulloch C. Back to the future: smoking in movies in 2002 compared with 1950 levels. Am J Public Health 2004;94:261–3.

[33] Thompson KM, Yokota F. Depiction of alcohol, tobacco and other substances in G-rated animated feature films. Pediatrics 2001;107(6):1369–74.

[34] Goldstein AO, Sobel RA, Newman GR. Tobacco and alcohol use in G-rated children's animated films. JAMA 1999;281(12):1131–6.

[35] Everett SA, Schnuth RL, Tribble JL. Tobacco and alcohol use in top-grossing American films. J Community Health 1998;23(4):317–24.

[36] Dalton MA, Tickle JJ, Sargent JD, et al. The incidence and context of tobacco use in popular movies from 1988 to 1997. Prev Med 2002;34(5):516–23.

[37] Escamilla G, Cradock AL, Kawachi I. Women and smoking in Hollywood movies: a content analysis. Am J Public Health 2000;90:412–4.

[38] Sargent JD, Tickle JJ, Beach ML, et al. Brand appearances in contemporary cinema films and contribution to global marketing of cigarettes. Lancet 2001;357(9249):29–32.

[39] Sargent JD, Dalton MA, Beach ML, et al. Viewing tobacco use in movies: does it shape attitudes that mediate adolescent smoking? Am J Prev Med 2002;22(3):137–45.

[40] Mekemson C, Glantz SA. How the tobacco industry built its relationship with Hollywood. Tob Control 2002;11(Suppl 1):I81–91.

[41] Shields DLL, Carol J, Balbach ED, et al. Hollywood on tobacco: how the entertainment industry understands tobacco portrayal. Tob Control 1999;8(4):378–86.

[42] Distefan JM, Gilpin EA, Sargent JD, et al. Do movie stars encourage adolescents to start smoking? Evidence from California. Prev Med 1999;28(1):1–11.

[43] Tickle JJ, Sargent JD, Dalton MA, et al. Favourite movie stars, their tobacco use in contemporary movies, and its association with adolescent smoking. Tob Control 2001;10(1):16–22.

[44] Greenberg BS. Trends in use of alcohol and other substances on television. J Drug Educ 1979;9(3):243–53.

[45] Lowery SA. Soap and booze in the afternoon: an analysis of the portrayal of alcohol use in daytime serials. J Stud Alcohol 1980;41(9):829–38.

[46] Cafiso J, Goodstadt MS, Garlington WK, et al. Television portrayal of alcohol and other beverages. J Stud Alcohol 1982;43(11):1232–43.

[47] Breed W, DeFoe JR. Mass media, alcohol and drugs: a new trend. J Drug Educ 1980;10(2): 135–43.

[48] Breed W, DeFoe JR. The portrayal of the drinking process on prime-time television. J Commun 1981;31:58–67.

[49] Breed W, DeFoe JR. Drinking and smoking on television, 1950–1982. J Public Health Policy 1984;5:257–70.

[50] Wallack L, Breed W, DeFoe JR. Alcohol and soap operas: drinking in the light of day. J Drug Educ 1985;15(4):365–79.

[51] Wallack L, Breed W, Cruz J. Alcohol on prime-time television. J Stud Alcohol 1987;48(1): 33–8.

[52] DeFoe JR, Breed W. Response to the alcoholic by "the other" on prime-time television. Contemp Drug Probl 1988;15(2):205–28.

[53] DeFoe JR, Breed W. Youth and alcohol in television stories, with suggestions to the industry for alternative portrayals. Adolescence 1988;23:533–50.

[54] Wallack L, Grube JW, Madden PA, et al. Portrayals of alcohol on prime-time television. J Stud Alcohol 1990;51(5):428–37.

[55] Fernandez-Collado CF, Greenberg BS, Korzenny F, et al. Sexual intimacy and drug use in TV series. J Commun 1978;28(3):30–7.

[56] Signorielli N. Drinking, sex, and violence on television: the cultural indicators perspective. J Drug Educ 1987;17(3):245–60.

[57] Heilbronn LM. What does alcohol mean? Alcohol's use as a symbolic code. Contemp Drug Probl 1988;15(2):229–48.

[58] Cruz J, Wallack L. Trends in tobacco use on television. Am J Public Health 1986;76:698–9.

[59] Madden PA, Grube JW. The frequency and nature of alcohol and tobacco advertising in televised sports, 1990 through 1992. Am J Public Health 1994;84(2):297–9.

[60] Hazan AR, Glantz SA. Current trends in tobacco use on prime-time fictional television. Am J Public Health 1995;85(1):116–7.

[61] Hall CCI, Crum MJ. Women and "body-isms" in television beer commercials. Sex Roles 1994;31(5–6):329–37.

[62] Fedler F, Phillips M, Raker P, et al. Network commercials promote legal drugs: outnumber anti-drug PSA's 45-to-1. J Drug Educ 1994;24(4):291–302.

[63] Mathios A, Avery R, Bisogni C, et al. Alcohol portrayal on prime-time television: manifest and latent messages. J Stud Alcohol 1998;59:305–10.

[64] Golden J. A tempest in a cocktail glass: mothers, alcohol, and television, 1977–1996. J Health Polit Policy Law 2000;25(3):473–98.

[65] Long JA, O'Connor PG, Gerbner G, et al. Use of alcohol, illicit drugs, and tobacco among characters on prime-time television. Subst Abus 2002;23(2):95–103.

[66] DeJong W, Atkin CK. A review of national television PSA campaigns for preventing alcohol-impaired driving, 1987–1992. J Public Health Policy 1995;16(1):59–80.

[67] DeJong W, Hoffman KD. A content analysis of television advertising for the Massachusetts Tobacco Control Program media campaign, 1993–1996. J Public Health Manag Pract 2000; 6(3):27–39.

[68] DeJong W, Wolf RC, Austin SB. US federally funded television public service announcements (PSAs) to prevent HIV/AIDS: a content analysis. J Health Commun 2001;6(3):249–63.

[69] DeJong W, Atkin CK, Wallack L. A critical analysis of "moderation" advertising sponsored by the beer industry: are "responsible drinking" commercials done responsibly? Milbank Q 1992;70(4):661–78.

[70] Lavack AM. Message content of alcohol moderation TV commercials: impact of corporate versus nonprofit sponsorship. Health Mark Q 1999;16(4):15–31.

[71] Hackbarth DP, Silvestri B, Cosper W. Tobacco and alcohol billboards in 50 Chicago neighborhoods: market segmentation to sell dangerous products to the poor. J Public Health Policy 1995;16(2):213–30.

[72] Pucci LG, Joseph Jr HM, Siegel M. Outdoor tobacco advertising in six Boston neighborhoods: evaluating youth exposure. Am J Prev Med 1998;15(2):155–9.

[73] Mastro DE, Atkin CK. Exposure to alcohol billboards and beliefs and attitudes toward drinking among Mexican American high school students. Howard Journal of Communications 2002; 13(2):129–51.

[74] Stoddard JL, Johnson CA, Boley-Cruz T, et al. Tailoring outdoor tobacco advertising to minorities in Los Angeles County. J Health Commun 1998;3(2):137–46.

[75] DuRant RH, Rome ES, Rich M, et al. Tobacco and alcohol use behaviors portrayed in music videos: a content analysis. Am J Public Health 1997;87:1131–5.

[76] Markert J. Sing a song of drug use-abuse: four decades of drug lyrics in popular music, from the sixties through the nineties. Sociol Inq 2001;71(2):194–220.

[77] Thompson KM, Haninger K. Violence in E-rated video games. JAMA 2001;286(5):591–8.

[78] Sepe EP, Ling M, Glantz SA. Smooth moves: bar and nightclub tobacco promotions that target young adults. Am J Public Health 2002;92(3):414–9.

[79] Halpern JH, Pope HG. Hallucinogens on the Internet: a vast new source of underground drug information. Am J Psychiatry 2001;158(3):481–3.

[80] Hong T, Cody MJ. Presence of pro-tobacco messages on the Web. J Health Commun 2002; 7(4):273–307.

[81] Ribisl KM, Lee RE, Henriksen L, et al. A content analysis of Web sites promoting smoking culture and lifestyle. Health Educ Behav 2003;30(1):64–78.

[82] Ribisi KM, Williams RS, Kim AE. Internet sales of cigarettes to minors. JAMA 2003; 290:1356–9.

[83] Ribisi KM, Kim AE, Williams RS. Web sites selling cigarettes: how many are there in the USA and what are their sales practices? Tob Control 2001;10:352–9.

[84] Ribisi KM, Kim AE, Williams RS. Are the sales practices of internet cigarette vendors good enough to prevent sales to minors? Am J Public Health 2002;92(6):940–1.

[85] Bryant JA, Cody MJ, Murphy ST. Online sales: profit without question. Tob Control 2002; 11(3):226–7.

[86] Malone RE, Bero LA. Cigars, youth, and the Internet link. Am J Public Health 2000;90(5): 790–2.

[87] Winickoff JP, Houck CS, Rothman EL, et al. Verve and jolt: Deadly new Internet drugs. Pediatrics 2000;106(4):829–30.

[88] Wax PM. Just a click away: recreational drug Web sites on the Internet. Pediatrics 2002; 109(6):e96.

[89] Gerbner G, Ozyegin N. Alcohol, tobacco, and illicit drugs in entertainment television, commercials, news, "reality shows," movies, and music channels. New York: Robert Wood Johnson Foundation; 1997.

[90] Roberts DF, Henriksen L, Christenson PG. Substance use in popular movies and music. Washington (DC): Office of National Drug Control Policy; 1999.

[91] Christenson PG, Henriksen L, Roberts DF. Substance use in popular prime-time television. Washington (DC): Office of National Drug Control Policy; 2000.

[92] Roberts DF, Christenson PG. Here's looking at you kid: alcohol, drugs, and tobacco in entertainment media. Menlo Park (CA): Kaiser Family Foundation; 2000.

[93] Comstock GA. Influences of mass media on child health behavior. Health Educ Q 1981;8(1): 32–8.

[94] Dietz WH, Strasburger VC. Children, adolescents, and television. Curr Probl Pediatr 1991;21:8–31.

[95] Villani S. Impact of media on children and adolescents: a 10-year review of the research. J Am Acad Child Adolesc Psychiatry 2001;40(4):392–401.

[96] Brown JD, Witherspoon ED. The mass media and American adolescents' health. J Adolesc Health 2002;31(6 Suppl):153–70.

[97] Grube JW. Alcohol in the media: drinking portrayals, alcohol advertising, and alcohol consumption among youth. In: Institute of Medicine, editors. Reducing underage drinking: a collective responsibility. Washington (DC): National Academy Press; 2004. p. 597–624.

[98] Goldman LK, Glantz SA. Evaluation of antismoking advertising campaigns. JAMA 1998; 279(10):772–7.

[99] Sussman S. Tobacco industry youth tobacco prevention programming: a review. Prev Sci 2002; 3(1):57–67.

[100] Agostinelli G, Grube JW. Tobacco counter-advertising: a review of the literature and a conceptual model for understanding effects. J Health Commun 2003;8(2):107–27.

[101] Wakefield M, Flay B, Nichter M, et al. Effects of anti-smoking advertising on youth smoking: a review. J Health Commun 2003;8(3):229–47.

[102] Friend K, Levy DT. Reductions in smoking prevalence and cigarette consumption associated with mass-media campaigns. Health Educ Res 2002;17(1):85–98.

[103] Austin EW, Johnson KK. Effects of general and alcohol-specific media literacy training on children's decision making about alcohol. J Health Commun 1997;2:17–42.

[104] Baillie RK. Determining the effects of media portrayals of alcohol: going beyond short term influence. Alcohol Alcohol 1996;31(3):235–42.

[105] Austin EW, Chen YJ. The relationship of parental reinforcement of media messages to college students' alcohol-related behaviors. J Health Commun 2003;8(2):157–69.

[106] Austin EW, Pinkleton BE, Fujioka Y. The role of interpretation processes and parental discussion in the media's effects on adolescents' use of alcohol. Pediatrics 2000;105(2):343–9.

[107] Dalton MA, Ahrens MB, Sargent JD, et al. Relation between parental restrictions on movies and adolescent use of tobacco and alcohol. Eff Clin Pract 2002;5(1):1–10.

[108] Castiglia PT, Glenister AM, Haughey BP, et al. Influences on children's attitudes toward alcohol consumption. Pediatr Nurs 1989;15(3):263–6.

[109] Forsyth AJ, Barnard M, McKeganey NP. Musical preference as an indicator of adolescent drug use. Addiction 1997;92(10):1317–25.

[110] Hansen CH, Hansen RD. Constructing personality and social reality through music: individual differences among fans of punk and heavy metal music. Journal of Broadcasting and Electronic Media 1991;35(3):335–50.

[111] Bobo JK, Husten C. Sociocultural influences on smoking and drinking. Alcohol Health Res World 2000;24(4):225–32.

[112] Kear ME. Psychosocial determinants of cigarette smoking among college students. J Community Health Nurs 2002;19(4):245–57.

[113] Austin EW, Miller ACR, Silva J, et al. The effects of increased cognitive involvement on college students' interpretations of magazine advertisements for alcohol. Communic Res 2002; 29(2):155–79.

[114] Altman DG, Levine DW, Coeytaux R, et al. Tobacco promotion and susceptibility to tobacco use among adolescents aged 12 through 17 years in a nationally representative sample. Am J Public Health 1996;86(11):1590–3.

[115] Albers AB, Biener L. Adolescent participation in tobacco promotions: the role of psychosocial factors. Pediatrics 2003;111(2):402–6.

[116] Evans N, Farkas A, Gilpin E, et al. Influence of tobacco marketing and exposure to smokers on adolescent susceptibility to smoking. J Natl Cancer Inst 1995;87(20):1538–45.

[117] Pierce JP, Distefan JM, Jackson C, et al. Does tobacco marketing undermine the influence of recommended parenting in discouraging adolescents from smoking? Am J Prev Med 2002; 23(2):73–81.

[118] Pierce JP, Choi WS, Gilpin EA, et al. Tobacco industry promotion of cigarettes and adolescent smoking. JAMA 1998;279:511–5.

[119] Pierce JP, Gilpin E, Burns DM, et al. Does tobacco advertising target young people to start smoking? Evidence from California. JAMA 1991;266(22):3154–8.

[120] Atkin CK. Effects of drug commercials on young viewers. J Commun 1978;28(4):71–9.

[121] Atkin CK, Block M. Effectiveness of celebrity endorsers. J Advert Res 1983;23(1):57–61.

[122] Atkin CK, Neuendorf K, McDermott S. The role of alcohol advertising in excessive and hazardous drinking. J Drug Educ 1983;13:313–24.

[123] Atkin CK, Hocking J, Block M. Teenage drinking: does advertising make a difference? J Commun 1984;34:157–67.

[124] Atkin CK. Effects of televised alcohol messages on teenage drinking patterns. J Adolesc Health Care 1990;11(1):10–24.

[125] Atkin CK. Effects of media alcohol messages on adolescent audiences. Adolesc Med 1993; 4(3):527–42.

[126] Pierce JP, Gilpin EA. A historical analysis of tobacco marketing and the uptake of smoking by youth in the United States: 1890–1977. Health Psychol 1995;14(6):500–8.

[127] Pierce JP, Lee L, Gilpin EA. Smoking initiation by adolescent girls, 1944 through 1988: an association with targeted advertising. JAMA 1994;271(8):608–11.

[128] Fischer PM, Schwartz MP, Richards Jr JW, et al. Brand logo recognition by children aged 3 to 6 years: Mickey Mouse and Old Joe the Camel. JAMA 1991;266(22):3145–8.

[129] Austin EW, Nach-Ferguson B. Sources and influences of young school-aged children's general and brand-specific knowledge about alcohol. Health Commun 1995;7(1):1–20.

[130] King C, Siegel M. Adolescent exposure to cigarette advertising in magazines: an evaluation of brand-specific advertising in relation to youth readership. JAMA 1998;279(7):516–20.

[131] King C, Siegel M. Brand-specific cigarette advertising in magazines in relation to youth and young adult readership, 1986–1994. Nicotine Tob Res 1999;1(4):331–40.

[132] King C, Siegel M. Exposure of black youths to cigarette advertising in magazines. Tob Control 2000;9(1):64–70.

[133] Arnett JJ. Adolescents' responses to cigarette advertisements for five "youth brands" and one "adult brand". J Res Adolesc 2001;11(4):425–43.

[134] Krugman DM, King KW. Teenage exposure to cigarette advertising in popular consumer magazines. Journal of Public Policy and Marketing 2000;19(2):183–8.

[135] King C, Siegel M. The Master Settlement Agreement with the tobacco industry and cigarette advertising in magazines. N Engl J Med 2001;345(7):504–11.

[136] Gidwani PP, Sobol A, DeJong W, et al. Television viewing and initiation of smoking among youth. Pediatrics 2002;110(3):505–8.

[137] Tye J, Altman DG, DiFranza JR. Marketing adolescent tobacco addiction. Md Med J (Baltimore) 1995;44(10):767–73.

[138] Tye JB, Warner KE, Glantz SA. Tobacco advertising and consumption: evidence of a causal relationship. J Public Health Policy 1987;8(4):492–508.

[139] Warner KE, Goldenhar LM, McLaughlin CG. Cigarette advertising and magazine coverage of the hazards of smoking: a statistical analysis. N Engl J Med 1992;326(5):305–9.

[140] Wallack L, Dorfman L. Health messages on television commercials. Am J Health Promot 1992;6(3):190–6.

[141] Strasburger VC. Prevention of adolescent drug abuse: why "Just Say No" just won't work. J Pediatr 1989;114(4 Pt 1):676–81.

[142] Strasburger VC. Television and adolescents: sex, drugs, rock 'n' roll. Adolescent Medicine: State of the Art Reviews 1990;1(1):161–94.

[143] Strasburger VC. Adolescents, drugs, and the media. Adolesc Med 1993;4(2):391–415.

[144] Strasburger VC, Donnerstein E. Children, adolescents, and the media: issues and solutions. Pediatrics 1999;103:129–39.

[145] Strasburger VC. Alcohol advertising and adolescents. Pediatr Clin North Am 2002;49(2): 353–76.

[146] American Academy of Pediatrics Committee on Adolescence. Alcohol use and abuse: a pediatric concern. Pediatrics 1987;79(3):450–3.

[147] American Academy of Pediatrics Committee on Substance Abuse. Alcohol use and abuse: a pediatric concern. Pediatrics 1995;95(3):439–42.

[148] American Academy of Pediatrics Committee on Substance Abuse. Alcohol use and abuse: a pediatric concern. Pediatrics 2001;108(1):185–9.

[149] American Academy of Pediatrics. American Medical Association, American Academy of Child & Adolescent Psychiatry, American Psychological Association, American Academy of Family Physicians, and the American Psychiatric Association. Joint statement on the impact of entertainment violence on children. Presented at the Congressional Public Health Summit. Washington (DC), July 26, 2000. Available at: http://www.aap.org/advocacy/releases/jstmtevc.htm. Accessed November 1, 2004.

[150] Federal Trade Commission. Marketing violent entertainment to children: a review of self-regulation and industry practices in the motion picture, music recording and electronic game industries. Available at: http://www.ftc.gov/opa/2000/09/youthviol.htm. (See related follow-up reports and meetings at: http://www.ftc.gov/bcp/workshops/violence/index.html.) Accessed November 1, 2004.

[151] Smoke Free Movies. The solution. Available at: http://www.smokefreemovies.ucsf.edu/solution/r_rating.html. Accessed November 1, 2004.

[152] Mosher JF, Wallack LM. Government regulation of alcohol advertising: protecting industry profits versus promoting the public health. J Public Health Policy 1981;2(4):333–53.

[153] Ile ML, Kroll LA. From the Office of the General Counsel: tobacco advertising and the first amendment. JAMA 1990;264(12):1593–4.

[154] Kessler DA, Witt AM, Barnett PS, et al. The Food and Drug Administration's regulation of tobacco products. N Engl J Med 1996;335(13):988–94.

[155] Kessler DA, Wilkenfeld JP, Thompson LJ. The Food and Drug Administration's rule on tobacco: blending science and law. Pediatrics 1997;99(6):884–7.

[156] Gostin LO, Arno PS, Brandt AM. FDA regulation of tobacco advertising and youth smoking: historical, social, and constitutional perspectives. JAMA 1997;277(5):410–8.

[158] Gostin LO. Corporate speech and the Constitution: the deregulation of tobacco advertising. Am J Public Health 2002;92(3):352–5.

[159] Bayer R. Tobacco, commercial speech, and libertarian values: the end of the line for restrictions on advertising? Am J Public Health 2002;92(3):356–9.

[160] Signorielli N. Children and adolescents on television: a consistent pattern of devaluation. J Early Adolesc 1987;7(3):255–68.

[161] Klein JD, Brown JD, Childers KW, et al. Adolescents' risky behavior and mass media use. Pediatrics 1993;92(1):24–31.

[162] Thompson KM. KidsRisk media guide. Available at: http://www.KidsRisk.harvard.edu. Accessed March 1, 2005.

ELSEVIER
SAUNDERS

Child Adolesc Psychiatric Clin N Am
14 (2005) 491–508

CHILD AND
ADOLESCENT
PSYCHIATRIC CLINICS
OF NORTH AMERICA

The Play's the Thing:
A Clinical-Developmental Perspective on
Video Games

Holly S. Gelfond, EdD[a,b],
Dorothy E. Salonius-Pasternak, PhD[a,b,*]

[a]Harvard Medical School Center for Mental Health and Media, 271 Waverley Oaks Road,
Waltham, MA 02452, USA
[b]Department of Psychiatry, Massachusetts General Hospital, 55 Fruit Street, Boston, MA 02114, USA

Computer and video games have received increasing attention over the past few decades from players and professionals alike. The first computer and video games were invented in the 1960s and 1970s, respectively, and their growing prevalence first in arcades and then in homes throughout the industrialized world began in the late 1970s [1]. The first game that was considered to be controversial, "Death Race," was published as an arcade game by Exidy in 1976 [2]. Computer and video games and their possible effects on players have been studied in many fields of scientific literature, with areas of focus including whether games with violent content increase aggression or violence [3–7], whether these games lead to desensitization to real aggression or violence [8], physiologic responses to playing computer and video games [9], addiction [10,11], possible influences of computer and video games on cognitive skills and development [12], possible therapeutic or pro-social effects of computer and video games [13–17], and the use and efficacy of computer and video game ratings [18]. Despite this seeming variety of perspectives and foci, however, in

This project was supported by grant no. 2003-JN-FX-0078 awarded by the Office of Juvenile Justice and Delinquency Prevention, Office of Justice Programs, United States Department of Justice. Points of view or opinions in this document are those of the author and do not necessarily represent the official position or policies of the United States Department of Justice.

* Corresponding author. Harvard Medical School Center for Mental Health and Media, 271 Waverley Oaks Road, Waltham, MA 02452.

  E-mail address: dsaloniuspasternak@partners.org (D.E. Salonius-Pasternak).

the last two decades few researchers have focused on computer and video games as play [19–24]. We posit that computer and video games must be considered play media and that children and adolescents who engage in these media are, in fact, engaging in play.

There are several reasons for clinicians, researchers, and the general public to consider computer and video games as play. First, considering computer and video games as play puts them into a normative context, reflecting the fact that most American children and adolescents play video games [25,26]. This classification allows us to study them from a clinical-developmental perspective so that any issues of pathology can be understood from this normative frame of reference. Second, children and adolescents regard them as play [27]. Studying the phenomenon through their eyes is a necessary step throughout the research process, from designing protocols and measures to analyzing and interpreting the data. Third, computer and video games may enrich children's play by offering new ways for children to pursue developmentally appropriate experiences (ie, imaginative play, negotiating rules, and safe exploration of aggression). By developing a further understanding of the roles that computer and video games may serve in children's play, we can become better able to facilitate these positive play opportunities in children's everyday lives and in clinical settings.

In this article we focus primarily on school-aged children, and we pay particular attention to the most significant concerns documented in the literature regarding electronic play: aggression and violence. We first present some major perspectives on play and salient developmental issues. We then explore computer and video games, which we call electronic play [23], and discuss their similarities and differences with other kinds of play and their potential contributions to children's cognitive and socioemotional development. We conclude the article with recommendations for clinicians in their work with children and adolescents and their parents. We also provide a discussion of future directions for research.

Definitions and functions of play

Play is often easy to recognize, but ambiguity surrounds its definition [23,28,29]. Several criteria for defining play have emerged in the literature, including the facts that the games incorporate positive affect, are flexible, voluntary, egalitarian, nonliteral (ie, pretense) [30], and enjoyable, concern means over ends, and occur for their own sake [31]. Scarlett et al [23] proposed that we consider not the noun of play but rather the verb of playing ("something one experiences and makes happen") and suggested that play can be defined as what children see as play. Pellegrini [29] suggested that the "tenor" of the activity, and not necessarily the activity itself, is what makes something play. For example, two children who are wrestling and screaming could be either playing or fighting, depending on the context of their own intentions, feelings, and expression. Given the diversity of activities and experiences that might be considered to be play, it is important not to apply a rigid definition to all of these activities and experiences but rather to consider multiple criteria that can be applied with some degree of flexibility, relative to the context [23].

Several perspectives exist regarding the functions of play. Researchers interested in culture have described play as a way in which children are socialized in the context of their society's knowledge, values, and practices [23,32]. Psychoanalysts view play as the ego's attempt to create a "world of illusion" [33], in which the conflicts between conscious and unconscious desires and their prohibition in the external world can be resolved. Researchers have documented numerous contributions of play to areas of children's socioemotional, cognitive, and physical development, including emotion regulation, peer and familial relationships, attention, problem solving, creativity, fine- and gross-motor skills, and overall physical health [23]. Sutton-Smith [34] called this the "rhetoric of progress"—that play contributes to children's development through at least short-term, if not long-term, benefits.

Although these positive contributions of play have been documented, this is not to say that all children's play should be considered positive. We all have witnessed examples of "bad play" [23]: mean-spirited teasing, chronic misbehaving play, or destructive play. Other examples of play are more ambiguous. On the surface, they may arouse concern, but further exploration can show that they may be examples of play that have some kind of hidden value. Electronic play is an example of play that is more ambiguous. From a clinical-developmental perspective, we can consider play to be on a continuum: on the surface, the same play activity can serve purposes that are more or less normative or adaptive, depending on aspects of development, intrinsic and extrinsic motivations, and other contextual factors. Later, we discuss some issues of concern relating to electronic play and explore the characteristics of electronic play that show that it cannot be dismissed entirely as "bad play."

Salient aspects of development in play

For school-aged children, a salient aspect of development in play is their increased interested in the structure and rules of play [23]. Strictly following the rules and meticulously categorizing toys demonstrate the concreteness of their cognitive development, and negotiating about the rules before play with their peers is an example of their increasingly sophisticated social development.

In play that is more structured, such as games, children direct their impulses (eg, start, stop, fast, slow) and manage their emotions in tandem with ever more complex cognitive skills. These skills include planning, strategy, and stealth and more clearly defined outcomes of winning and losing. Play embedded in games draws on rules and parallels the cognitive development of the elementary school–aged child who desires to know more about the organization of the larger world via its social, cultural, and physical laws. The school-aged child desires a sense of mastery across organized domains—school, the arts, sports, and play. This desire reflects Erikson's [35] psychosocial developmental stage of industry versus inferiority. Similarly, a child's developing interest in rules that systematize and organize the world also corresponds with Piaget's [36] cognitive developmental stage of concrete operational thinking. In games that also incorporate fantasy, the symbolic world of pretense is integrated within the structured world of rules. Imagination and organization, limitless fantasy, and rule-bound worlds merge in play as children develop increasing cognitive capacities.

Socioemotional development in children's rule-based play is demonstrated by the differences in the play of younger versus older children and in the play of new acquaintances versus familiar friends. Negotiating and establishing the rules in play provide opportunities for children to develop a sense of fairness and learn how to handle disagreements with peers. As children grow increasingly accustomed to playing with rules, their rules become more complex. When children play with new friends, however, they tend to play with simpler rules until they feel more comfortable in these less familiar relationships [23].

When children reach middle school, rules can dominate even more in their play. Creating, breaking, and negotiating rules are all forms of play for middle-school children. These children often spend much of their playtime discussing and disputing the rules of a game. It is as if playing with the rules is the game. Boys tend to focus on the rules in terms of what is fair and just [37], whereas girls focus on rules of inclusion and exclusion [38]. Only when a child is old enough to know the rules, however, is it fun to play with breaking those rules.

Another aspect of school-aged children's play is imagination, or make-believe. One function of make-believe in play is to facilitate children's making sense of the world around them. According to Scarlett et al [23], "...dragons and superheroes may fly, but they do so because of conditions (wings) or motives (to fight bad guys) not altogether different from those in the real world." When children incorporate frightening or perverse themes into their imaginary play (eg, aspects of violence or sexuality), these themes sometimes arouse concern in the adults who care for them, who fear that these themes in play imply that children will carry them out in the real world. Singer [39] argued, however, that "...even some of the more outrageous forms of make-believe play may have an adaptive role in clarifying for child players some of the necessary distinctions they must make in confronting the genuine difficulties of daily living." In the context of normative development, frightening or perverse themes provide children with opportunities to distinguish further between fantasy and reality, make sense of real-world rules, and gain a sense of mastery over difficult issues.

The impact of societal issues on play

In addition to developmental aspects that influence children's play, larger societal concerns can have an effect on children's play. Increasingly, parents feel that their children are in need of protection in places that once were considered safe havens. Child kidnappings, shootings by children, and playground violence are just some of the events that make the notion of children roaming free and playing outdoors less appealing than it may have been a century ago. Although the actual occurrence of these events has not increased in recent years, changes in media coverage have led many people to believe that it has. One response to the resulting urge to protect children has been to restrict children's outdoor play [34]. Moving play indoors also has given birth to the notion of playtime as a more private and solitary endeavor, which is often more supervised than it has been in the past. Sutton-Smith [34] believes that this is part of a larger trend over the past 300 hundred years to "domesticate" and control children's play. Sutton-Smith defines the domestication of play as "the increasing control and supervision of play to get rid of physical dangers and its emotional licenses."

In recent years, this domestication has taken the form of supervising children's activities, including recess, organized sports, peer-group social sets, and play in the classroom [40]. Sutton-Smith [41] believes that the content of children's play has become restricted in the United States, as reflected in the cultural controversies regarding war play, toy guns, and whether certain play genres should be gender specific. With increased supervision, much of the freedom within children's play has been eliminated. Children's free time in general also has been reduced. Because of a heightened urgency to increase children's cognitive skills at the cost of supporting other forms of development (as evidenced by the emphasis on standardized tests to measure a child's educational success), many schools have curtailed play-related aspects of their curriculums, including physical education and the arts [42]. Sutton-Smith [41] wrote "strangely, it is quite easy to find educators and administrators and politicians who act in a practical way as if play is of no damn use whatsoever by closing playgrounds, by abolishing recess, and by organizing children's free time in every possible way." Free time after school also has diminished for some children because of increasing amounts of structured activities [43].

These various intrusions into children's daily lives may be impediments to the essential functions that freer, less structured play serves in supporting children's emotional, social, cognitive, and linguistic development. We put forth the theory that particular video games—as toys or as a form of play—may have the potential to restore some of the critical elements of children's play that may have been lost because of the restrictions on children's space and the structuring and control of their time and imaginations.

Characteristics and demographics of electronic play

Electronic play is the first qualitatively different form of play that has been introduced in at least several hundred years. With most forms of play media, the essence of the game exists in the interactions between the players and the physical media (eg, blocks, sticks, dolls, pinecones, paints). Unlike most forms of play media, the essence of electronic play exists in the interactions between the players and the distinctly intangible potential for a wide range of experiences, whose physical properties of hardware and software are less the essence of the game and more simply a means of accessing it.

Although it is difficult to give exact figures, most studies indicate that most American school-aged children are playing electronic games—on home computers, console game systems (eg, Nintendo, PlayStation, X-Box), or both [44]. This is also true for European and Japanese children [45]. In these industrialized countries, the older a child gets, the more likely the child is to play computer and console games and play them for longer periods of time. By adolescence, the most common pattern is playing electronic games for 30 to 60 minutes daily [25,26]. Boys outnumber girls in terms of who is playing computer and console games. This is true throughout the industrialized world. The reasons for and implications of this gap are not yet well understood, however. It simply may be that more games are designed especially for boys [19].

Currently, the most popular types of electronic play are console and hand-held games. Console games are played through a special game console used with a television (eg, X-box, PlayStation, Nintendo Game Cube). Hand-held games are played on Game-Boys, personal digital assistants, and mobile phones. This division becomes less distinct as the technology that supports each type merges, however, and as the same games are frequently produced for each type of technology. As for the games themselves, there are several category systems for describing different types of games. No one system has emerged to provide a common language. Table 1 offers an example of one of these category systems, which is used by game designers, and incorporates the language often used by the players themselves.

Computer and console games played in a stationary setting are what we traditionally think of when we consider electronic play, but electronic play has become increasingly portable, especially with the advent of Nintendo's Game Boy and, more recently, with the inclusion of games that can be played on mobile phones and personal digital assistants. The Nokia N-Gage, a combination mobile phone, FM radio, MP3 player, and game deck with high-resolution graphics, increases the potential even further for mobile game play. A recent study showed that Finnish children use their mobile phones more often for games than for talking [46].

There are several striking features about modern video games that differ from older games and other types of play: (1) their graphics and realism, (2) their levels or graded challenges, and (3) their ways of encouraging interaction. Together, these features may explain some of the reasons why children find electronic play so appealing. The graphics and realism in modern computer and console games are striking. Realism describes how real the game feels to its players, how vivid the depicted world seems to be. Sports games not only provide opportunities to play soccer, basketball, or any other sport a player can imagine but also provide realistic representations of well-known sports arenas, real-life "color" commentators (eg, John Madden plays himself in "John Madden Football"), and all the gestures that help define a player as being linked to a

Table 1
Types of electronic games

Type of game	Description	Examples
Real-time strategy	Fast-paced strategy games; often played online with other players	Warcraft, Starcraft, Command & Conquer, Age of Empires
First-person shooters	First-person perspective "shoot-em ups"; often played online with other players	Doom, Quake, Unreal Tournament, Halflife
Empire builders	Slow-paced games that are played out over weeks; players begin with a small village equivalent and promote technologic progress, expansion, conquest, and trade in order to rule the world of the game	Civilization, Alpha Centauri, Master of Orion
Simulations	Games that simulate reality, a period in history, a fictional setting; emphasis typically is not placed on winning or losing	SimCity, Rollercoaster Tycoon, Caesar-Pharaoh-Zeus
Adventure	Games that follow a linear story involving puzzles to solve	King's Quest, Space Quest, Prince of Persia, Myst
Role-playing games	Games in which players take on the role of a character and build upon its knowledge and skills as the storyline progresses; often involves tactical combat	Baldor's Gate, Final Fantasy, Ultima, Diablo
Massively multiplayer role-playing games	Role-playing games that are played online with hundreds or even thousands of other players	Everquest, Ultima Online, Anarchy Online, Dark Age of Camelot
Sports	Games that simulate various kinds of sports	Grand Turismo, John Madden Football, Tiger Woods Golf
Puzzles	Games that involve logic or reflexes in putting pieces together	Tetris, Crystalis

Data from Brett Levin, Impressions Software, personal communication, 2002.

particular sport (eg, soccer players throwing up their hands when receiving a yellow card, tired-looking basketball players leaning over and gripping the bottoms of their shorts). Simulation games turn children into bona fide city planners, nineteenth-century pioneers settling the American west, and many other roles that children find exciting.

It is important to remember that the concept of realism does not refer to the degree to which a game accurately represents real life. In fact, many games that include realism are fantastic in their content. One aspect of technology to power realism (and interaction) in games is "real-time 3-D," which allows images to be created instantaneously as players progress through a game, unlike the "pre-rendered" images of earlier technology, whose limited range of possibilities rarely allowed players to forget even for a moment that it is only an illusion. The enhanced graphics and freedom of movement of real-time 3-D can promote physiologic responses, such as motion sickness or even vertigo, to perceptions of realistic movement [47]. Another aspect of games' realism is enabled by haptics technology, through which players can experience some of the force and vibration that matches the depicted play. Currently, haptics technology is not as advanced as other aspects of game technology, but it may reach that level in the future [48].

In addition to realism, other features of computer and console games that seem to appeal to children are levels and graded challenges. The goals of the sports game "Grand Turismo," in which players immerse themselves in the world of auto racing, include passing several driving tests by racing around a track in a certain amount of time, participating in races to earn money, and handling business aspects, such as buying new cars and improving existing cars. At first, players begin the game at a basic level, without much strategy involved. At the next level, players make decisions that solve simple, concrete problems that deal with matching the features of their cars to the particular racecourse laid out before them. While racing, they must orient themselves by looking at a map and changing their view of the track to figure out where the competition is and when to speed up or slow down. To succeed at the highest level, players must use complex strategies and think abstractly to evaluate systematically the different options and plan carefully their approach to the game. At this level, players must figure out subtleties, such as the best timing and speed of braking for particular track conditions, so that their cars get around curves quickly and without crashing.

Still another feature of computer and console games that seems to make them attractive is their way of encouraging interaction. Most console game systems provide ways for more than one player to play at the same time, and the Internet encourages much more, for computer games as well. Although the first online game was created in 1969, it was not until the early 1990s and widespread use of the Internet that online gaming became popular [49]. As broadband Internet connections become increasingly common, the potential of online gaming also grows; higher bandwidth facilitates greater online complexity and sophistication in games [50]. Currently, children on different continents who have never met can play computer and console games together through several different types of games. Players often find that the game experience is richer when played with or against people rather than the computer [50]. The Internet also has created the virtually unlimited potential for players to trade tips and strategies, access demo versions of new games, and form friendships based on their shared interest.

Electronic play and children's development

As with any kind of play, electronic play has the potential to contribute positively to children's cognitive and socioemotional development, and there may be particular ways in which the benefits of electronic play are unique.

In this section we consider how electronic play may contribute positively to children's imaginative play, self-regulation of arousal, rule negotiation, morality, coping, and socialization through safe expressions of aggression. We also explore ways in which electronic play can be incorporated into therapeutic play and play therapy to help children overcome difficulties in clinical settings.

The mass marketing of toys to children and the bombardment of images from mass media grow increasingly pervasive [51]. According to Singer [39], "the very act of beginning to form individualized images...and anticipatory fantasies becomes, in our crowded and sensory-bombarded world, the last refuge for an experience of individuality and personal privacy." Some experts believe that the prepackaged images produced by television, cartoons, or video games are another kind of intrusion on children's imaginary play [52]. There may be aspects of sensory bombardment that are inherent in video games. Video games also incorporate children's imaginations, however. Children who immerse themselves in electronic play assume the roles of spies, wizards, policemen, skateboarders, and a host of other characters. Other aspects of certain popular video games (ie, games that allow a player to explore the environment) support a freer and more unstructured space for play where imagination can flourish.

Sutton-Smith [34] believes that although there are certain benefits to over-structuring and organizing children's time, that practice can have deleterious effects on children's play, including taking away important time spent with one's own imagination. The advent of particular video games, on the other hand, has taken an opposite approach. One of the most popular and controversial games of recent times, "Grand Theft Auto III," may owe some of its popularity with children (and perhaps adults) not to the antisocial behaviors and violence for which it has become known, but rather for its lack of rigid structure and opportunity for exploration in its form of play. In "Grand Theft Auto III," which was released as a PlayStation console game at the end of 2001 and released as a computer game midway through 2002, the main plot of the game involves "...walking around the city mugging, maiming, killing, and car jacking" [52a]. A unique and particularly appealing aspect of the game is its "fully realized and dynamic" free-form design. The design allows players to disregard entirely the main plot lines and instead explore the virtual city complete with a plethora of interactive details, including delivering pizza and driving the injured to the hospital in an ambulance, which make the game one of the most realistic games currently available. Unlike many other games, disregarding the violent plot line does not result in play ending through a character's death. Since the release of "Grand Theft Auto III," other games that incorporate these characteristics have been published, including "Grand Theft Auto Vice City," "True Crime: Streets of LA," "Driv3r," "Simpsons Hit & Run," "Jak II," "Tony Hawk Pro Skater 4," "Tony Hawk's Underground," "Mafia," and "The Getaway."

Expanding on the idea of electronic play as free and imaginative, McNamee [27] described the video game world as a "heterotopia" (using Foucault's term), in which "...the playing of video games by children can be seen as a strategy for contesting spatial boundaries" within the real world. McNamee further argued that because children's leisure time is increasingly supervised, "...playing video games may, then, provide those who play them with the adventures that they are no longer allowed to have, in spaces which they do not inhabit in any real sense."

From McNamee's perspective, children seek the adventure that video games provide because they like doing things that they are not ordinarily allowed to do and from which they have become more and more restricted. From the perspective of the developmental role of play in children's lives, we also argue that adventures within video games allow children to confront danger and the concomitant feelings of fear and anxiety, mastery and defeat, power and powerlessness in a world that arouses fear but is ultimately safe. As with other types of play, the aspect of safety that emerges from the fact that the danger confronted is only pretend or make-believe allows a child to self-regulate and calm those feelings of fear and anxiety associated with such danger. Goldstein [21] explained "One characteristic of rough-and-tumble play, war play, and other forms of potentially dangerous or frightening entertainment is that they occur within a framework of safety and comfort." Goldstein suggested that these types of play give children the opportunity to self-regulate their states of arousal and stated that switching between feelings of fear and safety may be an aspect of play that children find enjoyable.

With their interactive technology and virtual worlds, video games offer unique opportunities for children to play with rules within a make-believe setting. In the video game "Tony Hawk's Pro Skater 4," for example, children, by identifying with the main character, are able to transcend the rules of physical reality by leaping higher and turning faster on a skateboard than they could in reality. Not only do the children transcend the ordinary rules of physics but they also experience a sense of mastery—if only symbolically—over the physical world and themselves in it. In "Grand Theft Auto Vice City," children play with breaking other types of rules—societal laws. In this video game, children act as a character who can break the laws of society by driving a car through a red light or stealing the car he or she drives. This appeals to older children, who appreciate that laws govern society and who are just beginning to negotiate the expectations of adult society to follow such rules. Although these make-believe video games allow children to break the rules of ordinary daily life, they still must follow the rules of the game. There are limits and boundaries to this kind of play. It is not that there are no rules, it is simply that the nature and boundaries of these rules are rearranged. This rearrangement of reality, scholars argue [53–55], can be adaptive in a child's development. Not only is it pleasurable for children to have a chance to break rules that are continually imposed on them, but scholars also believe that make-believe play—including breaking the rules of the ordinary world in a make-believe setting—serves the important function of helping children to understand more about reality [53,55] and the laws that make it up. That is, make-believe play, which allows children to compare varied possibilities of the natural and social world, helps them to clarify reality while they are experimenting with altering it.

Aggression, violence, and electronic play

Aggression or violence in the context of or resulting from video games is a hot topic in the literature and is perhaps the most linked topic with video games. In their review of the empirical literature of video game violence, Dill and Dill [56] described the game "Killer Instinct" as "...a game that pits two macabre characters (or, more to the point, its two young players) against one another in harsh, bloody combat to the death." This presentation implies that the game's "two young players" would not understand that the depicted characters do not exist in reality outside the game and that they would see themselves, and not just the depicted characters, as engaging in "harsh, bloody combat to the death" in reality. This is not an implication that should be presented hastily, for it is precisely the players' understanding of reality versus fantasy in the game that is likely to influence whether they will be more likely to display aggression or violence after playing such a game.

In considering the research that has been conducted in the area of electronic games with violent content, it is important to remember that we are considering a type of play. Electronic games can be viewed as a form of aggressive play, which is inherently different from actual aggression because of its lack of intent or attempt to injure a living person [22,57]. This can be seen as analogous to Pellegrini's [29] clarifying comparison of rough-and-tumble play and aggression in school-aged children: although rough-and-tumble play may resemble real fighting, its play tenor clearly differentiates it for its participants.

Pellegrini [29,58] discussed the changing role of rough-and-tumble play for adolescents, who begin to use it as a way to learn about aggression through socialization processes, which establish peer status through dominance without causing physical harm to participants. It may be that electronic play with aggressive or violent themes may serve a similar purpose for adolescents. From this perspective, rather than promoting aggressive or violent behavior, playing electronic games with violent content may be a healthy way for children and adolescents to experiment safely or grapple with the complicated issues of war, violence, and death without any real-world consequences [57,59]. As with physical aggression, some children and adolescents deviate from normative uses of electronic play with aggressive or violent themes, or they may extend behavior inappropriately to other non-play contexts. This is likely more to do with the interactions between the individual characteristics of the players and the games themselves. Whereas some children and adolescents have no difficulty resulting from their electronic play experiences, others may. Further research is needed to clarify how characteristics of players and the games themselves may affect the risk of harm.

Research on violence in television has demonstrated that being exposed to this type of media violence can increase aggressive behavior, cognitions, and affect [60]. One meta-analysis of the literature on the effects of violent content in electronic games on aggression found that the effect size for violent content in electronic games was smaller than the effect size for violent content in television [5].

Perhaps the more active role that children and adolescents take in electronic play could enable them to develop a deeper understanding of the depicted violence through the exploration of characters' motivations, moral dilemmas, and consequences of action. This exploration could result in greater reflection about violence than exists in typical television watching, given players' active role in the game. Jenkins [24] pointed out that "No story-telling medium in the history of mankind has been free of violence and aggression because mankind is not free from them either. We need our story-tellers and artists to help us think about the nature of violence." Although not yet widespread, games increasingly are being developed that encourage and sometimes require players to consider the meaning and consequences of their actions—violent or otherwise—to succeed in the game. These games include "Neverwinter Nights," "Morrow Mind," "Black and White" [24], "Swat 3," and "Combat Mission" [61]. Jenkins suggested that games such as these could help us as a society to understand the nature of aggression and violence [24]. Future research and policy work in this area should allow for the possibility of positive influences of these games.

Electronic play in clinical settings

A small but growing body of research suggests that electronic play also may have positive contributions in clinical settings, including psychotherapy, the treatment of specific conditions, such as impulsivity and attention deficit disorders, and pain management during medical procedures. Therapists have reported that video games can be used from the beginning of the therapeutic relationship as an enjoyable activity that establishes a "middle ground" with child or adolescent patients. Video games can provide opportunities for clinicians to observe a child's problem-solving strategies, ability to foresee consequences of behavior, and self-regulation of arousal from satisfying and frustrating experiences. Video games also can be incorporated into behavior management techniques to improve motivation, encourage cooperative behavior, and raise self-esteem [14,62,63].

Video games may be particularly useful in treating children and adolescents with specific conditions, such as impulsivity and attention deficit disorders. Several small studies and anecdotal reports have shown that the use of games designed for these populations and commercially available video games, as they are sold or modified to incorporate biofeedback, have been effective forms of treatment for reducing impulsivity and teaching and rewarding sustained focus on the activity at hand. It is likely that video games' overall appeal with children and adolescents and their characteristic of immediate feedback are at least partly responsible for the treatment efficacy [64–67].

Video games also have been used in pediatric hospital settings. Because of their ability to serve as a cognitive/attentional distraction, they frequently have been used as a tool in pain management. Video games used for this purpose were selected based on children's expressed individual preferences. They may be particularly effective for pain management in children and adolescents with chronic conditions or limited mobility. Children who played video games while undergoing chemotherapy experienced less nausea and lower systolic blood pressure, and a lower amount of painkillers was required [14,68–70]. Video games also have been used in pain management for children undergoing treatment for sickle-cell disease and burns and children in wheelchairs [71–73]. In addition to these positive effects for children, the use of video games in pediatric hospital settings is recommended because of the ease of integrating them into most treatment settings and their cost effectiveness relative to other pain management programs [68].

Preliminary studies have shown that electronic play also may contribute positively in the contexts of physiotherapy, occupational therapy, and facilitating the development of social skills in children and adolescents with learning disabilities, mental retardation, and autism spectrum disorders [13,42,63,74,75].

When clinicians use computer or video games in the context of therapeutic play or play therapy, it is crucial to devise carefully a treatment plan that appropriately matches the themes of the games, player interface, duration of play, and other relevant characteristics of the games and the play experience with a child or adolescent's particular issues, needs, or condition [14]. For example, video games that emphasize rapid, repetitive responses may not be suitable for treatment in children and adolescents with impulsivity or attention deficit disorders [66].

As we discussed the role of electronic play in children's socioemotional and cognitive development, we presented numerous ways in which computer and video games may be beneficial in the context of therapeutic play and play therapy. These benefits include facilitating children's ability to make sense of the world around them, developing and refining their abilities to distinguish between fantasy and reality, considering and experimenting with aggression through aggressive play in a safe environment, and negotiating societal roles and rules. When we consider therapeutic play, we are referring to play that occurs naturally or spontaneously or is facilitated by clinicians. In either case, therapeutic play is naturally beneficial or is designed to be beneficial in some way by following a child's agenda. Play therapy is a more formalized approach that takes advantage of the inherent benefits of play in a clinical setting, with established goals of treatment [23]. We believe that electronic play has the potential be therapeutic without clinicians' facilitation in naturally occurring, normative play experiences. The responsibility of supervising play in these cases rests with parents and, in some cases, teachers.

Recommendations for further research

Currently, there are more questions than research-based answers—questions about whether electronic play promotes violence, the characteristics of potentially harmful versus potentially beneficial games and electronic play patterns, how the effects of electronic play influence families and parent-child relations, and how electronic play should be incorporated into clinical settings. Regarding electronic play with violent content, there are indications that children and adolescents who are already predisposed to aggressive or violent behavior who engage in electronic play with violent content may be at greater risk for aggression and violence [7,22,57]. Currently, these and other frequently asked questions have no clear, research-based answers that pinpoint causes and effects. Further research is needed to develop a better understanding of the complicated issues that seem to be involved in this area.

One gap in the research on computer and video games is the lack of well-designed, well-executed experimental studies with solid operational definitions of independent and dependent variables. This lack of clearly defined variables calls into question the construct validity of the independent and dependent variables [5], which makes it impossible to demonstrate causality. For example, studies often do not distinguish between aggression and aggressive play as outcome variables [57], although currently no evidence supports the claim that electronically depicted acts of aggression and violence in the context of electronic play are perceived and understood the same as actual acts of aggression and violence. Aggressive play and actual acts of aggression and violence differ, especially in terms of children's intent and motivation, and this difference must be considered when defining research variables [22].

There is also a lack of research with any subsets of the population that may bear particular predispositions to aggression or violence. Hypotheses point toward groups of people who may be especially vulnerable to any negative effects of games with violent content, yet we do not have any empirical basis for assessing these effects or taking appropriate action to handle them [57]. Another gap in the research is the lack of attention to the ways in which cognitive and socioemotional development may play a role in how players respond to games with violent content. The different ways in which young children and adolescents understand the distinction between fantasy and reality is one example of a developmental factor that is likely to influence how young players respond to electronic play. Adolescents display great interest in electronic play and a greater propensity for aggression in general. Studies that adopt a developmental perspective are necessary to further our understanding of groups that may be at particular risk [57,76].

Other gaps include the lack of research on the influences context, including socioeconomic status and culture [77]. Socioeconomic status and culture likely would influence the characteristics that players bring to the game experience and how the game experience fits into their lives. Families' socioeconomic status may influence parents' availability and resources for supervising children's electronic play. Games that incorporate attitudes and beliefs already dominant in a player's culture may encourage the acting out of game content in the real world. For instance, the amateur games that were circulated around the Internet after the terrorist attacks of September 11, 2001, in which players could shoot depictions of Osama bin Laden, could have been more likely to promote aggression or violence, particularly against Arab-Americans, because the games mirrored other aspects of our culture that were promulgating fear of and negative attitudes toward Arab-Americans after the attacks [24]. Further research is needed to develop our understanding of how macrosystemic influences such as socioeconomic status and culture could influence how children and adolescents respond to electronic games.

Summary

Electronic play has the potential to contribute positively to children's socio-emotional development by facilitating children's making sense of the world around them, developing and refining their abilities to distinguish between fantasy and reality, considering and experimenting with aggression through a safe environment, improving their self-regulation of arousal, and negotiating societal roles and rules. Electronic play also has the potential to benefit children and adolescents in clinical settings, including psychotherapy, treatment of impulsivity and attention deficit disorders, and pain management during medical procedures. As we further our understanding of the role of electronic play in children's lives, we can incorporate this knowledge into our clinical work to expand our application of effective tools and methods with children and adolescents.

Further research is needed in this area. Future studies should use clearly and carefully operationalized definitions of variables and constructs, focus on subsets of the population that may be at particular risk, incorporate a developmental perspective, and address issues that relate to culture and socioeconomic status. Future studies also should consider the possible benefits of electronic play in the everyday lives of children and adolescents and in clinical settings. Because our understanding of the role of electronic play in clinical settings is currently limited, clinicians should use particular care in developing a treatment that appropriately matches the relevant characteristics of the games and the play experience with a child or adolescent's particular issues, needs, or condition.

References

[1] Kent SL. The ultimate history of video games: from Pong to Pokemon. New York: Prima Publishing; 2001.

[2] Gonzalez L. When two tribes go to war: a history of video game controversy. Available at: http://www.gamespot.com/features/6090892/index.html. Accessed November 1, 2004.

[3] Cooper J, Mackie D. Videogames and aggression in children. J Appl Soc Psychol 1986;16: 726–44.

[4] Anderson CA, Ford CA. Affect of the game player: short-term effects of highly and mildly aggressive video games. Pers Soc Psychol Bull 1986;12(4):390–402.

[5] Sherry JL. The effects of violent video games on aggression: a meta-analysis. Hum Commun Res 2001;27(3):409–31.

[6] Gentile DA, Lynch PJ, Linder JR, et al. The effects of violent video game habits on adolescent hostility, aggressive behaviors, and school performance. J Adolesc 2004;27:5–22.

[7] Funk JB, Hagan J, Schimming J, et al. Aggression and psychopathology in adolescents with a preference for violent electronic games. Aggress Behav 2002;28:134–44.

[8] Funk JB, Baldacci HB, Pasold T, et al. Violence exposure in real-life, video games, television, movies, and the internet: is there desensitization? J Adolesc 2004;27:23–39.

[9] van Reekum CM, Johnstone T, Banse R, et al. Psychophysiological responses to appraisal dimensions in a computer game. Cognition & Emotion 2004;18(5):663–88.

[10] Salguero RA, Moran RM. Measuring problem video game playing in adolescents. Addiction 2002;97(12):1601–6.

[11] Phillips CA, Rolls S, Rouse A, et al. Home video game playing in schoolchildren: a study of incidence and patterns of play. J Adolesc 1995;18(6):687–91.

[12] Baird WE, Silvern SB. Electronic games: children controlling the cognitive environment. Early Child Dev Care 1990;61:43–9.

[13] Griffiths M. Can videogames be good for your health? J Health Psychol 2004;9(3):339–44.

[14] Griffiths M. The therapeutic use of video games in childhood and adolescence. Clinical Child Psychology and Psychiatry 2003;8(4):547–54.

[15] Chambers JH, Ascione FR. The effects of prosocial and aggressive video games on children's donating and helping. J Genet Psychol 1987;148:499–505.

[16] Anderson CA, Bushman BJ. Effects of violent video games on aggressive behavior, aggressive cognition, aggressive affect, physiological arousal, and prosocial behavior: a meta-analytic review of the scientific literature. Psychol Sci 2001;12(5):353–9.

[17] Wiegman O, van Schie EGM. Video game playing and its relations with aggressive and prosocial behaviour. Br J Psychol 1998;37(3):367–78.

[18] Haninger K, Thompson K. Content and ratings of teen-rated video games. JAMA 2004; 291(7):856–65.

[19] Cassell J, Jenkins H. From Barbie to Mortal Kombat: gender and computer games. Cambridge (MA): MIT Press; 1998.

[20] Goldstein J. Toys, play and child development. New York: Cambridge University Press; 1994.

[21] Goldstein J. Aggressive toy play. In: Pellegrini AD, editor. The future of play theory: multidisciplinary inquiry into the contributions of Brian Sutton-Smith. New York: State University of New York Press; 1995. p. 127–59.

[22] Goldstein J. Effects of electronic games on children. Available at: http://www.senate.gov/~commerce/hearings/0321gol.pdf. Accessed July 24, 2003.

[23] Scarlett WG, Naudeau S, Ponte IC, et al. Children's play. Thousand Oaks (CA): Sage Publications; 2004.

[24] Penny Arcade. A conversation with Henry Jenkins, Pt I–III. Available at: http://www.penny-arcade.com/lodjenkins.php3. Accessed August 23, 2003.

[25] Annenberg Public Policy Center. Media in the home: the fifth annual survey of parents and children. Philadelphia: Annenberg Public Policy Center; 2000.

[26] Kaiser Family Foundation. Key facts: children and video games. Available at: http://www.kff.org/entmedia/3271-index.cfm. Accessed August 1, 2003.

[27] McNamee S. Foucault's heterotopia and children's everyday lives. Childhood 2000;7(4): 479–92.

[28] Fein G. Pretend play in childhood: an integrative review. Child Dev 1981;52:1095–118.

[29] Pellegrini AD. Perceptions and functions of play and real fighting in early adolescence. Child Dev 2003;74(5):1522–33.

[30] Sutton-Smith B. War toys and childhood aggression. Play & Culture 1988;1:57–69.

[31] Pellegrini AD, Smith PK. Physical activity play: the nature and function of a neglected aspect of play. Child Dev 1998;69(3):577–98.

[32] Roopnarine J, Johnson J, Hooper H. Children's play in diverse cultures. New York: State University Press; 1994.

[33] Ritvo S. Play and illusion. In: Solnit A, Cohen D, Neubauer P, editors. Many meanings of play: a psychoanalytic perspective. New Haven (CT): Yale University Press; 1993. p. 234–51.

[34] Sutton-Smith B. Does play prepare the future. In: Goldstein J, editor. Toys, play, and child development. New York: Cambridge University Press; 1995. p. 130–46.

[35] Erikson EH. Childhood and society. 2nd edition. New York: Norton; 1963.

[36] Piaget J, Inhelder B. The psychology of the child. New York: Basic Books; 1969.

[37] Piaget J. The moral judgment of the child. New York: Free Press; 1965.

[38] Maccoby EE, Jacklin CN. The psychology of sex differences. Stanford (CA): Stanford University Press; 1974.

[39] Singer JL. Imaginative play in childhood: precursor of subjunctive thought, daydreaming, and adult pretending games. In: Pellegrini ADE, editor. The future of play theory: a multidisciplinary inquiry into the contributions of Brian Sutton- Smith. Albany (NY): State University of New York Press; 1995. p. 187–220.

[40] Buchner P. Changes in the social biography of childhood in the FRG. In: Chisolm L, Buchner P, Kruger H, et al, editors. Childhood, youth, and social change. London: Falmer; 1990. p. 71–84.

[41] Sutton-Smith B. Conclusion: the pervasive rhetorics of play. In: Pellegrini AD, editor. The future of play theory: a multidisciplinary inquiry into the contributions of Brian Sutton-Smith. Albany (NY): State University of New York Press; 1995. p. 257–95.

[42] Gardner H. The unschooled mind: how children think and how schools should teach. New York: Basic Books; 1991.

[43] Elkind D. The hurried child. Reading (MA): Addison-Wesley; 1981.

[44] Jordan AB, Woodard EH. Electronic childhood: the availability and use of household media by 2- to 3-year-olds. Zero-To-Three 2001;22(2):4–9.

[45] Beentjes JWJ, Koolstra CM, Marseille N, et al. Children's use of different media: for how long and why? In: Livingstone S, Bovill M, editors. Children and their changing media environment: a European comparative study. LEA's Communication Series. Mahwah (NJ): Lawrence Erlbaum Associates, Inc.; 2001. p. 85–111.

[46] Suoranta J, Lehtimäki H. Children in the information society: the case of Finland. New York: Peter Lang Publishers; 2004.

[47] Keegan P. Culture quake. Available at: http://www.motherjones.com/news/feature/1999/11/quake.html. Accessed June 1, 2002.

[48] Kushner D. With a nudge or vibration, game reality reverberates. Available at: http://www.nytimes.com. Accessed July 22, 2003.

[49] Mulligan J. Happy 30th birthday, online games. Available at: http://www.gatecentral.com/shared_docs/Timeline1.html. Accessed October 20, 2004.

[50] PS3Land.com. Online gaming and the future. Available at: http://www.ps3land.com/onlinegaming.php. Accessed October 20, 2004.

[51] Kline S. The promotion and marketing of toys: time to rethink the paradox? In: Pellegrini AD, editor. The future of play theory: a multidisciplinary inquiry into the contributions of Brian Sutton-Smith. Albany (NY): State University of New York Press; 1995. p. 165–85.

[52] Sutton-Smith B. Paradigms of intervention. In: Hellendoorn J, Kooij RVD, Sutton-Smith B, editors. Play and intervention. Albany (NY): State University of New York Press; 1994. p. 3–21.

[52a] Armchair Empire. PC reviews: Grand Theft Auto III. Available at: http://www.armchairempire.com/Reviews/PC%20Games/grand-theft-auto-iii.htm. Accessed August 14, 2002.

[53] Singer DG, Singer JL. The house of make-believe: play and the developing imagination. Cambridge (MA): Harvard University Press; 1990.

[54] Singer DG. Encouraging children's imaginative play: suggestions for parents and teachers. Presented at Play, Play Therapy, Play Research: International Symposium. Amsterdam (The Netherlands), September 1985.

[55] Leslie AM. Pretense and representation: the origins of theory of mind. Psychol Rev 1987;94:412–22.

[56] Dill KE, Dill JC. Video game violence: a review of the empirical literature. Aggress Violent Behav 1998;3(4):407–28.

[57] Bensley L, Van Eenwyk J. Video games and real-life aggression: review of the literature. J Adolesc Health 2001;29(4):244–57.

[58] Pellegrini AD, Bartini M. Dominance in early adolescent boys: affiliative and aggressive dimensions and possible functions. Merrill Palmer Q 2001;47(1):142–63.

[59] Goldstein J. Why we watch: the attractions of violent entertainment. New York: Oxford University Press; 1998.

[60] Huesmann LR, Miller LS. Long-term effects of repeated exposure to media violence in childhood. In: Huesmann LR, editor. Aggressive behavior: current perspectives. New York: Plenum Press; 1994. p. 153–86.

[61] Osborne S. Teaching violence or violence that teaches? Available at: http://www.gamespy.com/editorials/may01/teaching/index1.stm. Accessed August 23, 2003.

[62] Gardner JE. Can the Mario Bros. help? Nintendo games as an adjunct in psychotherapy with children. Psychotherapy 1991;28:667–70.

[63] Spence J. The use of computer arcade games in behaviour management. Maladjustment and Therapeutic Education 1988;6:64–8.

[64] Kappes BM, Thompson DL. Biofeedback vs. video games: effects on impulsivity, locus of control, and self-concept with incarcerated individuals. J Clin Psychol 1985;41:698–706.

[65] Clarke B, Schoech D. A computer-assisted game for adolescents: initial development and comments. Computers in Human Services 1994;11(1–2):121–40.

[66] Wright K. Winning brain waves: can custom-made video games help kids with attention deficit disorder? Available at: http://www.discover.com/mar_01/featworks.html. Accessed November 1, 2004.

[67] Roach J. Video games boost visual skills, study finds. Available at: http://news.national geographic.com/news/2003/05/0528_030528_videogames.html. Accessed November 1, 2004.

[68] Redd WH, Jacobsen PB, DieTrill M, et al. Cognitive-attentional distraction in the control of conditioned nausea in pediatric cancer patients receiving chemotherapy. J Consult Clin Psychol 1987;55:391–5.

[69] Kolko DJ, Rickard-Figueroa JL. Effects of video games on the adverse corollaries of chemotherapy in pediatric oncology patients. J Consult Clin Psychol 1985;53:223–8.

[70] Vasterling J, Jenkins RA, Tope DM, et al. Cognitive distraction and relaxation training for the control of side effects due to cancer chemotherapy. J Behav Med 1993;16:65–80.

[71] Pegelow CH. Survey of pain management therapy provided for children with sickle cell disease. Clin Pediatr (Phila) 1992;31:211–4.

[72] O'Connor TJ, Cooper RA, Fitzgerald SG, et al. Evaluation of a manual wheelchair interface to computer games. Neurorehabil Neural Repair 2000;14(1):21–31.

[73] Adriaenssens EE, Eggermont E, Pyck K, et al. The video invasion of rehabilitation. Burns 1988;14:417–9.

[74] Griffiths M. The therapeutic use of videogames in childhood and adolescence. Clinical Child Psychology & Psychiatry 2003;8(4):547–54.

[75] Demarest K. Video games: what are they good for? Available at: http://www.lessontutor.com/kd3.html. Accessed September 1, 2004.

[76] Kirsh SJ. The effects of violent video games on adolescents: the overlooked influence of development. Aggress Violent Behav 2003;8(4):377–89.

[77] Griffiths M. Video game violence and aggression: comments on "video game playing and its relations with aggressive and prosocial behaviour." Br J Soc Psychol 2000;39(1):147–9.

ELSEVIER
SAUNDERS

Child Adolesc Psychiatric Clin N Am
14 (2005) 509–522

CHILD AND
ADOLESCENT
PSYCHIATRIC CLINICS
OF NORTH AMERICA

Hollywood Portrayals of Child and Adolescent Mental Health Treatment: Implications for Clinical Practice

Jeremy R. Butler, MD[a,b],*, Steven E. Hyler, MD[a,b]

[a]Department of Psychiatry, Columbia University, New York, NY, USA
[b]New York State Psychiatric Institute, 1051 Riverside Drive, New York, NY 10032, USA

On an inpatient unit a psychiatry resident found himself in the midst of a discussion with a 15-year-old boy hospitalized for explosive outbursts and transient paranoia. The conversation centered on starting an antipsychotic medication. "You just want to turn me into a zombie," he said. "That's all you psychiatrists want to do." This sentiment did not come from a middle-aged schizophrenic in the era of typical neuroleptics but was the impression of an adolescent who was newly exposed to psychiatric treatment on a unit in which there were no such patients to be found. In a discussion with the patient's mother, she said, "He needs to be locked up—for a year...at least. I'll sign the papers."

These were the words of a fearful adolescent and a frustrated mother, and yet they expressed common public perceptions that became important issues in this patient's treatment. Successful confrontation of this imagery—mentally ill patients turned into zombies, psychiatrists with omnipotent control, indefinite hospitalization decided in a flash—would determine medication adherence, family support of treatment, and therapeutic alliance. To the treatment-naïve, however, where had these images come from? When asked, the patient responded "Nightmare on Elm Street."

By and large, the public has much less contact with true psychiatrists than with their media representations. Psychiatry, as practiced in the real world, remains a black box to most of the public, and to new parents the subspecialty of

---

* Corresponding author. New York State Psychiatric Institute, Mailbox 84, 1051 Riverside Drive, New York, NY 10032.
  E-mail address: jrb67@columbia.edu (J.R. Butler).

child and adolescent psychiatry is a complete mystery. Into this black box, what dreams may come? Those dreams, nightmares, and fantasies can be found where dreams have been played out for the last 100 years—at the movies. As has been shown in studies, although film is an art form and an expression of the conscious and unconscious, it also influences its audience's perceptions [1,2] and, consequently, the care delivered.

In recent years, several Hollywood films have depicted the treatment of psychiatric illness in adolescence and childhood. Some of the more popular films include "Don't Say a Word" (2001), "Girl, Interrupted" (1999), "The Sixth Sense" (1999), and "The Cell" (2000). These films vary in their intended audiences, the realism with which they depict mental illness and its treatment, and the genre of film to which they belong. These and other films that depict mental health treatment are seen repeatedly by a public that may or may not encounter the real-life counterpart. Consequently, they have little by which to judge the Hollywood mythology of psychiatry. This mythology has a long history that has evolved over the last 100 years and has been slow to update despite changes in clinical practice [3,4]. Understanding the history of the film child psychiatrist and the mythology of his craft is vital to a clinician's communication with child and adolescent patients and their parents.

This article is designed to educate clinicians about Hollywood's myths of what is and is not childhood mental illness, what psychiatry is, who practices it, and how it works. Positive and negative portrayals are identified with clinical examples of how treatment can be affected. Finally, Hollywood does nothing better than create spectacle, and the authors provide suggestions for using that spectacle to the advantage of the patient and his or her treatment.

A brief history of child and adolescent psychiatry at the movies

Leslie Rabkin's book "The Celluloid Couch" [5] provides a comprehensive catalog of movie summaries that depict psychiatric treatment, dating back to the advent of film itself. From these descriptions of films (largely lost to viewing), one finds that the child psychiatrist debuted nearly simultaneously with his adult counterpart. Early films such as "Andy and the Hypnotist" (1914), in which a young boy is hypnotized and put under the doctor's control, started a genre that was cemented with the release of "The Cabinet of Dr. Caligari" (1919). Similar themes were found in other movies that depicted psychologists performing experiments with children to create utopian societies. Movie reviews from the 1910s described psychiatrists treating one young woman's kleptomania with a brain operation and another woman's condition with psychotherapy. Disruptive multiple personalities were conquered with talk therapy, and libidinal inhibition was cured with brain fluid transplantation.

From these early films through modern ones, the role of the child psychiatrist is to curb behavior that is unacceptable to society rather than reduce subjective distress experienced by the child or adolescent. Although by the 1920s, Hollywood became enamored with psychological theory and film became a way to explore the question of sanity and subjective experience in adults, child psychiatry on film largely avoided this type of exploration and ignored personal experience for ideas of societal betterment.

Throughout the 1930s, 1940s, and 1950s, the screen was littered with images of the juvenile delinquent and his or her home—the reformatory. "The Wild One" (1954), "Rebel Without a Cause" (1955), and "The Wild Angels" (1966) are enduring examples of this genre as subjects mutated from individuals to street gangs to motorcycle gangs. Although "Rebel Without a Cause" does not depict the delivery of mental health treatment, the psychiatrist/psychologist played an intermittent role in other films, often with unorthodox treatments. In "Little Tough Guys in Society" (1938), a society matron, following a psychiatrist's advice, invites a street gang to her estate to toughen up her son. In these films, delinquency is often depicted as a conscious choice on the part of adolescents, with less interest shown in diagnosis or cause than in hard-line punishment.

By the 1960s and 1970s, with movies such as "David and Lisa" (1962), "Diary of a Schizophrenic Girl" (1970), and "I Never Promised You a Rose Garden" (1977), the psychiatrist finally emerged as a character who treated authentic adolescent mental illness and not one who merely tried to manage sociopathic conditions. To this day, the depiction of adolescent psychiatry on film diverges: one half reunites with the adult depictions of mental illness (eg, movies such as "Ordinary People" [1980]), whereas the other half continues to depict psychiatry in the role of behavior enforcer, most commonly found in the horror movie genre.

Per Hollywood, who is the mentally ill child?

The public perception of what is or is not mental illness is one of the fundamental issues of this topic. The psychiatrist in the audience easily recognizes and diagnoses psychopathology, but does the lay audience viewer react similarly?

The recent film "Thirteen" (2003) contained a graphic depiction of substance abuse, eating disorder, sexual promiscuity, and self-injury consistent with conduct disorder and possible onset of borderline personality disorder. (The film was co-authored by Nikki Reed, who was only 13 years old.) The title of the movie, however, is not "Crazy Girl" or "In Need of Help" but rather the age of the main character. At no point in the film does the character visit a psychiatrist or seek any kind of mental health treatment. Despite significant distress and self-injury, it is not clear that the audience associates the behavior with mental illness that requires psychiatric treatment at all, but rather associates it with the behavior of a 13-year-old girl reacting to peer pressure and social conformity. The movie's tagline, "It's happening so fast," further suggests that to its producers and marketers the movie is about development and not disorder. What does Hollywood teach an audience about what actual childhood mental illness looks like?

The most common distortion in Hollywood is its preference for the spectacular rather than the mundane. Hollywood rarely shows police officers doing deskwork or surgeons performing follow-up care. Similarly, psychiatrists are rarely shown treating common (and mundane) conditions. There is a skewed depiction of what mental illness is, what psychiatrists do, and how serious the illness must be to necessitate psychiatric assessment. The authors were hard-pressed to find a single example of identified attention deficit disorder in films. Treatments of dramatically presented psychopathologic conditions are likely to be aggressive and often are administered involuntarily. The film psychiatrist is often more restricting and "invasive" than any psychiatrist would be in the real world. As one patient stated, "[In the movies] you see everyone getting handfuls of medication or shots from big metal syringes with huge needles."

The discrepancy between portrayed and actual conditions is important because adolescence is a popular Hollywood topic; films frequently depict the various social pressures that teens must navigate. The long list of such films includes "Fast Times at Ridgemont High" (1986), "The Breakfast Club" (1985), "Heathers" (1989), "Dazed and Confused" (1994), and, more recently, the "American Pie" (1999) series. These films frequently depict alcohol or marijuana abuse, depression, social anxiety, and impulsive behavior, some of which—if presented clinically—would warrant diagnosis and mental health treatment. It is unlikely, however, that most of the viewing public considers biologic and psychological formulations for such behavior. As a result, it is unlikely that these often dynamic, popular, and beautiful characters are perceived as requiring mental health treatment.

In an online adolescent discussion of the film "Thirteen," in reaction to a suggestion that the behavior portrayed warranted concern, a 13-year-old girl stated, "No, it's not that young. I have friends younger than thirteen who have done worse things than in this film. One of my best friends did everything the girls did and worse when she was eleven." Her comment suggested that the behavior shown, pathologic or not, in the world of teen peer pressure becomes a glamorous benchmark to beat, not an indication of distress.

On the opposite end of the spectrum, the spectacular also can be a supportive teaching tool. A 17-year-old individual with bipolar disorder and antisocial behavior said of "Girl, Interrupted," "I love Angelina Jolie. She was so cool in that movie." The drama that makes a film enjoyable to watch can make a diagnosis exciting and acceptable. For this patient, who had symptoms and behaviors similar to Angelina Jolie's character in that film, identification with an attractive, rich, successful actress was empowering and made her more comfortable with her illness. The character's use of disdain, dishonesty, and wit was equally present in this patient's relationship with the treatment team, however. Although intermittently charming, she was difficult to confront or motivate to change.

Per Hollywood, who is a psychiatrist?

Alongside policemen and lawyers, physicians are among the most common film characters. In an examination of portrayals of just prominent physician characters, psychiatrists are second only to surgeons (26% of physician depictions) in frequency of depiction [6]. When one includes the number of films in which the mental health provider is not clearly delineated as psychiatrist or psychologist or therapist (a persistently blurred boundary, with minimal attention paid to differences among the three), the number of portrayals of mental health providers increases significantly. Psychiatry debuted onscreen in the era of silent film, and its earliest treatments involved the use of hypnosis, because it was the principal treatment available. Schneider [7], a clinician with a love for film, grouped the depiction of film psychiatrists into three separate stereotypes: Dr. Dippy, Dr. Wonderful, and Dr. Evil. Schneider's monikers have been used over the last 20 years in several papers and books and have held as an accessible way to understand the limited variety of movie psychiatrists [8].

Dr. Dippy appeared in 1906 in "Dr. Dippy's Sanitarium" and embodied "the familiar comical movie psychiatrist—the one who is crazier or more foolish than his patients...His treatment methods tend to be bizarre, impractical or unusual." Dr. Wonderful debuted in the 1940s, because filmmakers had more practical experience with psychiatrists. Schneider said, "He is invariably warm, human, modest and caring. Time is of no concern to him...patients can see him or talk to him at any time and for any length of time." The final avatar of movie psychiatry is Dr. Evil, whose birth is most commonly traced to "The Cabinet of Dr. Caligari" (1919). "The chief characteristic of Dr. Evil, whatever his nature or intent, is his willingness to use what have been viewed as the coercive tools available to psychiatry. These include commitment of patients to an institution, experimentation, ECT, lobotomy, heavy medication, and hypnosis. In his hands these become tools for control, manipulation, power, revenge and financial gain."

Although the role that filmmakers have allotted the child and adolescent psychiatrist has been more circumscribed than that of the adult counterpart, the influence of these three stereotypes is never far from the surface and is referenced as other myths that surround child and adolescent psychiatry are explored.

How child psychiatry works: Hollywood's mental health myths

Evolving from the ways in which early films portrayed mental illness and its providers, several myths have pervaded the film portrayals of mental illness. Whereas the stigma of adult mental illness has been discussed at length elsewhere [9], the myths of childhood mental illness and its treatment largely have been ignored. The authors have compiled five of these myths, tracing their origins through the history described previously and providing clinical correlation to the messages contained within.

Myth #1: a child with "mental illness" can be cured with enough love

This myth is one of the fundamental beliefs of the onscreen psychiatric treatment of children and is shown repeatedly for any number of illnesses. It is an interesting distortion created by the adoption of Dr. Wonderful for child and adolescent psychiatry. Although Dr. Wonderful represents the ideal—a wish by adult filmmakers for the perfect psychiatrist—there are other implications in introducing him to the care of children.

In the recent film "Don't Say a Word," Dr. Nathan Conrad (played by Michael Douglas), the expert's expert, is brought in as consultant on the case of young Elisabeth (Brittany Murphy), who has had "twenty different hospitalizations, twenty different diagnoses." She has been diagnosed with "selective mutism, obsessive-compulsive behavior, post-traumatic symptoms," a first schizophrenic break, posttraumatic stress disorder, Asperger's syndrome, cyclothymic disorder, expressive-language disorder, attention deficit disorder, oppositional-defiant disorder, and manic-depression. Elisabeth, it seems, meets all criteria from the "Diagnostic and Statistical Manual." Dr. Conrad has a disdain for medications, a disdain for hospitals, and a disdain for diagnoses. After a brief interview and review of the chart, Dr. Conrad hands down a different diagnosis: "She's overlaying, she's a brilliant mimic." Through the course of the movie, this young woman is alternately depressed, catatonic, and violent to the point of causing "one hundred and eleven stitches." By protecting her from a band of vindictive jewel thieves, however, Dr. Conrad provides the compassion and embraces necessary for a complete recovery. At the end of the film, Elisabeth even gets a new father: Dr. Conrad himself.

Several insinuations are made in this tale, namely that a psychiatrist cannot accurately diagnose children and that given enough love and attention (or adoption, if necessary), a young adult with refractory mental illness can be cured. In this example, the story goes much further: not only is it love that cures but also the psychiatrist literally substitutes himself for the parent when necessary.

In "The Sixth Sense" (1999), Bruce Willis portrays Dr. Malcolm Crowe, an eminent child psychologist who is the rightful heir to Dr. Wonderful's legacy. Over the course of the film, Dr. Crowe treats Cole (Haley Joel Osment), a young child who suffers from crippling anxiety. His treatment of Cole is shown as supportive with infinite amounts of time. He follows Cole wherever he goes and overcomes Cole's initial resistance with charm and patience. While his own marriage falls apart, he remains dedicated to his young patient and ultimately cures the child of the anxiety symptoms with which he had been suffering. Although the final plot twist skews some of this reality, the audience experiences most of the film under this rubric. Dr. Malcolm Crowe's treatment is that of parental love without medication, diagnosis, or structure, and the result is cure.

This myth has been perpetuated through other illnesses, including mental retardation, autism, and selective mutism. The myth is not limited to male therapists; more recently, Jennifer Lopez took a turn as a child psychologist in "The Cell" (2000), in which she entered her patients' minds (at her own peril!)

to help them overcome their fears. The myth is also not limited to therapists or persons with any formal training. In "Marvin's Room" (1996), Leonardo DiCaprio meets criteria from the "Diagnostic and Statistical Manual" for conduct disorder through lying, threatening, and setting fires. Although hospitalization and therapy help minimally, a supportive relationship with an aunt (played by Diane Keaton) makes quick work of his sociopathy and anger.

Although the myth trivializes the importance of psychiatric diagnosis or treatment, there are positive and negative associations with these depictions. There is some understanding that by having a positive therapeutic alliance and a stable relationship with support and consistency, positive emotional and behavioral changes can occur. The lengths to which these characters go are unrealistic, however, and they create wholly unachievable standards of self-sacrifice on the part of the clinician. Whereas the adult clinician's display of dedication, professionalism, and caring is largely positive, Hollywood frequently chooses to set up a competitive dynamic between the mental health provider and the adolescent patient's parents. By suggesting that mental illness is cured by love and support, the converse is that that mental illness is caused by lack of support. Whereas successful treatment gives credit to the psychiatrist, the parents of young patients are left with the responsibility for the illness. This model usurps the organic, genetic, and traumatic progenitors of mental illness in exchange for a harsher, more simplistic, and more blameful conception.

This is a myth that portrays and perpetuates parents' worst fears. Dr. Wonderful implies an accusation of bad or absent parenting as the cause of a child's suffering and suggests that the psychiatrist will take over as parent. When reviewing films that depict child and adolescent mental health treatment, the authors repeatedly were struck by the number of films in which the treater adopted (legally or symbolically) the young patient into his or her family. "Silent Fall" (1994), "Don Juan de Marco" (1995), "Antwone Fisher" (2002), and "Don't Say a Word" provide a handful of examples. This can provoke fear but also hope, as with the frustrated mother who wanted to sign her son over to a psychiatrist "for a year...at least."

Although Dr. Wonderful is something of a psychiatric ideal in his treatment of adults, his presence in the minds of parents could be a deterrent to seeking psychiatric consultation for their children for fear of losing them. This message also serves to warn clinicians that enacting the role of the wonderful clinician can evoke paranoid fantasies of competition and displacement.

Myth #2: there is nothing to psychiatry; anything can be considered treatment and anyone a psychiatrist

In adult psychiatry this message has been most clearly depicted in movies such as "The Couch Trip" (1988), "M*A*S*H" (1970), and "Down and Out in Beverly Hills" (1986). In these films, an inexperienced impostor is able to evoke radical change through an off-the-wall approach to mental illness. Sometimes the rebel treater is a psychiatrist, whose disdain for the establishment leads him or her onto the path of truth. The myth is not unique to psychiatry and is seen in other branches of medicine in movies such as "Patch Adams" (1998) and "Awakenings" (1990).

In child and adolescent psychiatry, this same misconception exists. In "Silent Fall," Richard Dreyfus plays such a rebel psychiatrist, Dr. Jake Rainer. When charged by the police chief to make an autistic boy talk, he comes head to head with the "accepted" psychiatrist, Dr. Harlinger (John Lithgow), who wants to use intramuscular lorazepam instead. When the medication is used the boy loses control, but when the boy is hugged he demonstrates radical change and communicates. As with the general medical version of this myth, it is the physician or treatment that errs on the side of love that evokes change; by default, science, diagnosis, and structure are the enemies.

This myth defies a single pedigree of psychiatrist and includes Dr. Dippy, Dr. Evil, and Dr. Wonderful. Dr. Dippy can be seen in Hugh Grant's portrayal of a child-fearing psychiatrist in "Nine Months" (1995), in which he plays an ineffectual child psychologist, or in scenes with Jeffrey Tambor sleeping through sessions in "Girl, Interrupted." Dr. Evil can be seen in the form of the pompous psychiatrist who is so much a part of the system that he fails to see the benefits when they are blatantly present, and Dr. Wonderful is he whose qualities evoke change in that cold and unhelpful system. In a positive way, this belief encourages a climate of exploration or experimentation. It acknowledges that there are few available answers and that other treatments may be helpful. On the negative side, it encourages a climate of skepticism and cynicism. It feeds the culture of unstudied alternative medicine or untested herbal supplements, because the regular system is perceived as ineffectual. At its worst, it suggests that because cure is achieved without systematic "real" treatment, there is no "real" condition being treated.

A mother of a young man spoke with a psychiatric resident during her son's first hospitalization for a psychotic break. She worked as a case manager for mentally ill patients and had worked for years with the issues surrounding treatment. To the resident she said, "I know the medications are important, I do. But do you think that acupuncture and relaxation might be enough"? This myth provides a defense against the hopelessness and demoralization that psychiatric diagnosis can bring, but it also provides fodder for a whole host of mistruths. At its best, it is a stance of empowerment; at its worst, it feeds an environment of doubt, controversy, and arguments.

Myth #3: if you do not do what we want, you will be locked up forever

"One Flew Over the Cuckoo's Nest" (1975) had a pervasive effect on American psychiatry and cast a broad skepticism on the practice of ECT. With the character of Nurse Ratched it portrayed mental health practitioners as punitive and dictatorial. Thirty years after its release, audiences have long since forgotten that the main character malingers to get out of prison, but the image of psychiatry destroying free-wheeling R.P. McMurphy endures.

Susanna Kaysen's book "Girl, Interrupted" is a first-hand account of bor-derline personality disorder symptoms, including identity diffusion, disunity of time and place, and acute psychotic symptoms. When the book was adapted for the screen, a different spin was placed on Kaysen's tale, one in which the po-litical context of the late 1960s played heavily into her symptoms and clinical course. The film asks: in that "crazy" world, who would not be crazy? The film takes a stance against adulthood and suggests that resisting your parent's wishes will land you in the loony bin. Despite Kaysen's significant suicide attempt ("a bottle of aspirin, washed down with a bottle of vodka"), when Winona Ryder's character reads about her diagnosis in a textbook, she says: "Borderline personality disorder: an instability of self image, relationships and mood. Uncer-tainty about goals. Impulsive in activities that are self-damaging, such as casual sex. Social contrariness and a generally pessimistic attitude of often observed. That's me." Angelina Jolie's "sociopathic" character responds, "That's every-body." Although Kaysen clinically improves after engaging in therapy with the female head psychiatrist, any benefit that psychiatric treatment garners from this depiction is soon undone. At the end of the film, instead of coming to understand the role of therapy in her improvement, Winona muses while re-flecting on her hospitalization, "Was I ever crazy? Maybe. . .or maybe life is."

The horror movie genre is produced almost exclusively for adolescents and young adults and has continued to use Dr. Evil regularly. In the movie "Night-mare on Elm Street 3: Dream Warriors" (1987), a group of adolescents are permanent residents in a psychiatric hospital. Each suffers from horrible night-mares of an undead serial rapist trying to kill them. The catch is that should they die in their dreams, they never will wake up. Although the adolescents try multiple times to explain the situation to adults, the only treatments they re-ceive are oral sedatives and injections, which are subsequently lethal. In these films, there is never discussion of dangerousness to self or others, simply the existence of unacceptable beliefs, which the audience knows are not delusional at all. Psychiatrists are portrayed simply as jailers for nonconformists. The mes-sage takes on a special meaning for adolescents and suggests that their entire future can be taken away by saying the wrong thing. From that vantage point, these films can be understood as a negotiation of moral and social standards, but it remains unfortunate that the psychiatrist is portrayed as the recurrent enemy in this battle.

Onscreen, the depiction of the "mental hospital" is often highly unrealistic and overly harsh, and its staff relies heavily on force. The images are dredged from the cinematic archive of the early century, when sanitariums were impene-trable castles, and Gothic or expressionistic versions of "One Flew Over the Cuckoo's Nest" (1975) and "The Silence of the Lambs" (1991). They bear little relation to modern psychiatric hospitals and are frequently dirty, poorly lit, and labyrinthine. In this way the psychiatric hospital has remained its own character in films despite changes in its real-life counterpart; given the endurance of the Dr. Evil stereotype, it seems unlikely to change in the near (or distant) future. For patients, these images persist. One woman, who had never been hospitalized, said in describing her impressions of what a psychiatric hospital is like, "rusty bedframes with stripped mattresses, and that mystery room in the basement where they took you when you were bad or didn't participate in group session."

Myth #4: mental illness is actually a gift; psychiatrists take away that gift

This myth is ultimately one of the most upsetting of the perpetuated Hollywood myths. It follows from the myth of mental illness as just a different way of seeing the world, but it further suggests that the other way of seeing the world has its own benefits and may even improve on accepted reality. The myth is largely an intellectual construct and almost never takes into account the emotional and social toll that mental illness costs its sufferers.

In recent years, autism has become one of the most commonly dramatized identified mental illnesses in the child and adolescent populations. Hollywood has shown interest in developmental delay disorders, which has paralleled media interest in the disorder. Extending from "Rain Man" (1988), the childhood version of this myth have been shown in "The Wizard" (1989), "Hellbound: Hellraiser II" (1988), "Silent Fall," and "Mercury Rising" (1998). In each of these films, a child with social impairment or mutism has incredible abilities with video games, mimicry, puzzles, or complex codes. The portrayal of the idiot savant is linked with autism, and it is more often the norm than the exception that the on-screen autistic child is extraordinarily gifted rather than impaired.

This myth need not apply simply to autism, however. In "Equus" (1977), Dr. Martin Dysart (played by Richard Burton) becomes entirely preoccupied with his adolescent patient Alan's delusional system. The further he explores, the deeper he delves, the more his own life pales in comparison. Envy is sparked by the passion and love Alan has for horses, a displacement of sexuality in a rigid Christian family. Alan's treatment ignites a crisis of faith for Dysart, who understands Alan's illness as a thing of incredible beauty and psychiatry as the force that must strip that beauty away. "The normal is the good smile in a child's eye. It is also the dead stare in a million adults. It both sustains and kills, like a god. It is the ordinary made beautiful, it is also the average made lethal. Normal is the indispensable murderous god of health, and I am his priest."

In more recent films, such as "The Sixth Sense" and "Donnie Darko" (2001), young men are haunted by hallucinations that turn out to have greater significance than appreciated. Although the character seeks mental health treatment, the treatment team fails to appreciate the visions for what they really are—a gift that has the power to save people's lives.

The positive valence of this myth is that there is a beauty or gift attached to mental illness; mental illness is not simply a curse but also a blessing. It makes the diagnosis somewhat easier to swallow and might even give a sense of pride. On the negative side, linking illness with near-genius skills or beauty can have consequences for parents who seek those qualities in their children or put up an argument against treatment for individuals with disorders.

Myth #5: mental illness and evil overlap in their presentations

A clear example of this myth can be found in the horror classic "The Exorcist" (1973). When Linda Blair's character, Regan, who is in the early stages of possession, is examined by her pediatrician, she undergoes a battery of neurologic and medical studies. In the end, the pediatrician diagnoses "a disorder of the nerves, at least I think it is. We don't know yet exactly how it works. It is often seen in early adolescence. She shows all the symptoms: hyperactivity, quick temper, performance in math...it affects your concentration. Now this is for Ritalin, ten milligrams a day." Although in the film canon the number of depictions of diagnosed cases of attention deficit disorder is otherwise nil, the most comprehensive depictions of evaluation, diagnosis, and treatment come in the context of demonic possession. As Regan's condition persists, the evaluation extends to include electroencephalography and arteriography, and the diagnosis of temporal lobe epilepsy is posited. After "eighty-eight" doctors evaluate Regan, the diagnosis remains unclear, and long-term psychiatric hospitalization is recommended. When this option is dismissed, the medical professionals suggest exorcism. Neither the clergy nor physicians alone can help Regan; ultimately only a psychiatrist-priest can delineate evil from psychosis and provide definitive treatment.

Although not starring an adolescent, the recent film "Gothika" (2003) seems to have had a significant impact on teenagers, largely because of the film's star, Halle Berry. In this film, Berry plays a forensic psychiatrist who is hospitalized on her own unit after she kills her psychiatrist husband. The irony of her situation is dramatized with gusto until it is shown that she committed the murder only while possessed by a murder victim. Once again, possession by an angry spirit is what is responsible for a diagnosed psychiatric condition, not brain chemistry.

If not evil, the psychiatric patient is often violent and antisocial. The link between violence and adult mental illness has been deeply ingrained by the likes of Hannibal Lecter and Norman Bates, but with adolescents these depictions are no less frequent, as shown in "Heavenly Creatures" (1994), "Disturbing Behavior" (1998), and "Don't Say a Word." The equation of violence with mental illness has been one of the more difficult public perceptions to overcome and remains the largest obstacle to mental illness advocacy.

In their study of 34 animated Disney movies, Lawson and Fouts [10] found that 85% of those films contained references to being mentally ill. Most of these characters "serve as objects of derision, fear, or amusement." Just as Snow White and Cinderella are embedded in the collective cultural consciousness, the authors suggested that "children watching could associate mental illness labels with people who are so frightening and dangerous that they must be chained and locked away from the rest of society." The message that mental illness is something to be feared is taught early and altogether too often by Hollywood.

Discussion

To the parents of children who are symptomatic, parents who might consider mental health evaluation for their children, and the public at large whose opinions influence policy and acceptance, Hollywood gives various strong—but confusing—messages about what mental health treatment involves. It feeds hopes that parents' children might be otherwise gifted, but it also feeds fears that parents are to blame, that psychiatrists will usurp their parental role, and that the profession itself is a sham. To the adolescents and children who might enter treatment and must reflect on their illness and their ongoing care, Hollywood's myths can have significant impact and spark concern about being controlled or functionally castrated by adults through restraint, archaic hospitalization, and sedation. Adolescents and children are more likely to encounter psychiatrists in horror movies than in other film genres geared toward the child and adolescent populations, and they are less likely to seek out films in the dramatic genre that have more well-rounded portrayals.

As depicted in the clinical examples, these myths affect the cornerstones of successful mental health treatment, including therapeutic alliance, medication adherence, perception of illness, and self-esteem. In conclusion, the authors provide several ways in which they have found films to be of positive therapeutic benefit, as long as these distortions are understood and used to the advantage of a patient's clinical care.

Have open discussions about movies, especially when resistance is an issue in treatment

Children and adolescents have difficulty describing feelings or thoughts in a direct way and frequently externalize them. Movies can be helpful to treatment when used as an intermediary in that discussion. On an inpatient unit, an adolescent girl's group therapy session was sluggish and the girls were largely disengaged until a discussion of "One Flew Over the Cuckoo's Nest" was raised. Feelings of fear and anger were accessed easily, and talk about the movie overlapped with a discussion about the unit's unlocked doors and the girls' distrust of staff. This technique can be successful when a movie becomes a way to access a prepackaged fantasy life, but it also can become dysfunctional when movies become an obstacle for more topical matter.

By asking a patient, "Have you seen any movies with psychiatrists?" a clinician can respond, "Well, if I remember, in that movie the psychiatrist is...." Similarly, one might ask "Have you seen any movies with children who see psychiatrists"? With a sufficient vocabulary and database of these films, a clinician can respond, "Isn't that the one in which the psychiatrist locks up the kids?" or "That child was quite sick; I don't think that's what you have at all." In this way, acknowledging the fears and hopes depicted in onscreen psychiatric treatment can be a springboard for discussion. Discussion can help to acknowledge the myriad anxieties a patient or parent feels and can facilitate a stronger engagement in treatment [11].

Recommend positive depictions of psychiatric treatment

Hollywood does nothing if not select for the dramatic. One way to combat the dramatic negative portrayals is to recommend the dramatic more positive ones. In this way, Hollywood showmanship can be used to clinical advantage. Although they are rarer, there are some positive treatment depictions that have fewer boundary violations and present a more three-dimensional psychiatrist than average. "Ordinary People," "Good Will Hunting," and "Antwone Fisher" are examples of supportive male treaters. Vanessa Redgrave's role as head psychiatrist and Whoopi Goldberg's role as charge nurse in "Girl, Interrupted" are positive depictions, although their success is more modest and murky by the end of the film. The benefit of these films is that the drama comes not with violence or self-injury but from a "eureka" moment when the character makes a breakthrough and heals. These films can create unrealistic expectations of treater and time course, which should be addressed openly, but they also can help model process and treatment outcomes.

Recommend movies with realistic depictions of psychiatric illness

Many excellent film portrayals of child and adolescent mental illness can be resources for patient and family education. Sondheimer [12] collected a catalog of nearly 100 commercial films to be used in the education of residents and medical students. Included in his list are examples of childhood mental illness and some films that simply show teenagers struggling with the developmental tasks of adolescence. It is a list recommended by the authors as a resource for clinicians who are looking for visual stimuli to educate and promote discussion with patients and their families.

The goal in selecting a film for viewing should be considered deliberately by the clinician. Some films can help bolster self-esteem in part by using the star power of the actor or actress to equate to a particular condition. As described with Angelina Jolie, when a movie star is depicted with a psychiatric condition, it can be empowering and can change perceptions about the acceptability of a diagnosis or treatment. Unfortunately, the value of any given film in this manner is time-limited because of the draw of a particular star to a particular viewer at a given time.

Another option involves using films that de-sensationalize treatment and disorders, especially in situations in which the patient or family is miseducated about a disorder. Special care should be taken to recommend films that portray dangerous behavior by the patient or films that could deflate a patient's hopes of improvement. A good intervention involves using short clips from films to illustrate certain circumscribed symptoms, behaviors, or issues and minimizing any extraneous material. The ideal intervention involves the clinician viewing the film clip together with the patient or family and discussing positive and negative aspects of the depiction. In this way, the clinician communicates wanting to share, listen, teach, and help in one intervention and is able to promote positive aspects and address the multitude of negative aspects.

References

[1] Wahl OF, Lefkowits JY. Impact of a television film on attitudes toward mental illness. Am J Community Psychol 1989;17(4):521–8.
[2] Pirkis J, Blood RW. Suicide and the media, Part II. Portrayal in fictional media. Crisis 2001; 22(4):155–62.
[3] Hyler SE. DSM-III at the cinema: madness in the movies. Compr Psychiatry 1988;29(2): 195–206.
[4] Hyler SE, Gabbard GO, Schneider I. Homicidal maniacs and narcissistic parasites: stigmatization of mentally ill persons in the movies. Hosp Community Psychiatry 1991;42(10):1044–8.
[5] Rabkin LY. The celluloid couch. Lanham (MD): Scarecrow Press; 1998.
[6] Flores G. Mad scientists, compassionate healers, and greedy egotists: the portrayal of physicians in the movies. J Natl Med Assoc 2002;94(7):635–58.
[7] Schneider I. The theory and practice of movie psychiatry. Am J Psychiatry 1987;144(8): 996–1002.
[8] Gabbard GO, Gabbard K. Psychiatry and the cinema. Washington (DC): American Psychiatric Association; 1999.
[9] Corrigan P. How stigma interferes with mental health care. Am Psychol 2004;59(7):614–25.
[10] Lawson A, Fouts G. Mental illness in Disney animated films. Can J Psychiatry 2004;49(5): 310–4.
[11] Hyler SE, Schanzer B. Using commercially available films to teach about borderline personality disorder. Bull Menninger Clin 1997;61(4):458–68.
[12] Sondheimer A. The life stories of children and adolescents. Acad Psychiatry 2000;24:214–24.

ELSEVIER
SAUNDERS

Child Adolesc Psychiatric Clin N Am
14 (2005) 523–553

CHILD AND
ADOLESCENT
PSYCHIATRIC CLINICS
OF NORTH AMERICA

Media Literacy for Clinicians and Parents

V. Susan Villani, MD[a,*], Cheryl K. Olson, SD[b,c], Michael S. Jellinek, MD[d]

[a]Department of Psychiatry, Johns Hopkins School of Medicine, Kennedy Krieger Institute,
1750 East Fairmount Avenue, Baltimore, MD 21231, USA
[b]Harvard Medical School Center for Mental Health and Media, Department of Psychiatry,
Massachusetts General Hospital, 271 Waverley Oaks Road, Suite 204, Waltham, MA 02452, USA
[c]Department of Psychiatry, Harvard Medical School, Boston, MA, USA
[d]Department of Psychiatry, Massachusetts General Hospital, 55 Fruit Street, Boston, MA 02114, USA

The growth of technology over the past decades has created an environment rich in media opportunities for children and adults. From the first popular radio broadcasts in the 1920s through the widespread use of the Internet in the 1990s, electronic media clearly have been established as a dominant global influence. During this time, clinicians and researchers have sought to examine the impact of various types of media on children and adolescents. The research results have been scrutinized and debated heavily by the professional community, manufacturers and creators of media, government agencies charged with protecting children, and parents. Research in the field is complex; studies often attempt to imitate media exposure, but not in the context of a child's life that includes a long list of individual, developmental, family, cultural, and economic variables.

The field of media literacy has emerged and is defined as the ability to access, analyze, and evaluate media content [1]. Clinicians have struggled with how to integrate media literacy into clinical practice, and parents are torn between supporting the autonomy and learning opportunities electronic media make possible, and protecting their children from harmful influences. They need to know how to integrate research findings and expert opinion into the everyday world of parenting.

This article discusses media literacy for clinicians and parents through four lenses: (1) the interaction between tasks of development and media exposure,

---

* Corresponding author. Kennedy Krieger Institute, School Programs, 1750 East Fairmount Avenue, Baltimore, MD 21231.
 E-mail address: villani@kennedykrieger.org (V.S. Villani).

1056-4993/05/$ – see front matter © 2005 Elsevier Inc. All rights reserved.
doi:10.1016/j.chc.2005.03.001
childpsych.theclinics.com

(2) the "socialization" of media through the family, (3) special clinical circumstances and potential therapeutic uses of media, and (4) electronic media rating systems, monitoring and blocking devices, and guidelines from professional organizations.

The interaction between tasks of development and media

How young children perceive and use media

A basic understanding of developmental tasks at various ages helps to frame the debate about the use of media in a child's life. It is also important to note that aside from interactive games and some experimental television programs, electronic media provide one-way visual or auditory input. The reaction of a child who is watching or listening has no effect on what comes next, so cause and effect is passively learned through observation. Although many experts have suggested that the media merely provide entertainment, it is clear that they teach through repetition, with the ability to shape values and influence language and behavior. This passivity and potential receptivity are important underlying principles that should be borne in mind at each stage of child development.

Infancy through toddlerhood

During infancy (0–6 months), the primary tasks are adjusting to the world outside the womb, eating and sleeping to facilitate growth, and the beginning social interaction through smiling, cooing, and reaching for people and objects. Physical touch is essential, with soft cuddling and comforting important to the actual facilitation of eating and growth. Input to the brain as it is wiring itself and continuing to grow is crucial; it is highly likely that these early touch points with the environment influence neuronal pathways. The human voice and soft music are known to soothe and stimulate interaction, whereas loud voices and noises produce full-body startle response, interfere with an infant's ability to eat, and raise stress hormone levels. The media—especially music—may have a role in soothing and calming; parents naturally sing to their babies to quiet and comfort them.

From 6 months to 1 year, infants continue to grow and interact with others. Exploration of the world around them through touch and feel is essential. Language starts through reciprocal interactions, and children begin to understand cause and effect. All of these tasks require an interactive process. The nonreciprocal way in which the media operate does not provide the feedback loop necessary for children at this age. Infants need to explore through their senses, get feedback that is immediate, and then repeat these interactions over and over to learn from them. It is highly likely that at this early age cognitive and emotional learning are synergistic, that learning to pick up and eat "finger food' is developmentally optimized if the activity takes place with a warm, encouraging adult rather than in front of a television screen that presents images and words unrelated to an infant's behavior or feelings.

Aside from music, the best use of electronic media at this stage may be none at all. The American Academy of Pediatrics (AAP) discourages television watching for children under age 2 and encourages adult-child interaction (eg, talking, singing, or reading together) that promotes healthy brain development [2]. Surveys of parents suggest that many infants and toddlers spend time in front of the television, however [3]. A survey by the Kaiser Family Foundation found that 39% of children under age 4 live in homes in which a television is on all or most of the time, even if no one is watching [4]. (In the case of infants, it is difficult to know how "watching" is defined, because they do not seem to attend to television for more than brief periods.) The effects of television exposure may vary based on a child's temperament.

Moving on to children aged 1 to 2 years, the development of motor skills and language with purpose continues. Children begin to scribble, throw a ball, feed themselves, walk, and run. Media can play a role in teaching language; studies have found that television programs that promote language (as when characters "talk to" the viewing child and encourage responses or label objects) [5] and music have a role soothing. Visual images are fascinating, yet the ability to understand them is not developed and needs adult explanation. The ability to learn from a video image is limited [6]. Optimal learning at this stage depends on interaction with someone who is able to modify his or her response continuously and adjust to what a child has done and how a child is feeling (eg, frustrated, eager, tired, anxious). This interaction allows toddlers to figure things out in small incremental ways and build a step at a time in knowledge and self-esteem at their own pace. Television, even if played in the background, may disrupt this interaction and play with parents [6]. Because toddlers will be surrounded by and using television and computer screens throughout childhood and adulthood, however, too much emphasis on "protecting" them from media arguably could be counterproductive.

Preschool years

As exploration continues from age 2 to 5 years, children are moving more into the world of socializing with others through play. The play skills of sharing, taking turns, and following simple rules begin to emerge. Many skills acquired gradually over these 3 to 4 years are actually school readiness skills. Some media content is specifically geared toward promoting school readiness, primarily public television shows such as "Sesame Street," "Reading Rainbow," and "Between the Lions" and some newer commercial cable television programs with restricted advertising breaks, such as "Blue's Clues" and "Dora the Explorer." They often combine developmentally appropriate cognitive challenges, pacing, and repetition with characters that have feelings and values [6–8]. Many commercial network programs, however, are not geared to children's developmental stage and emphasize sales of program-related toys. Frequent viewing of such programs can hinder later academic performance [9]. The accompanying commercial advertisements for food, toys, and games also may be detrimental. Children at that age see little difference between program and commercial content and do not understand the persuasive intent of advertising [10]. The consumer-oriented push of enticing food ads requires close adult monitoring, lest a child be trained early in life to sit and eat. Increased hours of watching television and the presence of television in a child's bedroom contribute to preschoolers' increasing risk of being overweight [11]. This trend is especially concerning because of children's increasingly sedentary lifestyle at home and school and greater access to fast food and junk food.

At this stage, television, movies, and videos are the primary sources of media content, although computers and computer games come into play as children develop the necessary motor skills to manipulate input through a mouse, buttons, or a joystick-like implement. A child may sit on a parent's lap and play with the computer at age 2.5 and start pointing and clicking with a mouse at age 3.5 [12]. Currently, systems are being marketed for preschoolers that mimic video game consoles (eg., the VSmile by VTech) and hand-held game systems (eg, Leapster by LeapFrog) and have larger and simpler controls. As with television, effects of interactive media on cognitive development seem related to the appropriateness of software and parent involvement [13].

Although interactive games have greater capacity to teach cause and effect, they may limit fantasy play within the structure of the software rather than being derived from or related to a child's own life. Children benefit in their social and emotional growth when their own experiences and feelings can be acted out with creative materials. Dress-up, pretend worlds created with toys, drawings, paintings, and clay and cardboard creations are but a few examples of how play promotes self-expression at this stage. Although research is limited, a study of kindergarten children found that when played cooperatively, video games could enhance social skills [14].

One concern about children's media consumption is that children aged 8 and younger typically cannot reliably tell fantasy from reality and cannot comprehend complex motives and intentions. Researchers who study advertising have demonstrated that children younger than age 8 are perceptually dependent and focus more on how something looks than what is said about it [15,16]. If the visuals of a game contradict the semantic meaning, young children attend to the visuals. It becomes difficult for media literacy information to counteract the messages children get at this age through visual stimuli.

Studies by Cantor [17,18] have shown how children at this age become fearful upon seeing images that they think are real. Whereas the research demonstrated transitory fright responses, a small proportion of viewers had more debilitating reactions. Cantor's research of first, fourth, seventh, and eleventh graders regarding their reactions to televised coverage of the Persian Gulf War showed how children at different ages were upset by different aspects, with younger children being more upset by the visual images and older children being upset by the more abstract conceptual aspects [19].

Although these results are of concern, we also know from daily experience that children have a growing sense of what is real and what is not from an early age. When parents read fairy tales at bedtime, although there may be transient fright, few children suffer long-term harm or attempt the stunts related in the story. Few children have jumped out of windows to mimic Superman, Super Grover, or Spiderman. In our clinical experience, children who have taken serious risks come from chaotic and often abusive or neglectful homes. They know reality and try to escape it. Research cannot capture easily the interplay between a developing child and the thousands of increasing complex and confusing images they see through television, video games, computer animation, and movies, some of which are exciting, fun, or brutally realistic live coverage of a horrific event.

How school-aged children and adolescents perceive and use media

A national survey of children's media use found that children aged 8 to 13 spend more time with media than any other age group [20]. Children rapidly acquire new information during the early school age years with an accompanying understanding of time and motion and greater understanding of cause and effect. During this time, they move from concrete thinking and the world of fantasy to abstract thinking and the ability to understand more complex thought. They develop a greater ability to learn from electronic media. There are also gains in academic and social skills, membership in peer groups, and development of important friendships. Entertainment media begin to shape children's understanding of social relationships and expectations about behavior and appearance, but the learning is limited because it does not occur through children's personal interactions. There is also wide variability from child to child as to how they process information, particularly at the early phase of this stage from age 6 to 10, before the development of abstract thinking. Rather than attempt to summarize the body of research that addresses media influences on the development of older children and adolescents, this article focuses on areas of particular concern to parents and mental health professionals: the effects of violent and sexual content and the relatively new medium of video games.

Potential effects of media violence

One concern at this stage is how exposure to media violence may affect attitudes and later aggressive and violent behavior. A recent comprehensive study of broadcast and cable television—the National Television Violence Study 3 [21]—found that during a typical week, 61% of programs contained some violence. The most violence was found on premium cable channels, particularly in movies. As with earlier National Television Violence studies, the consortium of researchers agreed that exposure to violence had the potential to affect children adversely and that the risk of learning aggressive behavior increased when (1) the perpetrator was attractive, (2) the violence was seen as justified, (3) the violence was seen as realistic and involved a real-life weapon, (4) the violence was rewarded, or at least not punished, (5) the violence had little or no harmful consequences, or (6) the violence was seen as funny. (For children younger than age 7, most exposure to high-risk portrayals of violence came from cartoon programs.) Other research suggested that even portrayals of indirect aggression (eg, spreading rumors or secretly destroying someone's property) can inspire imitation [22]. Another concern is that exposure to violent content may increase fear of being victimized (particularly graphic, realistic, unjustified, or rewarded violence against appealing characters). Extensive graphic violence and humorous violence are believed to desensitize children to violence [21].

In the National Television Violence studies, violence was defined as "any overt depiction of credible threat of physical force or the actual use of such force intended to physically harm an animate being or group of beings." This category also included physically harmful consequences that resulted from unseen violent means. One difficulty in interpreting media violence research involves differences in how content is defined as violent and measures of exposure to violent content. This difficulty can be seen in two longitudinal studies of television violence. Johnson et al [23] followed children for 17 years and found that watching 3 or more hours a day of television at age 14 was associated positively with fights, assaults, and other aggressive acts at age 16 and 22. In a 15-year study by Huesmann et al [24], watching violent programs, professing belief in realism of content, and identifying with same-sex aggressive characters at ages 6 to 9 predicted young adult aggressive behavior.

The study by Johnson et al compared effects of watching 3 or more hours of television per day versus watching 1 hour or less per day. The content of programming was not assessed, based on the assumption that more television watched meant greater exposure to violence. The study by Huesmann et al did not measure directly the amount of exposure to either television or violent content. Instead, researchers presented children with an annual series of eight lists, each of which named ten programs, and asked them to mark their favorite on each list. Children also were asked whether they watched that show "every time it's on," "a lot, but not always," or "once in a while." These results were interpreted based on researcher rankings of these shows on a five-point scale that represented the amount of violence portrayed. (Examples of "very violent" shows included "The Six Million Dollar Man" and "Roadrunner" cartoons.) Belief in realism and identification were assessed by asking children whether selected violent live and cartoon shows were true in "telling what life is really like" and asking children how much they "acted like or did things like" specific characters.

Effects of video and computer games

Several recent studies have focused on the effects of violent content in video games. The availability and use of interactive games has increased dramatically over the past decade. Surveys suggest that boys spend an average of 30 minutes to 1 hour a day playing video games, with girls playing significantly less often [25,26]. (Of note, the appearance of games with greater appeal to girls, such as "The Sims" and "Dance Dance Revolution," may be closing this gap.)

At their worst, video and computer games allow children to sit in isolation for many hours immersed in a world of explicit sexual and violent aggression. Some experimental studies and surveys have found that exposure to game violence is linked with greater aggression, poor school grades, or desensitization to violence [25,27]. Other studies have found that a preference for violent games was linked to reduced aggression or that longer playing times were linked to less aggression than short playing times [28,29]. Several factors, including cultural differences and developmental stage of subjects, may partially account for these differences.

Popular press reports have linked violent games (along with fighting and gore in other media) to extreme acts or an epidemic level of violence [30]. It is worth noting, however, that in the period between 1994 and 2001—a time of extraordinary media growth and heightened concern about violence in the media— the rate of juvenile arrests for violent crimes fell 44%, to the lowest level since 1983. In terms of property crimes, the rate in 2001 was the lowest level in more than 30 years [31–34]. Media violence also is rarely put into context with other factors known to contribute to violence, such as abusive or antisocial parents, family poverty, and substance abuse [30].

As with television violence, varying definitions and measures of violent content and aggression make interpretation of research difficult. Because these are correlational studies, the direction of causality is also unknown [25,30]. Aggressive or hostile youths may be drawn to violent games, which might increase or decrease acting out for an individual student. Students who fare poorly in school may turn to games as a way to demonstrate competence. Until more evidence is available, it seems wise for parents to monitor the content of games, television, and movies and limit hours of use.

Some studies have examined the effects of interactive games on other aspects of children's development. Depending on the content, interactive games may promote the development of cognitive skills, such as spatial representation, interpreting diagrams (iconic skills), and visual attention [35]. Studies of how interactive games may promote or limit social development and friendships have had mixed results, perhaps related to variation in measures. This area needs further study [28].

Potential effects of media on self-image and sexuality

Exposure to unrealistic and often unhealthy body ideals from television, movies, and magazines affects children's self-image, aspirations about appearance, and efforts to control weight. A large prospective study of children aged 9 to 14 found that making efforts to look like same-sex media images predicted the development of weight concerns and constant dieting in girls and boys [36].

The movement through adolescence is characterized largely by the emergence of sexuality and the search for identity. There is increased independence from the family and more focus on the social group and the culture. Experimentation emerges and is paired with a belief in indestructibility. With these issues in mind, the widespread sexuality and portrayal of high-risk behaviors on television, in the movies, in music videos, and in video games—although appealing to the basic instincts and drives of teenagers—are also potentially overstimulating and encourage dangerous behaviors. A Kaiser Family Foundation study [37] found that 64% of television programs in 2001/2002 included some sexual content. Those programs averaged 4.4 scenes involving sex per hour. A related survey found that 72% of teens aged 15 to 17 think that such content influences sexual behaviors of teens "somewhat" or "a lot" [38].

In a 1987 in-home survey of 2760 14- to 16-year-old youths [39], the amount of exposure to radio, music videos, movies, and favorite type of music (eg, heavy metal) was associated with greater participation in eight potentially risky behaviors—sexual intercourse, drinking, smoking cigarettes, smoking marijuana, cheating, stealing, cutting class, and driving a car without permission—regardless of parental education level. A recent national longitudinal survey of 12- to 17-year-old youths found that watching programs with greater sexual content (ie, discussion or portrayal) predicted initiating intercourse and progressing to more advanced noncoital activities, even when controlling for other factors associated with earlier sex [40]. Among African-American youths in the sample, exposure to content that addressed sexual risks or safety reduced the odds of initiating intercourse or increasing noncoital activities. Sexual activity was not related to average number of hours of television exposure, which reinforced the importance of how sexual activity and its consequences are portrayed. (See the article by Collins elsewhere in this issue.) As with violence, it is important to put concerns about media influence on risky sexual behaviors into context. According to National Youth Risk Behavior Survey data from 1991 to 2003 [40a], fewer high school students are initiating sexual intercourse; those who are sexually active have had fewer sex partners.

Another 1-year follow-up study, which focused on African-American girls aged 14 to 18, found that hours of watching rap music videos were associated positively with several unhealthy behaviors, including having multiple sexual partners, getting in trouble with the law, using drugs or alcohol, and becoming infected with a sexually transmitted disease [41]. Viewing rap videos also was associated with less parental monitoring and unemployment, but the relationship held even when controlling for these covariates. Many other factors may contribute to or mediate these behaviors, such as poverty, exposure to violence in the home, quality of parenting, and quality of schools. We also do not know if individuals who chose to watch more rap videos would have exhibited the same dysfunctional behaviors regardless of media exposure.

Other health risk behaviors are also affected by mass media. A longitudinal study of children aged 10 to 15 found a dose-response relationship between hours of television watching and initiation of smoking [42]. Youths who watched 5 or more hours per day were six times more likely to start smoking than individuals who watched less than 2 hours, even after controlling for some other risk factors.

The role of temperament and traits

All development occurs on the substrate of inborn temperament and traits. As established by Thomas et al [43], children come into this world with styles and traits that are persistent throughout childhood into adulthood. Some babies are easier to manage and learn self-regulation more quickly. Other babies become easily overwhelmed, overreact to stimuli, and require a longer time to be soothed. As infants grow into toddlers, their characteristics of shyness, natural curiosity and ready exploration, and even aggressiveness become more apparent. The effect of watching a scary movie on a shy 3-year-old child or shy 7-year-old child might be different from the effect on a 3-year-old child who already exhibits aggressive tendencies or a 7-year-old child who is known for her daring behavior.

Media researchers have tried to take traits into account, particularly in the area of aggression and violence. Measures of trait hostility and aggression are used to determine if there is a differential effect. Some studies have found greater effects of violent content in video games for subjects high in trait hostility; others have not. More studies are needed to see how children's traits or temperament might moderate media effects [44]. Children with trait hostility and aggression may be drawn to more violent activities, whether they be contact sports (eg, football or wrestling), more aggressive school yard play, or more violent media. It is unclear whether playing football or a violent video game reinforces aggressive behavior for some children or provides a "release" of hostility that is socially acceptable for others. Research data that describe risk factors for groups of children do not take into account individual variability, parental interactions, and a host of other factors that should be a part of parents' daily decision making.

Discussion

Although this is not a comprehensive discussion of the interaction between media and the tasks of development, it highlights how the issues vary at different ages. Media literacy efforts must take into account the age of children and their developmental levels. It is clear that electronic media have the power to teach; it is a matter of what the programs and ads are teaching, the effects of these messages in the context of children's lives, and whether time spent with media unduly limits the necessary time for hands-on learning, first through play and later through age-appropriate social interactions. The reasonable balance between the passivity of television, interaction with electronic games, use of the Internet, one-to-one peer activities, group activities, and family time probably varies with every child based on age, personality, temperament, social or environmental factors, and more.

Family context and media

American children are growing up surrounded by media. At the end of the twentieth century, the typical child had three televisions, a video game console, a computer, and multiple VCRs/CD players in the home [20]. The rapid changes in media access are taking place within a family unit and culture that are also rapidly evolving. For example, because of divorce and remarriage, death of a parent, out-of-wedlock births, foster care, and imprisonment, fewer children are raised from birth to 18 in a traditional, two-parent nuclear family. (During 2003, 68% of children under 18 were living with two married parents, down from 77% in 1980 [45].) The number of children in day care and the number of hours children spend in care per week have increased, in parallel with the number of families with mothers who want to or have to work. (It is estimated that 41% of children younger than age 5 with employed mothers spend 35 or more hours per week in nonparental care [46].) Media literacy, the rapid evolution of media, and efforts to assess the impact of media are all happening quickly within a context of unstable family life and a society that in many of its actions does not value children.

It is difficult for children to avoid the influence of mass media. They face peer expectations to keep up with the most recent sports story, the hottest music video, and related fashion trends. School assignments encourage them to search the Internet. Many children own a portable music player that allows downloading of popular songs. Friends discuss the latest television event before the school day starts. Children play video-simulated sports against each other or join a worldwide game on the Internet.

What are reasonable family policies regarding the media? Parents may be tempted to shout, "Stop! I do not want my children exposed to all of these sights and sounds streaming into my home. I do not want their development harassed or hurried by media." Even if one could be successful in exerting the control necessary to limit media exposure, however, would that approach optimize a child's development? Appropriately limiting autonomy and peer relationships is good parenting when confronting substance use, gang behavior, or delinquency or protecting a younger child from a friend's irresponsible parents or peer who is a bully or demeaning. How great must the danger be to rationalize limiting children's developmental trajectory toward autonomy and the free flow of information among peers—preparation for the next stage of life, high school, and college?

It is also tempting to say, "The horse is out of the barn. I have no control and they are going to see it and hear it no matter what. I want my child to have friends and not be 'out of it.' I want my child to like me. And who has the time for all this monitoring? So, go to R-rated movies and watch MTV…I've got my own life to lead." Parents can feel caught in the dilemma of over-controlling their children's lives or surrendering control to the prevailing winds of our culture. Ultimately, parents must decide what is best for their children based on knowledge of each particular child's strengths, weaknesses, or vulnerabilities and the context of their chosen family values.

Family approaches and rules concerning media literacy and exposure should be consistent with what parents do to encourage autonomy in the many other areas of a child's life. Parents assess children's readiness, strengths, and weaknesses, determine the risk associated with the developmental step, prepare children, provide guidance, set rules or boundaries, cope with their own anxiety, and then launch the next step. For example, is a child ready to walk to school on his or her own? Can the child find the way? Should he or she go with a friend? Does the child understand the risk of going off the path or talking to a stranger? Can he or she follow traffic safety rules? Reckless or impulsive children may not be ready and must be older to safely accept this autonomy, whereas anxious yet competent children may benefit from encouragement to be among the first in the class to achieve this landmark. For most middle-class children in the United States, it certainly would be "safer" to wait and maybe never allow a child to walk to school (or be among the last in a class). If a child is ready, however, many parents would take the risk; the act of walking away is a metaphor for growing up, being trustworthy, and ultimately gaining self-esteem. Thousands of these little gains form the basis of productive adulthood and generative parenting.

The same process of gradual movement toward autonomy, guided by parental involvement, applies to media decisions. Children benefit, given our culture and being at the appropriate developmental step, from some decision-making authority about what they watch on television, what they do to "relax," how they balance leisure time with homework, what video games they play, and how they use the Internet. Parents who live in a safe neighborhood let a 6-year-old child walk to school after initially walking with him but do not let a child go downtown on a public bus. Similarly at this age, a child would be allowed to go to G-rated or maybe PG movies but not PG-13 or R-rated movies. Parents set a range of acceptable options and let children make some choices, the boundaries being set by the advantages of building autonomy and the risks of choices. In addition to limiting rental or purchase of materials, new technologies are available to help parents block some media content or restrict time spent with media. (See the description at the end of this article.)

The pervasive presence of violence or sexually inappropriate content in media unfortunately has created a general negative tone regarding its influence on children and family life. As researchers try to help parents manage the potential risks of excessive and unsupervised media use, the positive ways that media can be used within the family are often neglected. Television can bring family members together for shared recreation and as a trigger for relevant discussions. On the recreational side, cheering on a favorite sports team or just spending time together is special and creates important shared memories. In terms of building character, rooting for a team that does not often win but continues to play hard and embodies local pride can teach patience, anger management, and tolerance. On a more serious note, television can provide many hours of enjoyable time through educational shows, especially shows on history, science, hobbies, or current issues relevant to families. Watching entertainment programs as a family can have unexpected benefits.

For example, it can be fun to watch a pop culture show such as "American Idol" with a teenager and compare ratings of the contestants. This is also an opportunity to discuss unrealistic expectations, overdependence on other people's opinions or adoration, and coping with defeat. Discussion of the songs can lead to an appreciation of music favored by the younger or older generation that would not otherwise have been heard. Similarly, watching family dramas such as "American Dreams" can lead to an Internet search about the Vietnam War, the civil rights movement, and meaningful discussions of substance use, racism, premature and premarital sexuality, abortion, over- and under-controlling parents, grief, anger, and forgiveness. In a recent national survey, one in three teens aged 15 to 17 reported that television content had triggered a discussion about a sexual issue with a parent [38].

Just as they learn the alphabet or English grammar, children in the elementary grades can start to understand the technical and content aspects of television and movies [47]. The technical side includes the electronic workings of televisions as explained through interesting books, programs, and websites, such as "The Way Things Work" series, and the commercial aspect of television, including how programs are paid for by companies selling their products. Children also can learn about the different types of programs (eg, comedies, dramas, news, documentaries) and how to tell the "real" from the pretend. Finally, parents can describe the technical aspects of producing a program, from casting actors and making costumes and sets to camera angles and special effects. Parents can search for television programs and websites (including "Nova" on PBS) that explore topics such as these.

As children get older, they are more able to understand subtler aspects of program content, such as plots, themes, and historical or geographical setting and how these aspects combine with technical elements to affect how the program makes us feel. They also can explore motivations for characters' behaviors (from interpersonal relationships to substance use) and aspects of their appearance (eg, clothing or weight) and identify common—perhaps harmful—stereotypes (eg, the portrayal of grandparents, scientists, or "crazy people").

These types of questions can form the underpinnings of discussions with older children as you watch television programs or commercials together [48]:

- Who created this message and why are they sending it? Who owns and profits from it?
- What techniques are used to attract and hold attention?
- What lifestyles, values, and points of view are represented in this message?
- What is omitted from this message? Why was it left out?
- How might different people interpret this message?

With older teens, watching a program such as the F/X channel's "Nip/Tuck," a graphic and intense drama that deals with the personal lives of two plastic surgeons and their patients, creates an opportunity to discuss unrealistic expectations and desperation, promiscuity, dread about aging, and complex marital issues such as infidelity and damaging secrets. Although the scenes may be uncomfortable to watch with a teenager, it is likely that these same scenes will be watched with peers in their homes or at the movies with no adult available to help put the behaviors and feelings in context. Discussion of these topics without the show as a substrate or facilitator would be difficult at best and unlikely to occur at all.

Beyond television, experience with the Internet also can be positive. Use of the computer, access to the Web, "instant messaging," and games are all relevant to our culture, education, fun, and peer interaction. Although there is the real worry that X-rated material or a "stranger" lurking on the Web creates danger, when one weighs this potential risk against the gains of autonomy, access to information, and communicating with a group of friends, the benefits greatly exceed the risk, provided that parents have assessed the degree of autonomy their child is ready to manage and have discussed the dos and don'ts of online behavior.

GetNetWise, a website supported by a coalition of industry and advocacy groups, has an online safety guide that provides advice tailored to children's ages and likely activities (including chat, email, instant messaging, and newsgroups) [49]. For example, as preteens begin to master abstract thinking and are able to explore more content on their own, it is important to talk about the credibility of Web content and how to determine the quality or biases of what they find. This site also has links to sample "rules of the road" contracts that parents and children can review and agree to—from never giving out a full name, location, or password to alerting adults to messages that use bad language or seem threatening. (See later discussion for technologies that parents can use to limit Internet time or access.) The Federal Trade Commission also has helpful information for children, parents, and teachers [50].

These media risks are happening in the home, where there are opportunities to listen, observe (gently and at a distance), explain, and reassess. The key to media literacy is ongoing parental involvement that is geared to children's developmental levels, with gradual movement toward more autonomy as children mature.

Special clinical circumstances

Because of the focus on the potential negative effects of media, the special clinical circumstances in which media can serve a specific therapeutic role for a child and family are often neglected. Electronic media can be used as creative tools to address important issues, such as the capacity for play and relaxation, the development of self-esteem, and the development of peer relationships.

The striving family

Some families are on overdrive in terms of work, daily schedules, expectations, and achievement orientation. Any time focused on an activity, either individual or group, has to be productive or a step to a more evolved "useful" activity. Even fun is defined as a lesson or practice that is part of making progress. These families resist any "downtime" or "senseless fun." Often children in these families, if given a bit of permission, readily wish for or identify media opportunities through television, Internet, video games, or movies to take time off or feel more in tune with peers. These children state that their parents would never allow them to watch a desired television show or watch with them. Such parents assume a kind of elite status in their blanket condemnation of virtually all media.

These circumstances may call for a family prescription that mandates a regular hour of senseless fun watching a sitcom or drama to encourage a slight change in expectation or intensity of the striving. Sometimes families reject this single hour as the beginning of a moral decline, whereas others have discovered a show or a video game that has had a positive effect. (It is often an added benefit to have children tutor parents in a video game that reverses the common pattern in the striving family of parents constantly teaching and tutoring children.)

Many striving families are also controlling. In a recent visit to an upper-class urban community, parents were asked how many allow their sixth grade children to have a computer in their room with Internet access. It was stunning that only 3 of nearly 100 families permitted this access, although many had installed screening software. They all wanted their about-to-be teenagers to use the Internet in public view, in a hallway or kitchen, rather than privately. These children were among the most sophisticated and accomplished, were least likely to get into trouble, and lived in a safe community. It is doubtful that these parents really could control Internet access—or that they were as computer literate as their children. They still argued vigorously that this level of control was essential. Will these children ultimately feel better about themselves or be any safer for this scrutiny, or might this oversight have exactly the opposite effect?

Difficulties with peer relations

Some children have difficulties with peer relationships and need some structure to facilitate time with friends. Often this structure can be an activity, such as playing sports, being in band, or joining scouting. Some children do not participate in activities or groups, and media can serve this bridge function. Going to a movie is among the most structured of activities, as is watching television or playing video games. Children who are socially awkward may be masters at certain video games. Inviting a potential friend over for the newest version of a game can feel safe and facilitate a relationship.

Children with attention deficit hyperactivity disorder

Children with attention deficit hyperactivity disorder (ADHD) are frequently particularly devoted to media, including television, video games, and computers. Many of these children find school stressful, demanding, and—even with a customized treatment plan—not supportive of their self-esteem. Coming home from school and immediately starting on homework can be overwhelming. Children with ADHD seem to benefit from an after-school activity, especially a sport, and a little "down time" watching a television show as a transition to homework or as a break. Electronic games and the Internet are forgiving, can be reset, can be turned on and off, and do not criticize. Children are in control of the computer, video game and television, errors are private and reversible, and there is always another chance. Some children with ADHD are adept at video games and computers, which can provide a highly valued source of self-esteem. Research suggests that judicious use of interactive games can enhance social relationships and classroom learning for boys with ADHD [51].

Children with developmental disorders

Children who are developmentally delayed often use media in ways similar to children with ADHD. Television, videos, and computer games can occupy large amounts of time and fill the void of social contact. This population is at risk, however, of having difficulty distinguishing the fantasy world from the real world. In particular, some children mimic what they have seen and heard in the wrong social context and put themselves potentially at risk. An example of this is the young teenager with Asperger's syndrome who watches the Comedy Central show "South Park," then enters school the next day and calls another student a name used in the show. The guiding principles for parents with developmentally delayed children involve being aware of their children's ability to tell fantasy from reality and their tendency to mimic what is seen or heard in socially inappropriate ways. Children who are developmentally delayed may have trouble in these areas into their teenage years and beyond; parents must consider their children's developmental age versus chronologic age when using the age-based media rating systems.

Understanding rating systems, monitoring devices, and guidelines

Rating systems

Rating systems have been designed by each area of the entertainment industry for the ostensible purpose of helping parents to choose age-appropriate media for their children. They have done so in response to pressure from the public through grassroots efforts, from Congress, and from regulatory agencies, such as the Federal Communications Commission and the Federal Trade Commission. Note that in most of the world, government regulation (eg, the Australian Office of Film and Literature Classification) or close cooperation among government, industry, and consumer groups (eg, the new Pan European Game Information age rating system for interactive games) is the norm. This section first presents the ratings systems for television, movies, computer/video games, and music/

recordings. A discussion of the issues that have been debated among professional organizations, parents, and entertainment industry representatives follows.

Television

The "TV Parental Guidelines" were developed in anticipation of V-chip technology, a device mandated by the Telecommunications Act of 1996 to be installed in television sets (of 13 inches or larger) manufactured after January 2000. After the act was passed, entertainment industry executives began to plan a ratings system, which went into effect in 1997 [52]. The V-chip allows parents to program the television set such that shows designated to have violent content are not shown. The ratings are TV-Y (all children), TV-Y7 (directed to older children), TV-Y7-FV (directed to older children-fantasy violence), TV-G (general audience), TV-PG (parental guidance suggested), TV-14 (parents strongly cautioned), and TV-MA (mature audience only; unsuitable for children under 17). Programs in these last three categories also may have letter ratings, such as S for sexual situations, D for suggestive dialog, L for coarse language, and V for violence. Confusingly, the meaning of these letters is not the same for TV-PG, TV-14, or TV-MA; they represent progressively stronger content (Fig. 1).

Movies

The first modern US media ratings system—and the template for the rest—began in 1968 as a joint venture of the Motion Picture Association of America and the National Association of Theater Owners [53]. The Classification and Ratings Administration determines ratings and provides a brief explanation for those films not rated G (e.g., "rated R for violence and language"). The Classification and Ratings Administration rating board has 8 to 13 anonymous paid members; the Motion Picture Association of America president selects the chairman, but it is unclear how other members are selected. Producers or distributors who submit their movies for review pay fees that fund the board. According to the Motion Picture Association of America's website, there are no specific qualifications for board members other than parenting experience and "intelligent maturity." The criteria used to determine various categories are vague and are based on "theme, violence, language, nudity, sensuality, drug abuse and other elements" [54].

The established ratings are as follows: G (general audiences), PG (parental guidance suggested), PG-13 (parents strongly cautioned), R (restricted: under 17 requires accompanying parent or adult guardian), and NC-17 (no one 17 and under admitted) (Fig. 2).

Computer/video games

In response to congressional hearings and proposed legislation, a consortium of game producers founded the Interactive Digital Software Association (currently the Entertainment Software Association) in 1994. In turn, the Interactive Digital Software Association created and funded a self-regulatory body called the Entertainment Software Rating Board (ESRB) [53]. According to

The following categories apply to programs designed for the entire audience.

TV-Y
TVY All Children.
This program is designed to be appropriate for all children. Whether animated or live-action, the themes and elements in this program are specifically designed for a very young audience, including children from ages 2 - 6. This program is not expected to frighten younger children.

TV-Y7
TVY7 Directed to Older Children.
This program is designed for children age 7 and above. It may be more appropriate for children who have acquired the developmental skills needed to distinguish between make-believe and reality. Themes and elements in this program may include mild fantasy violence or comedic violence, or may frighten children under the age of 7. Therefore, parents may wish to consider the suitability of this program for their very young children. Note: For those programs where fantasy violence may be more intense or more combative than other programs in this category, such programs will be designated TV-Y7-FV.

The following categories apply to programs designed for the entire audience.

TV-G
TVG General Audience.
Most parents would find this program suitable for all ages. Although this rating does not signify a program designed specifically for children, most parents may let younger children watch this program unattended. It contains little or no violence, no strong language and little or no sexual dialogue or situations.

TV-PG
TVPG Parental Guidance Suggested.
This program contains material that parents may find unsuitable for younger children. Many parents may want to watch it with their younger children. The theme itself may call for parental guidance and/or the program contains one or more of the following: moderate violence (V), some sexual situations (S), infrequent coarse language (L), or some suggestive dialogue (D).

TV-14
TV14 Parents Strongly Cautioned.
This program contains some material that many parents would find unsuitable for children under 14 years of age. Parents are strongly urged to exercise greater care in monitoring this program and are cautioned against letting children under the age of 14 watch unattended. This program contains one or more of the following: intense violence (V), intense sexual situations (S), strong coarse language (L), or intensely suggestive dialogue (D).

TV-MA
TVMA Mature Audience Only.
This program is specifically designed to be viewed by adults and therefore may be unsuitable for children under 17. This program contains one or more of the following: graphic violence (V), explicit sexual activity (S), or crude indecent language (L).

Fig. 1. Television ratings. Actual TV Parental Guidelines Monitoring Board rating symbols can be viewed at http://www.tvguidelines.org.

the ESRB website, it consists of three (anonymous) trained raters who have no ties to the industry. (An application can be submitted on the ESRB website; prior experience playing games is not required.) Although academics and educators were involved in the founding of the ESRB and its first director was a child psychologist, experts are not currently known to be involved, and the ratings protocol is not made available.

The rating system consists of two components: an age symbol to be placed on the front of the game and a "content descriptor" to be placed beside the age symbol on the back. According to the ESRB, more than 550 publishers have submitted games to be rated, and more than 1000 are rated each year. In 2004,

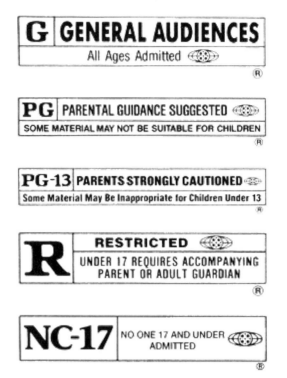

Fig. 2. Voluntary movie rating system. (Courtesy of the Motion Picture Association of America, Encino, CA; with permission.)

54% of the games received an E (everyone), 33% a T (teen), 12% an M (mature), and less than 1% were rated EC (early childhood). (There is also an AO or Adults-Only rating, but this is seldom used.) Sales figures are similar, with 53% of games sold rated E, 30% rated T, and 16% rated M [54a]. Ratings or sales data by content descriptors was not reported (Fig. 3; Box 1).

Music and recordings

In 1985, the Recording Industry Association of America reached an agreement with the National Parent Teacher Association and the Parents' Music Resource Center to place the logo "Parent Advisory" on music that has strong language or graphic references to violence, sex, or substance abuse. The nature of the explicit content is not stated on the label, and the industry does not provide lyrics to parents for review. There are no age-based guidelines, and it is up to individual retailers to decide whether to stock labeled recordings or edited versions, to attempt to restrict sales to minors, or to do nothing to limit minors' access (Fig. 4) [53,55].

Music labeling is a self-regulatory process; individual record companies and their artists decide whether to add the label [53]. According to the Recording Industry Association of America website (http://www.riaa.com), the "Parent Advisory Label lets parents take that responsibility for their families and respects

EC

EARLY CHILDHOOD
Titles rated **EC - Early Childhood** have content that may be suitable for ages 3 and older. Contains no material that parents would find inappropriate.

E

EVERYONE
Titles rated **E - Everyone** have content that may be suitable for persons ages 6 and older. Titles in this category may contain minimal violence, some comic mischief and/or mild language.

T

TEEN
Titles rated **T - Teen** have content that may be suitable for persons ages 13 and older. May contain violent content, mild or strong language, and/or suggestive themes.

M

MATURE
Titles rated **M - Mature** have content that may be suitable for persons ages 17 and older. Titles in this category may contain mature sexual themes, more intense violence and/or strong language.

AO

ADULTS ONLY
Titles rated **AO - Adults Only** have content suitable only for adults. Titles in this category may include graphic depictions of sex and/or violence. Adult Only products are not intended for persons under the age of 18.

RP

RATING PENDING
Titles listed as **RP - Rating Pending** have been submitted to the ESRB and are awaiting final rating.

Fig. 3. Video and computer game ratings. Actual Entertainment Software Rating Board rating symbols can be viewed at http://www.ESRB.org.

the core American value of freedom of expression that tolerates unpopular speech and frowns upon censorship." The Recording Industry Association of America does offer voluntary marketing and advertising guidelines that encourage prominent display of the label in advertising and during the sales process, including during online searches and sales. The new music downloading services vary considerably in how they label or describe content on the Web and during download. Some services do provide links to parentalguide.org, as Recording Industry Association of America guidelines recommend [55,56].

Rating systems discussion

Although the rating systems provide parents with useful information, all ratings are assigned subjectively by board members whose training and expertise are unknown using instruments and methods that are not publicly available. Greater transparency in the process and greater involvement of child development experts (especially experts with children who play such games) would reassure parents. For example, an independent review of ESRB content descriptors found many areas of disagreement [57].

Parents also are confused by the differing categories used by each industry. Is TY-14 the same as PG-13 and the same as T? Some professionals and parents advocate for a simplified, content-based media rating system that crosses all types of media [58]. Such a system would include descriptors in areas of concern to parents, such as violence, sex, nudity, strong language, and drug use. A review of systems used in other countries may be helpful; for example, the EU game ratings system [59] includes icons for fear (material that might scare young children) and

Box 1. Entertainment Software Rating Board content topics

- Alcohol reference
- Animated blood
- Blood
- Blood and gore
- Cartoon violence
- Comic mischief
- Crude humor
- Drug reference
- Edutainment
- Fantasy violence
- Informational
- Intense violence
- Language
- Lyrics
- Mature humor
- Mild violence
- Nudity
- Partial nudity
- Real gambling
- Sexual themes
- Sexual violence
- Simulated gambling
- Some adult assistance may be needed
- Strong language
- Strong lyrics
- Strong sexual content
- Suggestive themes
- Tobacco reference
- Use of drugs
- Use of alcohol
- Use of tobacco
- Violence

Data from Entertainment Software Rating Board. Understanding ratings. Available at: http://www.ESRB.org.

discrimination (content that depicts or may encourage discrimination). Comprehensive labeling of media would be analogous to food labels that explain content.

The Federal Trade Commission has raised concerns about the marketing of violence to youth and has published a series of reports [51,53,60]. These reports included results of "mystery shopper" sting operations to see if children aged

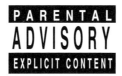

"The Parental Advisory is a notice to consumers that recordings identified by this logo may contain strong language or depictions of violence, sex or substance abuse. Parental discretion is advised."

Fig. 4. Music industry rating logo (Recording Industry Association of America, Washington, DC).

13 to 16 were able to purchase or view mature-content media. In the 39-state 2003 survey, 36% of the "mystery shoppers" were able to buy a ticket for an R-rated movie, 81% could purchase an R-rated film on DVD, 83% bought an explicit content–labeled music CD, and 69% acquired an M-rated video game. Approximately half of the children were asked their age at the movie theaters; fewer than one fourth were asked when purchasing DVDs, CDs, or games. The movie and video game figures showed improvement from the initial 2000 survey, but access to explicit-content music did not change. (DVD purchases were not previously measured.)

There is also concern about whether information about the ratings systems is readily available. Although movies and video games advertisements show the rating, there are no accompanying reminders of what the system is. For example, retailers that sell video games seldom prominently post a display that reminds parents of the ESRB rating system and cautions them about purchasing violent games. There have been some legislative efforts to require more prominent signs and explanations of the rating system, most recently in California [61]. The rating systems are nicely summarized at the website http://www.parentalguide.org. This site is sponsored by the entertainment industry groups; it also links to each of their sites, on which frequently asked questions about the rating systems are answered. The Federal Trade Commission's website also provides information and allows parents to file complaints [62].

Another issue involves "ratings creep," or stretching of the boundaries of acceptability in various rating categories [63]. This practice has been particularly apparent in the Motion Picture Association of America rating system for PG and PG-13 categories. What was once R content currently passes for PG-13, which concerns parents but benefits the movie industry, because it broadens a film's potential audience. This slide toward PG-13 inadvertently was encouraged by the Federal Trade Commission, which slammed Hollywood for marketing R-rated movies to children under 17 and theaters for allowing young teens to buy tickets [53]. A more restrictive rating (PG-13 versus PG or G) actually may make films more attractive to teens [64].

The Classification and Ratings Administration sponsors a website, http://www.filmratings.com, that allows parents to search for a movie by name and get brief information on its rating (eg, "Matrix Reloaded" is "rated R for sci-fi violence and some sexuality"). For persons who want additional information, websites with no connection to the motion picture industry are available, and they provide the user with extensive detail about a given movie (eg, http://www.kids-in-mind.com, http://www.gradingthemovies.com, and http://www.moviemom.com).

Some nonprofit media literacy groups also maintain useful websites. For example, the National Institute on Media and the Family, founded by David Walsh, PhD (http://www.mediafamily.org) provides extensive information for parents on video games, movies, and television shows. This information include "KidScore" game reviews with details on playability, graphics, reading level, entertainment and educational value, and age appropriateness. Common Sense Media (http://www.commonsensemedia.org) also provides "family friendly" ratings based on developmental criteria from respected experts. Other media education sites recommended by the AAP are as follows:

Annenberg Public Policy Center: http://www.annenbergpublicpolicycenter.org (research reports on media issues)

Center for Media Literacy: http://www.medialit.org (resources, training, and curricula for media literacy, including programs for school use)

Coalition for Quality Children's Media: http://www.cqcm.org/kidsfirst (a source of media reviews and quality children's media)

Kaiser Family Foundation: http://www.kff.org/entmedia/index.cfm (fact sheets, surveys, reports, news, and links)

LimiTV: http://www.limitv.org (advocacy for reducing children's television use)

Lion & Lamb Project: http://www.lionlamb.org (advocacy to stop the marketing of violent toys, games, and entertainment to children)

Media Education Foundation: http://www.mediaed.org (produces and distributes video documentaries to encourage critical thinking and debate around media content, media ownership, and diverse representations of ideas and people)

New Mexico Media Literacy Project: http://www.nmmlp.org (produces videos and CD-ROMs on media literacy; provides speakers and workshops)

TV-Turnoff Network: http://www.tvturnoff.org (encourages reducing television use to promote healthier lives and communities, including a "More Reading, Less TV" school program)

TV Parental Guidelines Monitoring Board: http://www.tvguidelines.org (from the television industry; provides information on ratings, guidelines, and the V-chip; links to education and advocacy organizations)

Monitoring and blocking devices

Many thoughtful parents struggle on a daily basis with how to monitor the media their children are consuming. For television and computers, there are technologies that may help. The V-chip allows parents to use a "parental lock code" as a password to activate or change V-chip settings. Programs can be blocked by age category or content label. For example, a parent could block all programs rated TV-14, but if the family's primary concern is violence, the block can be specific to TV-14-V shows. The V-chip also can be set to block unedited movies on premium cable channels via the Motion Picture Association of America film rating system. Unfortunately, the V-chip is not seen as user friendly; parents find it difficult to locate and complicated to program, especially given their often-limited understanding of the ratings system. Some parents also feel that they can supervise children's viewing adequately without the V-chip [65]. A 2001 survey found that only 7% of parents had used a V-chip [66].

Other technology is available for homes with cable television. Cable providers are required by law to offer "lockboxes" for sale or lease upon customer request. Some cable set-top boxes or keypads come already equipped with parental controls. More advanced digital equipment may allow multiple options, including blocking by date, time, channel, program title, and television or film rating [67].

Home computers are another portal of entry for material inappropriate for children, particularly in the realm of pornography. The speed at which technology advances and the adeptness of its makers and hackers have been daunting. The burden is unfortunately on parents, because the message from regulators essentially is that the rate at which technology develops far surpasses the rate at which laws and governmental monitoring can take place. The 1998 Children's Online Privacy Protection Act requires that website operators post their privacy policy, obtain parental consent before collecting, using, or disclosing personal information about a child, and allow parents to review personal information collected on their children and choose to revoke consent and delete the information. Information on policies and advice for parents, teachers, and children on safe Internet use is available on the Federal Trade Commission website [68].

GetNetWise.org reviews the technologies available to families to block or limit access to Internet content. GetNetWise permits a search for all of these tools by function, technology to be controlled, and computer operating system. (They suggest that parents first check with their Internet service provider or online service provider to see what child safety tools or features they offer free or at a discount.) Options include:

- Special Web browsers or search engines geared to children's interests and abilities
- Tools that block outgoing content to prevent children from sending personal information
- Tools that limit time spent online (either total time or times of day) to reduce excessive or unsupervised Internet use
- Tools that monitor children's online activity, such as storing addresses of websites visited, which can be used surreptitiously or with the child's knowledge
- Tools that filter or block content by website address (URL), human review of Web pages, key words (such as "sex" or "breast"), or "context sen-

sitive" key words that avoid overzealous blocking of innocuous pages with information on "breast cancer" or "chicken breast" recipes. Some filters allow parents to override the filter for certain sites

Filtering software is particularly controversial because it can over-block and prevent access to innocuous sites or under-block and allow offensive material to slip through. A 2000 survey found that approximately one third of parents with home Internet access had used a filtering device [69]. No technology can replace parental monitoring or discussions with children of how to handle the inevitable exposure to inappropriate or upsetting material.

Finally, parents have some limited ability to block inappropriate content in interactive games. For example, the Xbox game console has parental controls that can prevent playing of games based on rating (for example, all M-rated games). A few computer games offer an option to block mature content, although this may make the game or its plot more confusing.

Guidelines from professional organizations

Professional organizations that focus on children have researched the impact of media on children and adolescents for the past 40 years. The lead organizations have been the American Medical Association (AMA), the AAP, the American Psychological Association, and the American Academy of Child and Adolescent Psychiatry. Each organization has issued policy statements, published guidelines, brochures, and fact sheets for use by clinicians and parents.

The American Medical Association

In publications, on their website, and at public forums such as congressional hearings, the AMA has promoted greater awareness of media violence as a risk factor that affects the health of young people. They published a "Physician Guide to Media Violence" [70] in 1996 and a "JAMA Patient Page on Violence in the Media" in 2000 [71]. The AMA's most recent policy statement on the topic of media (H-515.974, Mass Media Violence and Film Ratings) addressed what it describes as the shortcomings of the current ratings systems. In sum, it stated that the AMA will do the following:

1. Speak out against the excessive portrayal of violence in media
2. Urge the entertainment industry to make fundamental changes in the rating system to contain more precise content information
3. Work with the entertainment industry to reduce media violence
4. Urge the entertainment industry to develop a uniform ratings system across all media forms
5. Use physicians to counsel parents about the known effects of media violence

6. Monitor changes in the current ratings systems
7. Urge consideration for the potential development of a television violence code
8. Support all other appropriate measures to address and reduce television, cable, and motion picture violence

The American Academy of Pediatrics

The AAP has been particularly active in addressing media effects on children. The AAP encourages pediatricians to incorporate questions about media use into their routine visits, including use of their "Media History Form" (available for purchase from the AAP). The form is designed to help youth and parents examine their media use habits and allow pediatricians to offer advice and support on areas of concern.

The AAP's Media Matters national public education campaign was launched in 1997 to "help pediatricians, parents and children become more aware of the influence that media (television, movies, computer and video games, advertising, popular music, etc.) have on child and adolescent health." The AAP website provides handouts and brochures for parents and professionals, such as "The Ratings Game: Choosing your Child's Entertainment," "Television and the Family," "The Internet and the Family," and "Understanding the Impact of Media on Children and Teens." The AAP also published a series of research-based policy statements in their journal *Pediatrics*, which is available in full text from the Media Matters section of their website (http://www.aap.org/advocacy/mmpolicy.htm). The series are as follows:

February 1995: Children, adolescents, and advertising [72]
August 1999: Media education [73]
July 2000: Joint statement on the impact of entertainment violence on children [74]
January 2001: Sexuality, contraception, and the media [75]
February 2001: Children, adolescents, and television [76]
November 2001: Media violence [77]

What follows is a summary of AAP guidelines for pediatricians to share with parents, drawn from "Children, Adolescents, and Television" and other policy statements:

• Limit children's total media time (with entertainment media) to no more than 1 to 2 hours of quality programming per day
• Remove television sets from children's bedrooms (create an "electronic media-free" environment in children's rooms)
• Discourage television viewing for children younger than 2 years and encourage more interactive activities that promote proper brain development, such as talking, playing, singing, and reading together

- Monitor the shows children and adolescents are viewing. Most programs should be informational, educational, and nonviolent
- View television programs with children and discuss the content. Use controversial programming as a stepping-off point to initiate discussions about family values, violence, sex and sexuality, and drugs
- Use the videocassette recorder wisely to show or record high-quality, educational programming for children
- Support efforts to establish comprehensive media-education programs in schools
- Encourage alternative entertainment for children, including reading, athletics, hobbies, and creative play
- Be good media role models by selectively using media and limiting their own media choices
- Alert and educate parents when positive media opportunities arise, either educational or informative

(It should be noted that some AAP statements on media effects have been criticized for inaccuracies or exaggerations [78]. As a general rule, researchers and clinicians are advised to read the original sources that are cited in research reviews.)

The American Psychological Association

The American Psychological Association, like the AMA, has focused predominantly on the area of violence prevention. American Psychological Association children and media policy briefings, congressional testimony, and article reprints can be found at http://www.apa.org. The American Psychological Association recently turned its attention to the health risks that children face from advertising [79], increasing the amount of "educational/informational" programming for children of various ages and backgrounds [80], and concerns about the effects of violent video games [81].

The American Academy of Child and Adolescent Psychiatry

The American Academy of Child and Adolescent Psychiatry has continued to publish advice for parents through its Facts for Families series (available at: http://www.aacap.org). Currently, five series deal with the media: "Children and TV Violence" (1999), "The Influence of Music and Music Videos" (2000), "Children and Watching TV" (2001), "Children Online" (1997), and "Children and the News" (2002). As a smaller member organization, the American Academy of Child and Adolescent Psychiatry works collaboratively with the other physician groups (AAP and AMA) and with the American Psychological Association on policy statements, supports grass roots efforts, and lobbies government for more active involvement.

Summary

Media literacy is a young field that has evolved over the last two decades in response to growing concern about how mass media affect children. This article has outlined an approach for clinicians and parents that is highly individualized and family based. Larger school-based approaches logically would have some appeal, but actual research in this area is scant. One randomized, controlled school-based study used a 6-month, 18-lesson curriculum to encourage second- and third-grade children to monitor and limit their media use and be "intelligent viewers" [82,83]. As a group, the intervention school students were found to have reduced their television use and perhaps videotape and video game use (parent and child reports differed or changes were nonsignificant); they also showed reductions in some measures of aggression at post-test relative to controls (peer-rated aggression and verbal aggression observed on the school playground). Other measures showed no significant changes, however. Because results were reported at the school level, it is hard to know what might have accounted for any changes at the individual level (eg, amount of exposure to the curriculum, changes in use of various media, or parent education about media use).

The content of television programs, videos, and video games was not assessed. Influencing choices about media content may be as important as limiting amount of media consumption, except when it comes to physical health, weight gain, and displacement of healthier activities. The Robinson study looked for effects of media consumption on weight and found that reducing meals eaten in front of the television and time sitting watching television promoted a healthier body weight. Future studies might provide useful insights for parents and health professionals on the relative influence of school-based and parent education on media literacy and changes in media choices and home routines.

Differing definitions, perspectives, and methodologies add to the challenge of translating existing media research into advice on which parents can act. The availability, content, and interactivity of media are evolving so fast that research conducted even a few years ago may offer little guidance. We also know little about how the dose of media, context of media use, and children's temperament, experiences, and relationships might mediate any positive or negative effects. We can, however, draw some comfort from the knowledge that children are influenced overwhelmingly by the values and behavior of their parents (and how they are treated by others, especially caregivers and teachers). In general, children are resilient and have an amazing capacity to adapt to the world. Parents, as they do for many areas of a child's life, must assess their own values and experiences, listen to various experts, and then guide children toward productive autonomy.

On a societal level, concerns about media's influence—especially on violence and social isolation—can be mitigated by addressing issues known to affect children's healthy development, such as day care, educational opportunities, after-school activities, adequate health care, access to mental health services, and protection from violence in the home. Efforts to give parents and families more time together and provide high-quality care for children when parents are absent are the positive supports that will help children and families cope with rapid cultural change.

References

[1] Thoman E, Jolls T. Media literacy: a national priority for a changing world. Am Behav Sci 2004;48(1):18–29.
[2] American Academy of Pediatrics. Committee on Public Education. Children, adolescents, and television. Pediatrics 2001;107(2):423–6.
[3] Certain LK, Kahn RS. Prevalence, correlates and trajectory of television viewing among infants and toddlers. Pediatrics 2002;109(4):634–42.
[4] Vandewater EA, Bickham DS, Lee JH, et al. When the television is always on: heavy television exposure and young children's development. Am Behav Sci 2005;48(5):562–77.
[5] Linebarger DL, Walker D. Infants' and toddlers' television viewing and language outcomes. Am Behav Sci 2005;48(5):624–45.
[6] Anderson DA, Pempeck TA. Television and very young children. Am Behav Sci 2005;48(5):505–22.
[7] Crawley AM, Anderson DR, Wilder A, et al. Effects of repeated exposures to a single episode of the television program Blue's Clues on the viewing behaviors and comprehension of preschool children. J Educ Psychol 1999;91(4):630–7.
[8] Anderson DR. Educational television is not an oxymoron. Ann Am Acad Pol Soc Sci 1998;557:24–38.
[9] Wright JC, Huston AC, Murphy KC, et al. The relations of early television viewing to school readiness and vocabulary of children from low-income families: the Early Window Project. Child Dev 2001;72(5):1347–66.
[10] Valkenburg PM. Media and youth consumerism. J Adolesc Health 2000;27S:52–6.
[11] Dennison BA, Erb TA, Jenkins PL. Television viewing and television in bedroom associated with overweight risk among low-income preschool children. Pediatrics 2002;109:1028–35.
[12] Calvert SL, Rideout VJ, Woolard JL, et al. Age, ethnicity, and socioeconomic patterns in early computer use. Am Behav Sci 2005;48(5):590–607.
[13] Li X, Atkins MS. Early childhood computer experience and cognitive and motor development. Pediatrics 2004;113(6):1715–22.
[14] Shimai S, Masuda K, Kishimoto Y. Influences of TV games on physical and psychological development of Japanese kindergarten children. Percept Mot Skills 1990;70:771–6.
[15] Bruner JS. On cognitive growth I & II. In: Bruner JS, Oliver RR, Greenfield PM, editors. Studies in cognitive growth. New York: Wiley; 1966. p. 1–67.
[16] Hoffner C, Cantor J. Developmental differences in responses to a television character's appearance and behavior. Dev Psychol 1985;21:1065–74.
[17] Cantor J. Studying children's emotion reactions to mass media. In: Dervin B, Grossberg L, O'Keefe B, et al, editors. Rethinking communication (vol. 2): paradigm exemplars. Newbury Park (CA): Sage; 1989. p. 47–59.
[18] Cantor J, Omdahl BL. Effects of fictional media depictions of realistic threats on children's emotion responses, expectations, worries, and liking for related activities. Commun Monogr 1991;58:384–401.
[19] Cantor J, Mares ML, Oliver MD. Parent's and children's emotional reactions to the televised coverage of the Gulf War. In: Greenberg B, Gantz W, editors. Desert Storm and the mass media. Cresskill (NJ): Hampton Press; 1993. p. 31–53.
[20] Rideout VJ, Foehr UG, Roberts DF, et al. Kids and media @ the new millennium: executive summary. Menlo Park (CA): Kaiser Family Foundation; 1999.

[21] Smith SL, Wilson BJ, Kunkel D, et al. Violence in television programming overall: University of California, Santa Barbara study. In: Federman J, editor. National television violence study 3. Thousand Oaks (CA): Sage; 1998. p. 5–220.
[22] Coyne SM, Archer J, Eslea M. Cruel intentions on television and in real life: can viewing indirect aggression increase viewers' subsequent indirect aggression? J Exp Child Psychol 2004; 88:234–53.
[23] Johnson JG, Cohen P, Smailes EM, et al. Television viewing and aggressive behavior during adolescence and adulthood. Science 2002;295:2468–71.
[24] Huesmann LR, Moise-Titus J, Podolski L, et al. Longitudinal relationships between children's exposure to TV violence and their aggressive and violent behavior in young adulthood: 1977–1992. Dev Psychol 2003;39(2):201–21.
[25] Gentile DA, Lynch PJ, Linder JR, et al. The effects of violent video game habits on adolescent hostility, aggressive behaviors and school performance. J Adolesc 2004;27:5–22.
[26] Roberts DF, Foehr UG, Rideout VJ, et al. Kids and media @ the new millennium: a comprehensive national analysis of children's media use. Menlo Park (CA): Kaiser Family Foundation; 1999.
[27] Funk JB, Buchman DD, Jenks J, et al. Playing violent video games, desensitization, and moral evaluation in children. J Appl Dev Psychol 2003;24:413–36.
[28] Colwell J, Kato M. Investigation of the relationship between social isolation, self-esteem, aggression and computer game play in Japanese adolescents. Asian Journal of Social Psychology 2003;6:149–58.
[29] Sherry JL. The effects of violent video games on aggression: a meta-analysis. Hum Commun Res 2001;27(3):409–31.
[30] Olson CK. Media violence research and youth violence data: why do they conflict? Acad Psychiatry 2004;28:144–50.
[31] Snyder HN, Sickmund M. Juvenile offenders and victims: 1999 national report. Pittsburgh (PA): National Center for Juvenile Justice, Office of Juvenile Justice and Delinquency Prevention; 1999.
[32] Snyder HN. Juvenile arrests 2001: juvenile justice bulletin. Washington (DC): Office of Juvenile Justice and Delinquency Prevention; 2003.
[33] Blumstein A, Rivara FP, Rosenfeld R. The rise and decline of homicide, and why. Annu Rev Public Health 2000;21:505–41.
[34] Buka SL, Stichick TL, Birdthistle I, et al. Youth exposure to violence: prevalence, risks and consequences. Am J Orthopsychiatry 2001;71(3):298–310.
[35] Subrahmanyam K, Greenfield P, Kraut R, et al. The impact of computer use on children's and adolescents' development. J Appl Dev Psychol 2001;22:7–30.
[36] Field AE, Camargo Jr CA, Taylor CB, et al. Peer, parent, and media influences on the development of weight concerns and frequent dieting among preadolescent and adolescent girls and boys. Pediatrics 2001;107:54–60.
[37] Kunkel D, Biely E, Eyal K, et al. Sex on TV 3: a biennial report. Menlo Park (CA): Kaiser Family Foundation; 2003.
[38] Kaiser Family Foundation. Survey snapshot: teens, sex and TV. Available at: http://www.kff.org. Accessed March 31, 2005.
[39] Klein JD, Brown JD, Childers KW, et al. Adolescents' risky behavior and mass media use. Pediatrics 1993;92:24–31.
[40] Collins RL, Elliott MN, Berry SH, et al. Watching sex on television predicts adolescent initiation of sexual behavior. Pediatrics 2004;114:e280–9.
[40a] Centers for Disease Control and Prevention. National youth risk behavior survey: 1991–2003. Trends in the prevalence of sexual behaviors. Fact sheet. Available at: http://www.cdc.gov/yrbss. Accessed March 31, 2005.
[41] Wingood GM, DiClemente RJ, Bernhardt JM, et al. A prospective study of exposure to rap music videos and African-American female adolescents' health. Am J Public Health 2003; 93(3):437–9.
[42] Gidwani PP, Sobol A, DeJong W, et al. Television viewing and initiation of smoking among youth. Pediatrics 2002;110:505–8.

[43] Thomas A, Chess S, Birch HG. Temperament and behavior disorders in children. New York: New York University Press; 1968.

[44] Kirsh SJ. The effects of violent video games on adolescents: the overlooked influence of development. Aggress Violent Behav 2003;8(4):377–89.

[45] Federal interagency forum on child and family statistics. America's children in brief: key national indicators of well-being. Available at: http://childstats.gov. Accessed March 31, 2005.

[46] Capizzano J, Adams G. The hours that children under five spend in child care: variation across states. New federalism national survey of America's families (Series B, No.B-8). Washington (DC): The Urban Institute; 2000.

[47] Singer DG, Singer JL. Developing critical viewing skills and media literacy in children. Ann Am Acad Pol Soc Sci 1998;557:164–79.

[48] Kaiser Family Foundation. Key facts: media literacy (publication #3383). Menlo Park (CA): Kaiser Family Foundation; 2003.

[49] Internet Education Foundation. GetNetWise. Available at: http://www.getnetwise.org. Accessed March 31, 2005.

[50] Federal Trade Commission. Kidz privacy. Available at: http://www.ftc.gov/bcp/conline/edcams/kidzprivacy/. Accessed March 31, 2005.

[51] Houghton S, Milner N, West J, et al. Motor control and sequencing of boys with attention-deficit/hyperactivity disorder (ADHD) during computer game play. Br J Educ Technol 2004;35(1):21–34.

[52] Cantor J. Ratings for program content: the role of research findings. Ann Am Acad Pol Soc Sci 1998;557:54–69.

[53] Federal Trade Commission. Marketing violent entertainment to children: a review of self-regulation and industry practices in motion picture, music recording and electronic game industries. Washington (DC): Federal Trade Commission; 2000.

[54] Motion Picture Association of America. Movie ratings. Available at: http://www.mpaa.org/movieratings/about. Accessed March 31, 2005.

[54a] Entertainment Software Association. Computer and video game software sales reach record $7.3 billion in 2004 (January 26, 2005). Available at http://www.theesa.com. Accessed March 31, 2005.

[55] Federal Trade Commission. Report to congress. Marketing violent entertainment to children: a fourth follow-up review of industry practices in the motion picture, music recording and electronic game industries. Washington (DC): Federal Trade Commission; 2004.

[56] Recording Industry Association of America. Parental advisory program guidelines. Available at: http://www.riaa.com/issues/parents/advisory.asp. Accessed March 31, 2005.

[57] Haninger K, Thompson KM. Content and ratings of teen-rated video games. JAMA 2004;291:856–65.

[58] Walsh DA, Gentile DA. A validity test of movie, television and video-game ratings. Pediatrics 2001;107:1302–8.

[59] Pan European Game Information. Available at: http://www.pegi.info/home.jsp. Accessed March 31, 2005.

[60] Federal Trade Commission. Report to congress. Marketing violent entertainment to children: a one-year follow-up review of industry practices in the motion picture, music recording and electronic game industries. Washington (DC): Federal Trade Commission; 2001.

[61] Yee L, Lieber SJ, Montañez C, et al. Assembly Bill 1793. Available at: http://democrats.assembly.ca.gov/members/a12/press/p122004074.htm. Accessed March 31, 2005.

[62] Federal Trade Commission. Entertainment ratings guide. Available at: http://www.ftc.gov/bcp/conline/edcams/ratings/ratings.htm. Accessed March 31, 2005.

[63] Federman J. Rating sex and violence in the media: media ratings and proposals for reform. Menlo Park (CA): Kaiser Family Foundation; 2002.

[64] Bushman BJ, Cantor J. Media ratings for violence and sex: implications for policymakers and parents. Am Psychol 2003;58(2):130–41.

[65] Jordan A. Parents' use of the V-chip to supervise children's television use. Philadelphia: Annenberg Public Policy Center; 2003.

[66] Kaiser Family Foundation. Parents and the V-chip 2001: a Kaiser Family Foundation survey. Menlo Park (CA): Kaiser Family Foundation; 2001.

[67] Federal Communications Commission. Consumer facts: how to prevent viewing objectionable television programs. Available at: http://www.fcc.gov/cgb/information_directory.html. Accessed March 31, 2005.

[68] Federal Trade Commission. How to protect kids' privacy online. Available at: http://www. ftc.gov/bcp/conline/edcams/kidzprivacy/. Accessed March 31, 2005.

[69] Annenberg Public Policy Center. Media in the home. Philadelphia: Annenberg Public Policy Center; 2000.

[70] Walsh D, Goldman LS, Brown R. Physician guide to media violence. Chicago: American Medical Association; 1996.

[71] Pace B. JAMA patient page. In: Glass RM, editor. Violence in the media. JAMA 2000; 283(20):2748.

[72] Committee on Communications. Children, adolescents, and advertising. Pediatrics 1995;95(2): 295–7.

[73] Committee on Public Education. Media education. Pediatrics 1999;104(2):341–3.

[74] Cook DE, Kestenbaum C, Honaker LM, et al; American Academy of Pediatrics, American Academy of Child & Adolescent Psychiatry, American Psychological Association, American Medical Association, American Academy of Family Physicians, American Psychiatric Association. Joint statement on the impact of entertainment violence on children. Presented at the Congressional Public Health Summit. Washington (DC), July 26, 2000.

[75] Committee on Public Education. Sexuality, contraception, and the media. Pediatrics 2001; 107(1):191–4.

[76] Committee on Public Education. Children, adolescents and television. Pediatrics 2001;107(2): 423–6.

[77] Committee on Public Education. Media violence. Pediatrics 2001;108(5):1222–6.

[78] Free Expression Policy Project. Exchange of letters between AAP and the Free Expression Policy Project. Available at: http://www.fepproject.org/news/aapletter.html. Accessed March 31, 2005.

[79] Wilcox BL, Kunkel D, Cantor J, et al. Report of the APA task force on advertising and children. Available at: http://www.apa.org. Accessed February 20, 2004.

[80] Children's Media Policy Coalition. In the matter of children's television obligations of digital television broadcaster [MM docket no. 00-167]. Testimony presented before the Federal Communications Commission. Washington (DC), April 21, 2003.

[81] Anderson CA. Violent video games: myths, facts and unanswered questions. Available at: http://www.apa.org/science/psa/sb-anderson.html. Accessed March 31, 2005.

[82] Robinson TN. Reducing children's television viewing to prevent obesity: a randomized controlled trial. JAMA 1999;282(16):1561–7.

[83] Robinson TN, Wilde ML, Navracruz LC, et al. Effects of reducing children's television and video game use on aggressive behavior: a randomized controlled trial. Arch Pediatr Adolesc Med 2001;155(1):17–23.

ELSEVIER
SAUNDERS

Child Adolesc Psychiatric Clin N Am
14 (2005) 555–570

CHILD AND
ADOLESCENT
PSYCHIATRIC CLINICS
OF NORTH AMERICA

The Functional Assessment of Media in Child and Adolescent Psychiatric Treatment

Caroly Pataki, MD*, Jeff Q. Bostic, MD, EdD,
Steven Schlozman, MD

*Department of Psychiatry, David Geffen School of Medicine, University of California at Los Angeles,
12-105 Center for Health Sciences, Box 957035, Los Angeles, CA 90095-7035, USA*

Young people in Generation 2000 are the embodiment of the proliferation in modern culture of multimedia communication. Youth throughout the United States and much of Europe spend a significant portion of their time engrossed in interactive CD-ROMs, complex computer video games, electronic mail (E-mail), instant text messaging through cell phones, two-way pagers, and Internet Web-sites and chat rooms. More traditional forms of media, such as television (TV), telephone, music via compact discs, TV music videos, radio, magazines, news-papers, and movies remain available, although perhaps they are less appealing to this generation. Several years ago, it seemed shocking that by the end of high school, United States students had spent more time watching television than they had in school [1]. A recent survey concluded that youth from elementary school through high school spend 6 to 8 hours per day immersed in old and newer forms of media [2]. Increasingly, a case can be made that we indulge ourselves tech-nologically in products without the necessary safeguards to measure and ensure that our quality of life is enhanced by their use. This phenomenon could be viewed as systemic; one need only examine our complex relationship with food, dieting, and obesity to point out that abundance has the potential to prove dam-aging. Whereas obesity currently plagues our children because of chronic expo-sure to unhealthy food choices, the current glut of media arouses images of mechanized children with scant experience in real, face-to-face social exchanges that require feelings such as empathy and compassion. The impact of this evolv-ing technologic media expanse on child and adolescent development frequently has been debated, although not well documented. With the substantial daily youth

* Corresponding author.
   E-mail address: cpataki@mednet.ucla.edu (C. Pataki).

childpsych.theclinics.com

media diet, however, it undoubtedly provides a powerful effect on a youth's social, cognitive, and emotional growth. Like food, however, the evidence does not imply that more necessarily is better.

Media exposure creates neither a "positive" nor "negative" circumstance per se. Instead, media exert a potentially helpful influence on developing youth by modeling effective coping techniques, but they also have a potentially deleterious impact on shaping youth self-esteem, peer relationships, and risk-taking behaviors by presenting larger-than-life media images that youth accept as normal or typical. Published literature has paid particular attention to the impact of "violence" in the media on youth [3]. Recently, reports of increased risk-taking behaviors have been documented among adolescent chat room users [4]. Little concrete data exist to inform our overall interpretation of media's effect on youth. What we do know is that the media are pervasive and influence nearly every area of life for children and adolescents. Evidence also suggests that the amount, variety, and intensity of all forms of media will continue to increase before the quality of media is reviewed adequately and matched to its developmentally appropriate audience. Efforts to determine how the media impact individual youngsters may provide us, as clinicians, with insights to recommend healthier media diets for our patients. It may be useful for clinicians to use a paradigm for assessing the function of the media in a given youth's life. The "functional assessment of media" paradigm should aid in clarifying the effects of one's media consumption, so that media might be harnessed to illuminate its effect on social, cognitive, and emotional development.

Media exposure for American youth: dateline 2004

The overwhelming amount of media available with few guidelines set for quality has become a potential public health hazard. A recent national survey of more than 2000 randomly selected adolescents found that more than 97% of the households in the sample have TVs, video cassette recorders, and audio systems and more than 75% of households have video game systems and personal computers [2]. A typical home contains [2]:

- Three TV sets
- Three audiotape players
- Three radios
- Two video cassette recorders
- Two compact disc players
- One video game player
- One computer

At the same time, the likelihood of a given child or adolescent having a TV, video cassette recorder, or video game player in his or her bedroom is inversely related to the family income [2], which suggests that the lower socioeconomic households were more likely to provide children with more private, personal access to TV media. Numerous sociologic explanations are available for these developments, including the important facts that quality childcare is expensive and that parents often work long hours at multiple jobs. One of the implications of these findings is that because parents are elsewhere, the media often have become virtual childcare workers. Consumer pressure, advertisements, peer pressure (on children and parents), prestige factors around owning newer gadgets and games, and the decreasing prices for media equipment add to the pervasive home use of these media.

Finally, important age-related differences in media exposure can inform our understanding of the ways in which media affects youth. Current data among young people show increased TV viewing time up to age 13. Adolescents aged 14 through 18 replace TV viewing with increased exposure to movies, video games, and computer activities. The amount of exposure to music also doubles from early to late adolescence [2].

Influence of the media on youth development and behavior

Media and physical activity among youth

"My So-called Life"

Youth are known to be profoundly influenced by the appearance, habits, and behavior of admired peers and by media figures whom they idolize. The complexity of identification among young adolescents leads some to emulate harmful behaviors, such as smoking cigarettes, or imitate the potentially unhealthy eating habits of those whom they admire [5]. Media influences on adolescence also can promote positive behaviors, however. A survey of approximately 1000 boys and girls between the ages of 9 and 16 years revealed that approximately half of the girls and nearly one third of the boys make some effort to look like admired media personae [6]. The older adolescents particularly reported increased frequency and intensity of exercise to look like one of their idols [6]. The association between wanting to look like media idols and increased physical activity among adolescents has implications to be used as a model for more "healthy" behavior, yet it is also important to remember that the developmentally expected pattern of "imitation" among adolescents does not possess its own intrinsic limits. Youth may not know the boundaries for physical exertion of their age compared with their icons and, perhaps more importantly, they may not understand limitations of their body habitus as they try to transform into their icons or their icon's "body double." Adolescents who are infatuated with idols may not be prepared to distinguish healthy from unhealthy imitation. Adolescents are potentially faced with the almost impossible task of emulating personae who seem to achieve almost super-human standards consistently. To engage in what seems to be extreme behavior by emulating admired figures is a nearly universal experience among youth. A typical example occurs frequently among adolescent girls who begin to view themselves as too heavy after perusing models in fashion magazines. Consequently, they undertake an extreme diet in the service of becoming more like the models who have become their idols of beauty and societal representations of health. As clinicians are acutely aware, adolescents are uniquely vulnerable to carrying out their imitations to self-destructive proportions, so it stands to reason that the youth with "extreme" role models are at greater risk of engaging in more potentially dangerous imitative behaviors. Recognizing this vulnerability among youth has led clinicians and researchers to advocate that the media should cultivate and reinforce realistic expectations, particularly in the areas of physical activity and body image [6].

Media and the development of self-esteem, feminine identity, and body image among girls

"The Swan"

The media have become some of the dominant influences on adolescents' internalization of ideal body image and satisfaction or dissatisfaction with themselves. For girls, "appearance magazines" (such as *Teen*, *Cosmo Girl*, and *Seventeen*) are reported to influence their ideas of perfect body image for most girls, and for at least half of adolescent girls, magazine pictures have induced them to diet [7]. Early adolescent girls from Latino, white, and black cultural backgrounds gravitate toward appearance magazines to examine and communicate with each other about their evolving sexual and feminine identities. The latest fashions, which are important to adolescents who are trying on identities separate from their parents, are coupled with the body types modeling these fashions. Although insidious, an adolescent's attention to the shape and look of a model often exceeds the attention they give to the costume.

Influence of erotic media on adolescents' sexual attitudes and behaviors

"Sex and the City"

Many forms of current media contribute to adolescent notions of sexuality by providing essentially perpetual access to a wide range of sexual information and erotica. Video games, Internet chat rooms, and Websites (too often cloaked by seemingly innocuous names such as spikelee.com) provide a smorgasbord from which adolescents can choose for their sexual media diet [4,8,9]. Although sufficient data are not available to identify optimal sexual education for adolescents, consideration of the vast array of sexual material that bombards adolescents on a daily basis may lead to guidelines for positive sexual attitudes and diminished high-risk sexual behavior among adolescents. It is fair to assume that teens choose media that resonate with their developing sense of sexual identity. In this light, establishing sexual values, attitudes, and behaviors is a central part of the process [8], and the process is likely to include desires to emulate certain peers and media figures and distinguish oneself from others. Some evidence suggests that initial frequent exposure of young adults (not children) to erotic and sexually graphic stimuli leads to diminished feelings of guilt, repulsion, or disgust toward sexual behavior and an increase in enjoyment, whereas prolonged exposure tends to lead to seeking more novel, possibly deviate, forms of sexual interactions [9]. Repeated exposure to erotic media leads to the perception among young people of exaggerated sexual activity among adults [9]. Recent surveys documented that adolescents who regularly visit chat rooms are four times more likely than non–chat room users to experience online sexual solicitation [10]. Trends in the emerging literature also suggest that frequent exposure of young people to graphic sexual media is associated with more callous attitudes toward victims of forced sexual encounters.

Given the lack of evidence-based sexual education parameters that promote healthy sexual identity among youth and the recognition that advertising or marketing agendas often predominate over healthy sexual development prerogatives, the National Commission on Adolescent Sexual Health [11] devised suggested guidelines for media portrayal of sexual images: (1) Eliminate the stereotype that all adolescents engage in sexual intercourse. (2) Provide diverse images of appearance and body shape and form in portraying sexual relationships, not only "beautiful people." (3) Portray interactions between men and women as respectful and not exploitative. (4) Present use of contraceptives. (5) Provide dialogue that portrays parent-child communication about sexuality and relationships.

Multiple venues and opportunities are available for the media to include overt and subtle messages to youth that may promote healthier sexual attitudes, such as TV shows, music videos, movies, magazines, and video games, to name a few. Media can be instrumental in promoting realistic, positive, and respectful attitudes toward the opposite sex in numerous forms. These positive images may be incorporated by teens into their repertoire of thoughts and feelings about sexuality.

Case 1: "Have you seen what's out there?"

A 16-year-old boy with a mood disorder and nonverbal learning disorder presented to his weekly therapy sessions with concerns about increased sexual self-stimulation. After the therapist assessed his concerns and reassured him regarding his normal adolescent behavior, he wondered whether the therapist was aware of the sexual material available on the Internet. "Have you seen what's out there?" the patient asked, and before the therapist could respond, the patient detailed his difficulty in deciding what, if any, Internet erotica was "appropriate" for his viewing. From there, the patient described a recent Internet foray in which he had been researching the movie "Star Wars," followed a link that promised more information about Princess Lea, and found himself viewing "naked" celebrities in various compromising positions. The patient seemed bothered by the extent of what he had discovered and the ease with which he found himself at "adult" Websites despite numerous Internet filters that his parents had installed on his personal computer. The session ended with reassurances from the therapist that having found such Websites did not automatically signify sexual deviance and acknowledgment that curiosity about sexual material is developmentally normal. Finally, the therapist was aware of the overall sense of guilt that the patient experienced at his own feelings regarding these sites and the need to address these issues in a nonjudgmental and empathic fashion.

Media violence and youth behavior

"CSI: Crime Scene Investigation"

Exposure to violence through the media seems ubiquitous in our society, and this exposure begins in early childhood. Young children are exposed routinely to movies that contain violent themes [12]. A survey of 1000 parents who brought their children to a pediatric visit found that 73% of families believed that their youngest child viewed TV violence at least once a week [12]. A recent school-based survey of 15 New England public schools found that a popular violent movie, "Scream," was viewed by two thirds of middle school students and more than 40% of fifth graders [12]. This survey revealed that substantial numbers of elementary school–aged children had viewed violent movies, including movies listed in Box 1.

The finding that a significant percentage of children and adolescents have been exposed to extremely violent media—many on a regular basis—is a confounding variable in understanding the effects of violent media on child development, because few children and adolescents have not been exposed. Although the effects of media violence on children are one of the most concerning issues among clinicians and researchers, it has not been easy to obtain persuasive data on the most vulnerable populations: children and adolescents. Another obstacle to studying the effects of violent media on youth is the obvious ethical dilemma

---

Box 1. Movies seen by more than 40% of early adolescents and more than 30% of fifth graders in 1998/1999

- "Scream"
- "I Know What You Did Last Summer"
- "Scream 2"
- "Con Air"
- "Face-Off"
- "Die Hard"
- "Halloween H20: Twenty Years Later"
- "Bride of Chucky"
- "Blade"

Data from Sargent JD, Heatherton TF, Ahrens B, et al. Adolescent exposure to extremely violent movies. J Adolesc Health 2002;31: 449–54.

when one considers exposing children to violent stimuli in a research setting. Few data are available on the effects of extremely violent media on children and young adolescents, although multiple studies of exposure to violent media in young adults are often cited [12]. Existing data regarding the effects of exposure to violent movies on children indicate the production of fear that may linger for long periods of time [3]. Young children tend to be frightened of disgusting and grotesque characters, whereas older children and adolescents more often are affected negatively by viewing threatening events, including sexual assaults or supernatural events [13].

One of the most pertinent questions to clinicians and parents is whether viewing extremely violent content of TV, movies, and video games leads to increased levels of interpersonal violent behavior. In this regard, data from research with young adults have supported several themes that generate profound concerns. Regular viewing of violence in media among young adults has been reported to be associated with (1) violent behavior toward property, (2) criminal violence, (3) acceptance of violent solutions to conflict, and (4) desensitization and reduced tendency to intervene in a fight or feel sympathy for a victim [3]. Even with limited data, it seems difficult to contend that media violence itself promotes any type of health in young viewers.

Case 2: "Fetal Death"

A 17-year-old boy with depression and some substance abuse was interested in "metal" music. When asked by his psychiatrist to describe these interests, the patient noted that "metal" comes in various forms, including goth-metal, heavy metal, and, his favorite, "death metal." He then described his own band, which he and his friends had titled "Fetal Death." He noted that although many of the lyrics that he and his friends composed were angry sounding, he did not worry that these lyrics necessarily reflected that he or others would act on their aggressive feelings. He argued that the lyrics were instead somewhat protective. "Sometimes we just get pissed off, you know?" He acknowledged that the music helps him to "get his feelings out" and avoid what might otherwise be aggressive altercations.

Media activities and their effect on peer relationships

While the media are often used by youth interactively as a form of communication, some youth seem to substitute media for peer relationships themselves. Given the high level of stimulation that can be derived even from playing many video games alone, a preference for the media is of concern for youth who already have difficulties making and keeping friends. For some children and adolescents, TV or video games come into play as surrogate babysitters, whereas for others, social isolation and peer rejection may further drive their fascination with video games. Concerns related to the presence of media in the lives of youth as standing in for either "babysitters" or friends are heightened by data provided by children and adolescence that substantiate how often they engage in media use "mainly alone" [2]. For example, music consumption doubles during adolescence and sometimes is used by youth to distinguish in-group and out-group members [14]. Whereas all forms of music may enhance peer affiliation [15], youths with lower self-esteem seem more likely to assail the musical choices divergent from their own.

Case 3: "I don't think there's a difference…"

An 18-year-old boy began spending increasing amounts of time online playing Internet poker. He started at sites on which no money was exchanged, but eventually he began playing for more and more cash. Although he was largely successful at winning, his parents discovered his behavior and became alarmed first at the amount of money being wagered and second at the extent to which this behavior came at the expense of social interactions. When his psychiatrist asked him to describe Internet poker, he seemed to grasp well the particulars of poker in general and said that he could easily tell when others were bluffing by noting the amounts and the ways that his online opponents placed their bets. The psychiatrist then pointed out that much of poker was a social interaction. The clinician argued that reading an opponent's motivations is based largely on studying the opponent's demeanor in person and not via an Internet transmission and an on-screen schematic. The patient considered this observation but then smiled and disagreed. "I don't think there's a difference," he explained. "Playing poker online seems exactly like playing poker in person."

Functional assessment of the media in the psychiatric evaluation of youth

The media diets of our patients warrant careful assessment. The existing data suggest strongly that the media our youths consume profoundly affects physical health and emotional development. Given these important concerns, a useful model for the examination of the influence—positive and negative—of media on youth may be provided by a functional assessment of media in their daily lives. An example of such an assessment tool is provided to clarify impacts of the media and identify specific functions of the media in a given youth's life.

What is functional media assessment?

Any functional assessment seeks to derive the function served by a given behavior. In this case, such an assessment scrutinizes the viewing or listening and the overall engagement in specific forms of media. Often used clinically with youth to understand undesirable behaviors that seemed unresponsive to adult redirection, functional assessments typically involve the identification of the settings or context in which the behaviors occur, including the antecedents to a behavior, the descriptions of the troubling behavior, and the actual consequences of that behavior [16–18]. For example, in classroom applications, a student with deficits in academic skills may engage in disruptive talking to other students during math class, which results in teacher reprimands but also accomplishes the secondary gain of diversion from academic tasks or attaining peer status, which sustains the behavior.

The functional assessment of media use is used more broadly because such an assessment seeks the potential constructive and destructive functions that the media serve. For example, when bored, a youth may channel surf through a multitude of TV programming, derive seemingly little from it, and then fail to complete school assignments, which results in conflicts with teachers and parents. Accordingly, in this scenario, the media function negatively by distracting the youth from responsibilities but perhaps positively by diminishing anxiety about schoolwork. Efforts by parents or clinicians to alter such viewing in this case likely will require attention to these "functions" for a change to be successful. Clinicians are faced with the often formidable task of identifying the differences in perceptions by adolescents, parents, and teachers and developing an integrated functional assessment and plan that takes into account the various views of family members. Attention to strengths and challenges and to overall motivation surrounding maladaptive behaviors remains paramount. For example, the individual mentioned previously may lack the academic skills to do homework or may lack time management or organizational skills. The youth may not perceive the homework as worthwhile ("I'll never recite lines from Beowulf, so I'm not wasting time reading it") and may be more motivated—and reinforced—to channel surf, because that particular activity might yield more immediate gratification than a specific academic task. The task of the clinician then becomes one of using the naturally occurring incentive of the media as a reward for completing academic work rather than an alternative to it.

The paradigm among youth of gravitating toward activities that provide immediate gratification over those that require effort and delayed reward is not particularly new. Children and adolescents have been watching TV and listening to music at the expense of their academic tasks almost since these media choices first became available. These issues are amplified for modern youths because of the overall quantitative changes in media availability and the qualitative characteristics of the media that compete for youth attention.

Components of a functional assessment of media

Arrested development

The components of a functional media assessment include identification of the media diet, what leads to consumption of various media, and the consequences of exposure to this media, both immediately (while viewing, listening, or game playing), and subsequently (impacts hours to weeks later). These components are summarized Table 1.

The media diet

The specific media preferences of a youth can be ascertained by questions about daily consumption patterns and about context surrounding consumption.

Table 1
Sample framework for a functional assessment of media in youth

Media exposures	Time spent (per day)	Context (alone/social)	Functions of these media	Consequences Negative	Positive
Television					
Movies					
VHS/DVD					
Radio					
Music (CDs)					
Music (downloads)					
Video games					
Internet searches					
E-mail					
Magazines					
Newspapers					
Telephone conversations					
Text messaging					

An assessment of the media diet might include the following questions to the youth and to parents or other reliable reporters in the youth's home:

- What forms of media are meaningful in the life of an adolescent?
- How much time is spent with various media modalities?
- Are media activities sought in isolation or interactively?
- Who monitors the media diet of the youth?
- What do parents watch, and what do they intend to teach their childre about media consumption?

To determine the forms and frequency of media consumption, youths can be asked what occurs outside of school hours. Practicing sports or music may be identified, but subsequent questions should focus on ascertaining the amount of time allocated daily to (1) TV viewing, (2) listening to music, (3) playing video or computer games, and (4) reading newspapers and magazines. Follow-up questions about regular (routine) practices (eg, playing a video game after school for 30 minutes, always watching certain shows, or having a certain show schedule on a particular day) usually reveal whether the diet is consistent (same shows, routine) or variable (various shows watched when bored). In some cases in which a youth cannot recall usual practices, a 1-week "media diary" can elucidate how much time is allocated to media involvements.

Context of media exposure provides clues to antecedents to media exposure and to social circumstances surrounding this exposure. Examples of antecedents might include "I play a video game after school to wind down," "I watch TV when there's nothing else better to do, usually from 4 to 6 PM," "I listen to music when I'm really angry," or "I listen to music 3 hours each night while I'm doing homework." Determining who else is present and what role they play during media exposure may reveal that a parent and child watch certain instructional TV shows and use the shows to stimulate discussion versus a youth watching violent or parent-warning programming in isolation. Similarly, "chat room" conversations may be the primary social encounters a youth has, may occupy hours with strangers, or may position vulnerable youths to the forays of sexual predators or drug dispensers.

The context and collection of others sharing in the media experience leads to querying about who in the family monitors the youth's media diet. Parents vary dramatically in terms of their awareness of what media their children are exposed to and their vigilance about what media exposures are acceptable and what are "off limits." Parent/guardian/sibling media consumption also is important, because youth often are aware of what others in the household are listening to or viewing. Finally, it is instructive to ascertain what aspirations guardians have, if any, in terms of what specific media they would prefer that their child digest.

It is important to note that parents may be taken by surprise by this line of inquiry. Many parents have not considered or decided what they wish to teach their children about media exposures, and efforts at investigating these issues initially may be resisted by family. With this in mind, such an assessment benefits from a nonjudgmental and empathic approach. Although clinicians naturally strive toward such an approach, the sheer enormity of media consumption among youth and their caretakers often leads families to feel somewhat daunted in their attempts to discuss all aspects of these issues. Ultimately, however, parents transmit—mindfully or by example—some message about media consumption, so clarification of their desired goals provides opportunities for parents to engage their children about appropriate media use and demonstrate appropriate media exposure in their own lives.

Functions of media

Once the influences, amount, and context of media exposure are identified, the clinician may determine what functions these media play in the lives of individual patients. Common functions served by media are provided in Table 2. The following discussions are useful in clarifying the functions of the media.

How does a youth's media diet impact his or her life?

At a most basic level, how do the media influence a youth's daily life? What problems occur because of these media exposures? For example, do the influences of media make a youth more anxious or less inclined to engage with peers, or do they interfere with school or home responsibilities? At the same time, which media exposures exert positive influences on a youth's life? For example, the youth may take pride in staying abreast of weather or sports information or may report feeling in a better mood after listening to or watching particular music or shows.

Table 2
Functional assessment of media in treatment planning

Media-related problem behaviors	Skills to be developed	Motivational factors	Evaluation	
			Adherence to intervention	Effectiveness of intervention
Example: too much time watching television leads to chore neglect				
Example: imitates "antihero" yelling, which annoys family members				
Example: breaks household items after listening to certain music				
Example: spends time searching Internet for gruesome photos, stays up all night, cannot wake up for school				

How does the media diet relate to a youth's development? Is this media diet developmentally appropriate?

Does the youth access media that are "designed" for his or her age group? Does the youth understand the messages provided by the medium, and do the messages enhance this youth's life? Too often, youths witness information for which they are ill prepared, and consolidation of this information can be difficult or even disturbing to them.

How does the media diet propel development (particularly identity formation)?

Does the media diet assist youths in making helpful choices about identity? Does the media information overwhelm the cognitive and emotional skills of youths so that confusion results, or does it stretch these skills in a way that promotes rather than hinders identity formation? Similarly, some media information may overwhelm the psychological defenses of a particular youth and result in increased anxiety or regression to more primitive defenses. For example, a youth might be exposed to imagery of violence or conflict that makes the youth fear and avoid people of different ethnic origins while simultaneously yielding stereotypes because of limited cognitive skills.

Much of an adolescent's struggle is to determine an identity apart from parents, so adolescents commonly "try on" different identities that are usually popular among their peers but sometimes are much different than their parents' identities. The issue is not always "who" they choose to emulate so much as "what" it is specifically about these icons that young people seek to portray. For example, whereas parents sometimes recoil at their youth's interest in "antiheroes," such as Eminem or Slipknot, sometimes the youth's interest is around desirable attributes these icons possess (eg, Eminem's dexterity with words and rhyme or the drumming of Joey Jordison from Slipknot). Conversely, adolescents sometimes perceive that they can, like Eminem, for example, on receiving MTV Awards in the United States and in Europe, make obscene gestures to society, and they believe that this strategy applies to many social situations. Although many adolescents may fantasize about making antisocial gestures with impunity, an important aspect of any young person's development is making sense of social standards as they fluctuate as a function of person and place. Eminem may be able and even expected to make obscene gestures to the world. Most of us, however, are not expected to do such, and the consequences of such actions for most people often are not portrayed clearly in popular media. Media portrayals in the absence of real-life examples have the potential to be confusing and at times even detrimental.

How does the media diet expand treatment opportunities and reveal issues for a patient?

Discussion of the media diet often can illuminate a youth's particular psychosocial challenges. Media choices occur for reasons, and preoccupations often suggest desires to master particular conflicts. As functions of various media unfold, the conflicts they address can provide an additional window to understanding a youth. Asking about a youth's "favorite" movies, TV shows, bands, icons, Websites, books, or magazines often accelerates and illuminates important aspects of the child's inner world. Simply being curious about and understanding as much as possible how a young person's media diet influences his or her daily life is enormously helpful in the therapeutic setting. We all use displacement and projection as potent tools to express feelings that we would rather not directly own, and the job of the clinician is to elucidate these feelings with empathy and understanding. In this light, a nonjudgmental curiosity about media choice often makes clear important information that otherwise would be substantially less forthcoming. As in any psychotherapy treatment, the themes and therapeutic targets that emerge via the media vary in each case. For some, issues pertinent to identity formation and self-esteem may emerge. For others, focus on the media may elucidate important challenges around competency in social situations, body image misperceptions, poor judgment, and difficulties with impulsivity. In other words, many of the issues that are particularly germane to children and adolescents are often most clearly elucidated by making use of the media in the clinical encounter.

How does the media diet enhance treatment options for a patient?

A functional assessment of the media often reveals targets for intervention. Youths are predictably influenced by the media habits of their parents, older siblings, and peers. The functional assessment is broadened by ascertainment of the context in which youths view media. The antecedents and contexts that lead to unhelpful media choices and the consequences that youths encounter through these choices allow interventions to be planned and even prioritized. For example, if a youth every day after school begins Internet chatting with strangers and then increases Internet chat time when an Internet chat room "friend" is identified such that homework is neglected and grades deteriorate, multiple intervention targets can be identified. Contexts or settings can be targeted to increase time and opportunities in the real world of the youth to have meaningful social encounters. This intervention could address skill deficits that sustain unhealthy behaviors. The consequences (limited relationship quality with a chat room persona, impacts from school failure) provide additional intervention targets. Similarly, motivations for continuing the Internet relationship at the expense of relationships in the youth's real world warrant attention.

A youth's media diet usually affords the clinician additional pathways to important themes. Adolescents who are resistant to working with adults often can discuss topics ordinarily intolerable by describing how characters or icons they admire would address such a topic. In this light, the media may provide a projective device for youth to address issues, much like play therapy in younger patients provides a communicative device for patients too young to examine verbally their distress (Table 2; Box 2).

Box 2. Common functions of the media in youths (examples provided)

- Information: news programs, History Channel, newspapers, magazines
- Stimulation: music videos, Discovery Channel, video games
- Pleasure: HBO, video games, situation comedies, music
- Distraction: talk shows (eg, Jerry Springer, Montel), soap operas
- Preoccupation: repetitive playing of Dungeons and Dragons, soap operas
- Imitation: The Cosby Show, choosing media icons to emulate (characters that represent Goth, Straight Edge)
- Communication: Internet "chat" interactions, text messaging, e-mail
- Education (Is this really different from information?): obtaining information about sexuality, medical problems via Internet
- Social connection: "chat" interactions
- Sense of accomplishment: X-Box, Playstation games with scores/points
- Comfort: music, TV
- Challenge: computer games

Clinical implications

Media diet information affords clinicians an additional lens through which to view their patients and additional modalities with which to engage and treat youths. Clinicians can be more effective in their communication with youths by becoming more media literate themselves and can be more adept at conducting their own functional assessment of media during the psychiatric interview. This assessment does not always occur during the initial evaluation because of the many other topics that must be addressed, but such an assessment should be considered around a youth's long-term "media health." This information potentially yields a useful gauge of the issues that impact youths and provides additional ways of connecting and aligning with youths.

A nonjudgmental inquiry about these topics with children and adolescents often reflects the ubiquitous influence of the media in their ideals, their fascination with heroes and antiheroes derived from movies, TV, musical groups, magazines and Internet exchanges, and the extent to which these preoccupations guide their psychological development. Supporting an adolescent's sense of boundaries—taking special care to recognize, respect, and not blindly condemn media choices—goes a long way toward allowing even the most troubled adolescents to examine their network of idols and the extent to which these idols inform their evolving self-concept.

Most youths are drawn to a range of icons, including those who hail from "mainstream" arenas (eg, movies and TV) and increasingly counterculture antiheroes who more commonly become media figures through the arts or music. This array of seemingly fragmented and contradictory loyalties attached to the gamut of "heroes" to "antiheroes" is a virtual representation of the textured emotions of developing adolescents. Clinicians who are familiar with some of the media diet youths are often positioned to examine or even help these young people substitute similar, but healthier, media diet choices.

Clinicians and parents share a responsibility to educate themselves in how young people communicate with each other and how it impacts on communication with the adults in their lives. The greater fluency that clinicians have with the world of youth—for example, the staccato language of instant messaging, the too-frequent combat mentality of video games, and the typically callous humor of current TV and movies—the easier it is to begin a meaningful dialogue with young people. Such a dialogue always has been the purview of clinicians interested in the developmental trajectory of their young patients. The sheer enormity of media exposure and the rapid and dizzying changes that characterize current media formats make such a dialogue particularly important and challenging. This line of inquiry is also particularly rewarding, however. From watching video clips to listening to music, this assessment affords clinicians a snapshot, which is often shared with patients themselves, into the milieu of the modern young world. The dialogue is "virtually" always well worth the effort.

References

[1] Comstock G, Paik H. Television and the American child. San Diego (CA): Academic Press; 1999.

[2] Roberts D. Media and youth: access, exposure and privatization. J Adolesc Health 2000; 27(Suppl):8–14.

[3] Cantor J. Media violence. J Adolesc Health 2000;27(Suppl):30–4.

[4] Beebe TJ, Asche A, Harrison PA, et al. Heightened vulnerability and increased risk-taking among adolescent chat room users: results from a statewide school survey. J Adolesc Health 2004;35:116–23.

[5] Brown JD, Cantor J. An agenda for research on youth and the media. J Adolesc Health 2000; 27(Suppl):2–7.

[6] Teveras EM, Ridas-Shiman SL, Field AE, et al. The influence of wanting to look like media figures on adolescent physical activity. J Adolesc Health 2004;35:41–50.

[7] Field AE, Cheung L, Wolf AM, et al. Exposure to the mass media and weight concerns among girls. Pediatrics 1999;103:36.

[8] Brown JD. Adolescents' sexual media diets. J Adolesc Health 2000;27(Suppl):35–40.

[9] Zillmann D. Influence of unrestrained access to erotica on adolescents' and young adults' dispositions toward sexuality. J Adolesc Health 2000;27(Suppl):41–4.

[10] Mitchell KJ, Finkelhor D, Wolak J. Risk factors for and impact of online sexual solicitation of youth. JAMA 2001;285:3011–4.

[11] Haffner D, editor. Facing facts: sexual health for America's adolescents. New York: SIECUS; 1995.

[12] Sargent JD, Heatherton TF, Ahrens B, et al. Adolescent exposure to extremely violent movies. J Adolesc Health 2002;31:449–54.

[13] Paik H, Comstock G. The effects of television violence on antisocial behavior: a meta-analysis. Commun Res 1994;2:516–46.

[14] Gowensmith WN, Bloom LJ. The effects of heavy metal music on arousal and anger. J Music Ther 1997;34:33–45.

[15] Thompson RL, Larson R. Social context and the subjective experience of different types of rock music. J Youth Adolesc 1995;24:731–44.

[16] Gable RA, Magee Quinn M, Rutherford Jr RB, et al. Addressing problem behaviors in schools: use of functional assessments and behavior intervention plans. Preventing School Failure 1998;42:106–19.

[17] Cheng TL, Brenner RA, Wright JL, et al. Children's violent television viewing: are parents monitoring? Pediatrics 2004;114:94–9.

[18] Harrison KS, Cantor J. Tales form the screen: enduring fright reactions to scary media. Media Psychology 1999;1:97–116.

**ELSEVIER
SAUNDERS**

Child Adolesc Psychiatric Clin N Am
14 (2005) 571–587

CHILD AND
ADOLESCENT
PSYCHIATRIC CLINICS
OF NORTH AMERICA

Visual Narratives of the Pediatric Illness Experience: Children Communicating with Clinicians Through Video

Michael Rich, MD, MPH*, Julie Polvinen, BA, Jennifer Patashnick, BS

*Center on Media and Child Health, Division of Adolescent/Young Adult Medicine,
Children's Hospital Boston, 300 Longwood Avenue, Boston, MA 02115, USA*

The pediatric health care system is in flux. Because of dramatic increases in medical knowledge over the last several decades, many formerly fatal diseases have been prevented, cured, or transformed into chronic conditions. Many lives have been saved, but the prevalence of chronic disease has increased. Asthma and obesity have reached epidemic proportions [1–3]. Other conditions, such as spina bifida and cystic fibrosis, require long-term management and increasingly complex technology. Our successes in acute intervention have been shadowed by a continuing struggle to understand and respond to the different needs of patients who live with chronic disease.

Every day, patients with chronic conditions must deal not only with their disease but also with how their families, communities, and they themselves understand and respond to their condition. Biomedically similar patients can have different symptomatology, levels of disability, and means of coping. Disease is a biologic dysfunction, but illness is a social construct [4–8]. Children and adolescents who live with chronic disease are often separated from their peer groups,

Project/Investigator Support: This work was supported by the Arthur Vining Davis Foundations, the Deborah Munroe Noonan Memorial Fund, the John W. Alden Trust, the William F. Milton Fund, and Leadership Education in Adolescent Health Project #5 T71 MC 00009-12 of the Maternal and Child Health Bureau (Title V, Social Security Act), Health Resources and Services Administration, Department of Health and Human Services. Dr. Rich is supported by the National Institute of Child Health and Human Development through grant K23HD1296.

* Corresponding author.

E-mail address: michael.rich@childrens.harvard.edu (M. Rich).

doi:10.1016/j.chc.2005.02.013
childpsych.theclinics.com

infantilized by parents and clinicians, and, because of care provided with the best of intentions, prevented from maturing normally and developing autonomy. The contexts in which these young people live with illness, the social environments, relationships, and attitudes of others that they experience, and the ways in which they understand and cope with their conditions have profound and varied effects on their physical and mental health outcomes [9].

The origins of Video Intervention/Prevention Assessment (VIA)

Disease cannot be understood fully outside the context of a patient's life. This is particularly true in children and adolescents who are working through the important tasks of development while managing a chronic condition. We need better knowledge of patients' experiences, understanding, and management of their conditions before we are able to treat them effectively. Video Intervention/ Prevention Assessment (VIA) originated in the realization that to gain a better understanding of the pediatric illness experience, we needed to ask the experts— children and adolescents with chronic conditions. Combining techniques of video therapy [10] and therapeutic self-expression [11–14] with established qualitative research methods [15–17], we developed VIA as a child-friendly tool with which young people could teach their clinicians about their illness experiences [18,19].

Human experience is complicated, subjective, and fleeting, which make it a difficult subject to investigate. Constructivism theorizes that human experience and social realities are best examined from multiple perspectives and most accurately communicated through various media, including words, sounds, and images [20,21]. Video was chosen as the data collection medium because most children and adolescents, who have been brought up with television, are comfortable with electronic technology and may have more ease and fluency in relating their personal narratives in an audiovisual rather than solely verbal mode. Video therapy was first developed in psychiatry as a "technological mirror" through which patients could see themselves as they appeared to others, a technique that worked particularly well with adolescent boys [22]. Therapeutic self-expression was an approach to chronic disease management that included writing about traumatic experiences as a means of establishing mastery over one aspect of life to build self-efficacy. Designed to serve both of these functions and allow patients to become equal partners in their medical management, VIA encourages young people to show and tell the stories of their day-to-day lives, create visual illness narratives from their own perspectives, and focus on what they perceive as important.

As a research method, VIA is based in visual anthropology [23–25], the study of people and the human condition through images of and by them, which range from cave paintings to broadcast television. Since the invention of image-making technology, still photographs [26] and motion pictures [27,28] have been used by outside observers as tools for ethnographic study. Recent improvements, miniaturization, and simplification of imaging technology allow researchers to place cameras in the hands of the people whose lives are being studied [29]. Because the patients' perceptions of their condition are as critical to their symptomatology and outcomes as objective factors [4–9,30], a unique strength of the VIA method lies in the fact that it reveals the illness experience from the perspective of each patient. Building on the concept of the illness narrative [31,32] and applying techniques of participant-created visual research developed by Worth and Adair [33] and Chalfen [34,35] first with the Navajo and later with adolescent girls in a Philadelphia mental health clinic, VIA asks patients to create visual illness narratives—"video diaries"—of their lives with chronic disease and focus on their experiences of illness, health, and health care. Trained only in the technical aspects of "making the camera work," study participants produce raw but powerful images that contain a first-hand rendering of their experiences. Through audiovisual self-documentation of their experiences living with illness, patients can communicate more important information about their life experiences and their perceptions of those experiences than may be found in data collected and controlled solely by researchers or clinicians.

In many ways, VIA is as straightforward as it sounds: patients document their illnesses in the context of their lives to share with their clinicians. As VIA has extended and enriched the medical history, it has shed light on obstacles faced by patients of which clinicians were not previously aware. VIA has proved to be a remarkably flexible investigative tool that can be focused on a wide variety of conditions that bear on the physical, mental, and social health of young people.

Health care professionals traditionally have investigated and treated illness "from the outside in," studying its external features and responding to them with tools that generate a measurable response. This approach has been effective in the treatment of acute medical problems in which, traditionally, the clinician defines, diagnoses, and treats the disease. Chronic conditions, particularly those such as asthma and obesity that are environmentally or socially mediated, have not responded well to our current approach of clinician-centered care, particularly when there are time-limited clinician-patient interactions. Communication suffers and adherence wavers. We must acknowledge that it is patients, not clinicians, who manage chronic disease. They know their condition better than anyone; they can monitor it constantly. If patients feel that they are being heard and their goals are being met, they can take ownership of their condition, trust that their clinician will bring his or her knowledge and skills to bear on their concerns, and develop a true partnership in their care. This kind of care cannot be done "from the outside in." It is our goal to introduce VIA as a powerful and effective tool that can be used by any clinician or researcher who is interested in understanding a patient's experience "from the inside out" and evolving a care paradigm for the future.

Participant recruitment

Audiovisual recording of a patient's experience of illness generates rich, complex data that require significant time to collect and analyze, which limits the number of research participants. Unlike large epidemiologic studies that achieve generalizability through large study populations and statistically significant findings, qualitative inquiry seeks the universal in the few. Participants are exemplars of the population affected by the condition, patients who meet clinical diagnostic criteria and represent the population's diversity of gender, race, ethnicity, culture, and socioeconomic characteristics [36]. Most VIA studies are conducted in collaboration with a condition-specific specialty clinic, in which the VIA field coordinator works in close collaboration with a clinical case manager who knows and is trusted by the patient population. Before each clinic session, the case manager reviews the list of expected patients and notes all who fit the VIA study criteria. As part of the clinic visit, the case manager briefs the patients and their families on the study to see if they are interested in the possibility of documenting their illness experience through VIA. If they are, the clinician introduces the patients to the VIA field coordinator in the hopes of transferring some of the patient's and family's trust and opening the door toward an effective working relationship for VIA.

During this initial meeting, the field coordinator explains the VIA process, the focus of the study, and what is required for successful completion. The field coordinator makes certain that the potential participants are interested in and confident of their capability to meet the objective, which is to teach their clinicians about their experiences and needs by making a visual illness narrative. After explaining the study in detail, the field coordinator answers any questions the potential participants and their family may have and then asks them if they are interested in being involved in the study. If the potential participants agree, a later date is set for enrollment, usually within 2 weeks of the initial contact. A comprehensive medical and psychosocial history is obtained either directly from the patient in a clinical interview or from the chart, depending on the study. This standard of care clinical history, termed the "condition-specific verbal report," is compared with other data in the analysis phase.

Ethical considerations

Using audiovisual recordings of participants' lives as data requires that several unique features be included in the VIA informed consent process. As with any research that involves humans, written informed consent is obtained from each participant and from a parent or guardian if the participant is under the age of 18 years. The VIA informed consent contains a paragraph that extends the clinician-researcher's role as a mandated reporter of child neglect or abuse to what is revealed in the study videos. The only significant risk of the VIA method is a loss of privacy for participants, family, friends, and others who are potentially recognizable in the videos. Video data cannot be stripped of all personal identifiers, as is required of most research protocols under current patient privacy rules. In an attempt to protect participants' privacy and give them maximum control of their image and voice recordings, the VIA informed consent that is obtained on enrollment permits only the research and clinical teams to view and analyze VIA video data. On completion of their visual illness narratives, participants are provided VHS copies of their visual narratives. After being allowed to view the tapes and request the editing of any material with which the participant is uncomfortable, participants are asked for a written release of their image and voice recordings for dissemination in any medium, which allows their audiovisual data to be used for publication in online or print journals or books, radio and television broadcast, research presentations, and educational settings. All VIA study protocols have been reviewed and approved by the Children's Hospital Boston Committee on Clinical Investigation.

Enrollment

Enrollment occurs at each individual's home, where privacy can be maintained. The field coordinator reviews the informed consent sheet and allows participants, parents, or guardians to read through and ask questions before signing. Health-related quality-of-life (HRQL) questionnaires are administered to obtain a validated measure of participants' functional status, which is compared to the general population. Participants are taught the basic operations of the small, easy-to-use, consumer MiniDV camcorder: how to record, pause, load tapes, change and charge batteries, and aim the camera at the subject they want to record. Techniques for optimizing the image and audio pickup are discussed. For example, the field coordinator demonstrates why participants should not shoot dark silhouettes in front of a bright light source and may suggest that participants turn off a nearby radio or TV while they are conducting an interview so questions and answers can be heard. Once participants are comfortable with the camera and feel that they have an understanding of the goals of the study, they are ready to begin recording their visual illness narratives. Participants are supplied with contact information so that they can reach the field coordinator or another VIA staff member at any time should questions or technical problems arise.

Visual illness narratives

The most important goal of the visual illness narrative is for participants to tell their stories, from their own perspectives, in their own ways. Participants decide what to record and how to record it. Once participants understand this and take control of their self-documentation, this approach yields important information about the ways that they perceive their illnesses, how they respond, and what is most important to them.

In our experience, however, many young people "stall out" at the beginning of the VIA process. Having grown up with camcorders in their homes, they are comfortable with video but believe that it is for recording important events, such as birthday parties and graduations. They feel that their everyday lives are boring and uneventful. As a result, even when encouraged to document their daily lives, participants often do not know what to tape when they start their visual illness narratives. At the request of participants, we have developed a guide, a list of general suggestions of what to shoot, such as "a tour of your home, in which you show each room and describe it," and "taking medications and explaining why you take them and how they make you feel." Participants have responded well to the guidance, which helps them get started and provides documentation of common life experiences that the analysis team can compare among participants (Box 1). These "VIA shooting suggestions" have not directed the participants toward a more "produced" look or disrupted the individuality of their visual illness narratives, allaying our concern when we introduced them. Participants are free to tape the suggestions in any manner in which they are comfortable. Although we ask participants to record each suggestion, the list is designed as a

---

Box 1. Sample Video Intervention/Prevention Assessment (VIA) shooting suggestions and prompts

Shooting suggestions

>   A tour of your home (show each room and describe it)
>   Playing, hanging out, or fooling around with your friends
>   Daily meals (breakfast, lunch, dinner, and snacks)
>   A doctor/clinic visit

Interview prompts (participants' medical conditions in parentheses)

>   What do you know about (obesity)?
>   Do you think my doctors have helped me deal with (spina bifida)?
>   What do you think has gotten most in the way of me
>   doing better?
>   Do you ever feel people treat me differently because of
>   my (asthma)?
>   What worries you most about my (sickle cell disease)?
>   How does my (HIV) affect you?

Monologue prompts

>   How do you feel about what happened today?
>   What has been on your mind?
>   What really annoys you?
>   Do you think your friends treat you differently because you have
>   (cystic fibrosis)?
>   What do you worry about?

springboard for their own ideas. We encourage them to move beyond or even away from the suggestions if they have a better way of telling their story. Participants are in total control of the content of each tape.

In addition to documenting their everyday life experiences, VIA participants are asked to interview family members, friends, teachers, school nurses, and anyone else who knows them well. Participants are asked to elicit those people's perceptions of and experiences with a participant's chronic condition. Although the participants are encouraged to make the interviews as conversational as possible and ask their own questions, many young people find it difficult to formulate appropriate interview questions. To assist them, VIA provides a standardized set of condition-specific interview questions as prompts (Box 1). These questions address the interviewee's understanding of the participant's chronic condition, attitudes toward and beliefs about people with the condition, and observations and feelings about how the participant manages.

Finally, so that the participants can share their internal lives, they are asked to set up the camcorder each evening and speak to it directly about their experiences, observations, thoughts, and feelings. They are encouraged to relate the day's events and whatever else comes to mind, speak out loud their responses to events of the day, and voice their concerns, hopes, and fears. It is from the "personal monologues" that VIA has elicited some of the most unexpected and important insights regarding the feelings about, responses to, and meaning of living with a chronic condition.

To facilitate the participants' creation of the visual narratives, the field coordinator schedules regular meetings with each participant. The field coordinator visits each participant's home at least every other week and maintains contact by phone or email on a weekly basis, if not more often. If a participant is admitted to the hospital, the field coordinator establishes daily contact to facilitate recording the inpatient hospital experience and lend support. At each visit, the field coordinator tries to make participants feel comfortable and reiterates that they are in full control of the recording process and the content of the videotapes. Discussing the participants' progress in the study, the coordinator asks the participants what was taped previously and what they intend to tape next. He or she also determines whether participants need help setting goals for future taping. The field coordinator collects completed tapes, provides new blank tapes for the next week's recording, and addresses any technical or study-related questions.

The field coordinator's relationship with participants is based on communicating clarity of purpose for the study and building trust. Successful field coordination entails being able to initiate conversation with sometimes nonverbal teens, asking questions, and having a genuine interest in the participants' lives. At each visit, the field coordinator asks how the participants are feeling—physically and emotionally. Intermixed with study-related activities, the field coordinator tries to become better acquainted with each participant by learning their likes and dislikes, discovering what activities they currently pursue, and discovering their personal goals. An ability to listen, openness, lack of judgment, and kindness go a long way in establishing trust. A sense of humor, patience, and genuine personal respect are essential to supporting participants in revealing their life and expressing themselves on camera.

The field coordinator supports and encourages participants to feel free to show and tell as much of their lives as they are comfortable. One 18-year-old participant felt that his life was boring and did not understand why we would want him to videotape himself spending time alone in his room. The field coordinator explained to him that everything in his life is important to the understanding of how chronic conditions affect young people. Only by showing his life as he lives it on camera and by telling us as much as he feels comfortable will he be able to teach us why he is bored, why he feels the way that he does, and what his life is like in the context of his chronic condition. When he understood that he provided a unique window into an experience that clinicians otherwise do not know and when he realized that we intended to respond to the needs and concerns that he expressed, he was able to produce revealing video of his life. He showed, with sometimes painful intimacy, the limitations of spina bifida and the beliefs surrounding his condition that motivated him and his family.

A balanced relationship between the field coordinator and a willing and communicative participant, in which both parties acknowledge and value the role of the other, promotes the production of an honest and open visual illness narrative. Participants have individual and sometimes changing needs as the study progresses. Constant communication is essential between both parties for a better understanding of what those needs may be and how to address them successfully. As the weeks progress, the working relationship grows and trust builds between participants and the field coordinator. Participants become more receptive to encouragement from the field coordinator and, in many cases, they become more willing to share more personal, unseen areas of their life. At the start of her visual illness narrative, a 28-year-old woman said she hated her father and never wanted to show him on camera. With the support and encouragement of the field coordinator, she was able to move through her anger enough to record him briefly at her birthday party and playing with her dog. These brief scenes not only fleshed out the nature of their relationship but also indicated the therapeutic effect of VIA as a process of self-examination and reflection.

Participants typically require 12 to 16 weeks to complete a visual illness narrative. Most VIA studies have been based on the creation of a single visual illness narrative, the participants' portrayals of their lives with chronic conditions. The current VIA study, which examines the process of patients with function-limiting conditions as they transition from pediatric to adult-oriented care, is longitudinal and is based on three separate visual narratives: when they are in pediatric care, when they transfer their care, and once they are in adult-oriented care or, if they have not transitioned successfully, approximately 1 year after the creation of the second visual narrative. As a result of their transition schedules and depending on their readiness to re-enter the study, participants have a break between visual illness narratives that lasts 4 months to 1 year.

A visual illness narrative is complete when a participant and the field coordinator believe that the participant's story is told. As participants complete their goals for the visual illness narrative to the satisfaction of the field coordinator, they are asked if they have shown and told everything necessary to portray their experiences, responses, and needs. More time is allowed if a participant has more to express; otherwise an agreement is reached for a date on which to conclude. Over the three VIA studies to date, participants' visual illness narratives have ranged in length from 4 to 78 hours.

When participants feel that their visual illness narrative is complete, the camera gear is collected and the HRQL instrument is administered to determine whether any changes in a participant's quality of life have occurred during the creation of the visual illness narrative. Participants in the VIA study of asthma demonstrated statistically significant improvements in the HRQL after the self-examination process of VIA but before they or their clinicians had viewed or responded to the visual illness narratives [37]. These intriguing findings indicated that VIA, like video therapy and written self-expression, had a therapeutic effect on study participants. Interviews of the VIA study of asthma participants revealed that most of them felt that the VIA process helped them to pay more attention to their asthma symptoms and management, reconciled what they did with what they knew they should do, and addressed the frequently observed discrepancies between patients' health-related knowledge and behavior. Several participants noted that being entrusted with communicating their experience through video gave them the confidence that they could take control of other aspects of their lives. Attaining mastery of VIA increased their self-efficacy, which may have expressed itself in improved self-management.

Copying, reviewing, and preparing visual illness narratives for analysis

At each field visit, the field coordinator collects finished tapes from participants. In the week that follows, the field coordinator makes three copies of each original MiniDV tape, including one DVCAM digital master tape, one VHS tape with superimposed numerical readouts of the participant identification number, tape number, and frame-specific video time code (used to locate data in the logging and data analysis process), and one "clean" VHS tape (without numerical readouts), which is given to the participant.

While the copies are being made, the field coordinator takes notes on the content of each original tape and highlights areas to be discussed with the participant at the next site visit. If a tape reveals any reason to be concerned for a participant's physical or mental health, the coordinator immediately screens it for the principal investigator, who is a practicing adolescent medicine physician. This viewing of visual illness narratives as they are being produced helps the field coordinator to understand what is going on in each participant's life, provides topics for discussion, and gives him or her an idea of what the participant may be able to expand upon during that week's tapings. As an example, one 19-year-old participant taped himself taking his medications with a glass of water. He showed the pills and how he swallowed them but never explained what they were or why he was taking them. At the next site visit, the field coordinator praised the participant for showing his medications and asked if he would feel comfortable explaining more about the pills and their uses. This discussion encouraged the participant to speak more about his medical condition but gave him control of whether and how he wanted to record it.

Analyzing visual illness narratives

More than 1000 hours of audiovisual data have been produced by participants in VIA studies to date. These data are dense with information on a diverse variety of health-related topics that range from tangible features of their lives, such as the environments in which they live and the medications they use, to behavioral and psychosocial influences on their conditions, including dysfunctional family relationships and counterproductive explanatory models of disease [38].

Formulating a flexible yet rigorous method to analyze the visual illness narratives has been a crucial step in the development of the VIA methodology. There is no precedent for examining the type of data generated by VIA. First, the sheer volume of high-quality audiovisual information that is collected precludes any attempt to maintain and access it solely from computer and server storage. Second, there exists no previous research using participant-controlled intermittent documentation of continuous human behavior. As one of our participants re- minded us, "Sometimes when the camera is off, you don't see what I do outside of the camera work. I let you see whatever I want you to see."

Despite the challenges that it presents for analysis, this first-person point of view is one of the strengths of the VIA method. Because patients create their own visual narratives, VIA elicits objective and subjective information about young people's lives with illness. The objective data that the video captures are enriched by the subjective dimension of the patients' perceptions. Because VIA par- ticipants have control over the process of documenting their experience and are aware that their video will be seen, heard, and responded to, many of them engage powerfully with the creation of their visual illness narratives. They document the activities and rhythms of everyday life with chronic conditions, some of it remarkably candid and revealing of information hitherto inaccessible to researchers and clinicians.

Because VIA data are singular and unpredictable, we take a qualitative approach to analyzing the salient features of the pediatric illness experience. VIA is based in grounded theory [16,39], which examines and structures data to build theoretical models rather than use data to test a predetermined hypothesis. To optimize the analyses of these complex, variable data, VIA uses a multidis- ciplinary research team composed of medical doctors, public health researchers, clinical social workers, psychologists, and anthropologists. To examine the data through these diverse theoretical frameworks, we sought an analytical strategy that generated a multidimensional document that could respond to queries and observations from each perspective. The data must be managed and displayed in such a way that the original video and the analyses performed by all members of the research team can be accessed, structured, and analyzed with an approach that is inclusive and cumulative.

The first step toward analyzing VIA visual illness narratives is to document what is on each tape through the process of logging. Essential to the organization of the data is the discrete identification of each frame of VIA videotape by means of the participant identification number, tape number, and a running video time code in hours, minutes, seconds, and frames. Using these numbers, researchers can note the locations of each observation on the videotapes.

The logging of VIA data is a carefully structured, detail-oriented procedure similar to the transcription of audio tape. It includes descriptions of what is seen, what is heard (on and off screen), and from whose perspective it is seen and heard (who is holding the camera). Loggers record a dual stream of "objective observations" and "subjective accounts" to transform the visual narratives into the text format necessary for optimizing computer-assisted qualitative data analysis.

Objective observations record emotionally neutral data that are audible or visible and on which most observers would agree—descriptions of participants' appearance and behaviors, where they are, whom they are with, and any dialog that occurs. If the topic of conversation is related to the focus of the study or health-related issues, loggers record the dialog verbatim. Loggers are specifically cautioned to avoid editorial comments in their objective observations and refrain from making assumptions about relationships between individuals until proof of identity of each individual is established in the visual narrative.

Subjective accounts are loggers' responsive interpretations of the emotional tone or psychosocial dynamics of the scene. The purpose of subjective accounts is to capture the multifaceted nature of human experience and record the spontaneous thoughts and feelings elicited in loggers by the visual narratives, in much the same way a therapist uses autognosis as a diagnostic tool with a patient [40]. Because of a logger's gender, age, ethnicity, and life experience, all viewers may not necessarily agree with specific subjective accounts. To optimize reliability, each visual narrative is logged at least twice by different loggers. When loggers pay attention to the biases that they and others bring to their observations, they can acknowledge and counteract them. Subjective accounts of participant-documented private events allow us to value and document the observer's empathic response to the experience of another human being.

Loggers are encouraged to be scrupulous and detailed about objective data with their first logging pass to develop a comprehensive narrative spine on which to build with future passes. Additional logging passes may flesh out logs with details unnoticed on the first pass, add observations on a particular feature or question for which researchers have returned to the audiovisual data, or enrich subjective observations with what has been learned from other scenes in the visual narrative. This allows evaluation of the logs for synchronic reliability (ie, the reproducibility of observations made by different loggers) and diachronic reliability (ie, the consistency of observations made at different times) [41].

When the logs are complete, they are imported into NVivo (Qualitative Solutions and Research, Pty. Ltd., Victoria, Australia) qualitative data analysis software. NVivo allows researchers to analyze VIA visual illness narratives as a whole, compare various loggers' observations on the same audiovisual material, and compare the log of each participant with others from the same study population to derive broad themes. Emerging themes are coded as "free nodes," which are defined, modified, and refined by the research team at weekly meetings.

At best, the transcription of audiovisual data is an incomplete representation; it is essential to have ready access to the raw data. Because sheer volume would make it difficult to have the entire set of visual narratives accessible on a computer, VIA makes use of a feature of NVivo known as a Databite. Databites allow internal and external annotation to be added to the documents. Appearing as hyperlinks in the text, these "electronic sticky notes" enable researchers to create notes within the data, link to a Web page, or attach a file. During VIA analysis, Databites are used to attach raw video data to the appropriate passage in the log. This process permits quick and easy access to crucial video segments whose essence may not be captured by even the most thorough logging.

Once the logs have been coded, NVivo allows researchers to build conceptual relationships between nodes and structure free nodes into conceptual "trees" of related themes. NVivo can be used to meta-structure the findings and identify areas in which themes overlap by querying the data to examine specific areas of interest. An infinite variety of questions about the pediatric illness experience can be explored by combining node searches with demographic attributes. For example, medical and public health researchers can evaluate the VIA visual narratives for health-affecting features of participants' physical and psychological environments, medical self-management, and the nature and quality of relationships with health care providers. Clinical social workers can identify and explore obstacles to and facilitators of health, such as personal and familial attitudes toward disease, participants' ability to pay for medications and medical care, and barriers to health care access posed by transportation, language, or culture. Psychologists can assess participants' responses to their chronic condition, coping mechanisms and skills, health-related behaviors, and interpersonal dynamics with family and peers. Anthropologists can "read" the visual narratives and apply visual anthropology to understand how participants see, synthesize, and make meaning of their illness experiences and their worlds.

With access to the logs and the original videotapes, the VIA research team triangulates the visual narrative data with information from the condition-specific verbal report and HRQL obtained at the outset of the study. The visual narratives are compared with the condition-specific verbal reports to evaluate the participants' quality of recall and the accuracy of the clinical medical history. The condition-specific verbal reports add explicit and implicit nonvisible information to what is revealed by the visual narratives. The HRQL instruments provide quantified measures of physical and psychological health status so that participants can be located in relation to young people from the broader population with and without their chronic condition, while the visual narratives provide a "real-life" context for the HRQL scores. Overall themes that emerge from the three data sources are identified and areas of consonance and dissonance noted.

Summary

The pediatric illness experience is a complex subject that requires a multidimensional, flexible, and patient-centered approach. The VIA method, with its diverse source data and multidisciplinary analytical frameworks, generates findings that can be examined from any number of perspectives simply by asking different questions. As an exploration of human experience, VIA can be applied to various medical and psychiatric conditions. It has been used to investigate the experiences of children and adolescents who live with asthma [9,38,42,43], obesity [44–46], spina bifida [47], and diabetes mellitus [48,49] (Box 2). VIA currently is being applied to a longitudinal examination of the transition to adulthood by pediatric patients with spina bifida, cystic fibrosis, sickle cell disease, and HIV. A multicenter study of adolescents with eating disorders is being planned.

Beyond research, VIA methods may be applied in certain clinical situations, such as when it is not affordable or practical to send an environmental specialist to a patient's home to survey for asthma triggers or infectious causes, when a patient wishes to show the clinician health-affecting features of his or her lifestyle, or when an in-depth evaluation of a patient's psychosocial situation is needed. In advancing patient-centered care, VIA visual illness narratives created by young people who live with chronic medical conditions have proved to be valuable resources for educating clinicians and advocating with insurers and legislators.

The experience of illness has a potent effect on one's health-related attitudes, behaviors, and outcomes. VIA allows patients to show and tell about their illness experiences on their own terms and in their own words and images, which brings valuable information to the clinical relationship. Understanding the pediatric illness experience "from the inside out," seeing patients' goals, challenges, and needs from their perspectives, and recognizing that patients ultimately manage their own disease can redirect clinicians toward care strategies that are sensitive to and effective for patients in the context of their lives. Patients and clinician bring resources, knowledge, and skills necessary but not sufficient, in and of themselves, to manage their care. By developing a care plan in collaboration, each party is invested in a positive outcome and is willing to work through challenges and setbacks together. With this mutual exchange of information,

Box 2. Examples of findings from Video Intervention/Prevention Assessment (VIA) studies

Asthma

Known asthma triggers not identified in medical history were observed in 95% of homes

One or more inappropriate uses of medications were observed in 89% of participants' visual narratives; two or more in 44% [43]

33% of participants overdosed on medications, 28% discontinued medications without informing clinician, 72% had ineffective inhaler technique [43]

With biomedically similar disease, illness presented with varying degrees of disability, denial, self-comforting, and ''specialness'' [9]

Patients' asthma knowledge was excellent, but self-management was guided more powerfully by explanatory models derived from personal experience, anecdote, and cultural beliefs [38]

Asthma-specific quality-of-life measures significantly improved after participants completed VIA visual illness narratives but before they or clinicians saw the tape or changed management plans [37]

Obesity

92% self-comforted with high-calorie snacks [45]

100% were heavy media users and watched television or played video games for more than 4 hours/day [45]

''Unconscious eating'' of foods with high salt, sugar, and fat levels was related to oral stimulation rather than to hunger satiation and was associated mostly with television watching [46]

Psychological responses included sadness, isolation from peers, family conflict over food/weight issues, resentment toward entertainment figures who define attractiveness, and tantrums because diets denied them favorite foods [46]

Spina bifida

Participants with involved parents were more likely have a handicapped-accessible home, participate in physical activities, and be capable of some health self-management [47]

All involved parents revealed varying degrees of parent-child enmeshment: ''We can't move or we pee.'' [47]

Diabetes

Greater parental involvement was associated with better metabolic control [48]

Adolescent boys were much more private about diabetes management than girls [48]

Adolescents of both genders found diabetes and its management to be stigmatizing [48]

---

trust, and respect, patients can become effective partners with clinicians in improving their care.

References

[1] National Center for Health Statistics. Asthma attack prevalence and lifetime asthma diagnosis by age, gender, race/ethnicity and region/division, 1998–2002. Available at: http://209.217.72.34/asthma/ReportFolders/reportFolders.aspx. Accessed December 27, 2004.

[2] Hedley AA, Ogden CL, Johnson CL, et al. Overweight and obesity among US children, adolescents, and adults, 1999–2002. JAMA 2004;291:2847–50.

[3] Ogden CL, Flegal KM, Carroll MD, et al. Prevalence and trends in overweight among US children and adolescents, 1999–2000. JAMA 2002;288:1728–32.

[4] Sargent CF, Johnson TM. Medical anthropology: contemporary theory and method. Westport (CT): Praeger; 1996.

[5] Currer C, Stacey M. Concepts of health, illness, and disease: a comparative perspective. New York: Berg; 1986.

[6] Radley A. Making sense of illness: the social psychology of health and disease. London: Sage; 1994.

[7] Twaddle AC. Sickness behavior and the sick role. Boston: GK Hall & Co.; 1979.

[8] Morse JM, Johnson JL. The illness experience: dimensions of suffering. Newbury Park (CA): Sage; 1991.

[9] Rich M, Taylor SA, Chalfen R. Illness as a social construct: understanding what asthma means to the patient to better treat the disease. Jt Comm J Qual Improv 2000;26(5):244–53.

[10] Danet BN. Videotape playback as a therapeutic device in group psychotherapy. Int J Group Psychother 1969;19(4):433–40.

[11] Smyth JM. Written emotional expression: effect sizes, outcome types, and modifying variables. J Consult Clin Psychol 1998;66:174–84.

[12] Smyth JM, Stone AA, Hurewitz A, et al. Effects of writing about stressful experiences on symptom reduction in patients with asthma or rheumatoid arthritis: a randomized trial. JAMA 1999;281:1304–9.

[13] Pennebaker JW, Kiecolt-Glaser J, Glaser R. Disclosure of traumas and immune function: health implications for psychotherapy. J Consult Clin Psychol 1988;56:239–45.

[14] Pennebaker JW, Beall SK. Confronting a traumatic event: toward an understanding of inhibition and disease. J Abnorm Psychol 1986;95:274–81.

[15] Denzin NK, Lincoln YS, editors. Handbook of qualitative research. Thousand Oaks (CA): Sage Publications; 1994.

[16] Glaser BG, Strauss AL. The discovery of grounded theory: strategies for qualitative research. Hawthorne (NY): Aldine de Gruyter; 1967.

[17] Rich M, Ginsburg KR. The reason and rhyme of qualitative research: why, when, and how to use qualitative methods in the study of adolescent health. J Adolesc Health 1999;25(6):371–8.

[18] Rich M, Lamola S, Gordon J, et al. Video Intervention/Prevention Assessment: a patient-centered methodology for understanding the adolescent illness experience. J Adolesc Health 2000;27:155–65.

[19] Rich M, Patashnick J. Narrative research with audiovisual data: Video Intervention/Prevention Assessment (VIA) and NVivo. International Journal of Social Research Methodology 2002;5(3): 245–61.

[20] Goodman N. Ways of worldmaking. Indianapolis (IN): Hackett Publishing Co.; 1978.

[21] Gardner H. Gifted worldmakers. Psychol Today 1980;13(9):92–6.

[22] Furman L. Video therapy: an alternative for the treatment of adolescents. Arts in Psychotherapy 1990;17(2):165–9.

[23] Collier Jr J, Collier M. Visual anthropology: photography as a research method. Albuquerque (NM): University of New Mexico Press; 1986.

[24] Hockings P. Principles of visual anthropology. 2nd edition. Berlin: Mouton de Gruyter; 1995.

[25] Banks M, Morphy H, editors. Rethinking visual anthropology. New Haven (CT): Yale University Press; 1997.

[26] Bateson G, Mead M. Balinese character: a photographic analysis. New York: The New York Academy of Sciences; 1962.

[27] Flaherty RJ (producer), Flaherty RJ (director). Nanook of the north. Pathé Exchange Inc.; 1922.

[28] Balcon M (producer), Flaherty RJ (director). Man of Aran. Gaumont British Picture Corporation of America; 1934.

[29] Asch T, Cardozo JI, Cabellero H, et al. The story we now want to hear is not ours to tell: relinquishing control over representation. Toward sharing visual communication skills with the Yanomami. Visual Anthropology Review 1991;7(2):102–6.

[30] Rich M, Ruth AL, Chalfen R. Explanatory models of asthma: are beliefs about management more important than knowledge of disease? J Adolesc Health 2000;26(2):101.

[31] Kleinman AM. The illness narratives: suffering, healing, and the human condition. New York: Basic Books; 1988.

[32] Kleinman AM. Local worlds of suffering: an interpersonal focus for ethnographies of illness experience. Qual Health Res 1992;2:127–34.

[33] Worth S, Adair J. Through Navajo eyes: an exploration in film communication and anthropology. Albuquerque (NM): University of New Mexico Press; 1997.

[34] Chalfen R. A sociovidistic approach to children's filmmaking: the Philadelphia project. Studies in Visual Communication 1981;7(1):2–33.

[35] Chalfen R, Haley J. Reaction to socio-documentary film research in a mental health clinic. Am J Orthopsychiatry 1971;41(1):91–100.

[36] Mishler EG. Validation in inquiry-guided research: the role of exemplars in narrative studies. Harv Educ Rev 1990;60(4):415–42.

[37] Rich M, Lamola S, Woods ER. Quality of life with asthma: Video Intervention/Prevention Assessment (VIA) as intervention. J Adolesc Health 1999;24(2):151.

[38] Rich M, Patashnick J, Chalfen R. Visual illness narratives of asthma: explanatory models and health-related behavior. Am J Health Behav 2002;26(6):442–53.

[39] Strauss AL, Corbin JM. Basics of qualitative research: grounded theory procedures and techniques. Newbury Park (CA): Sage Publications; 1990.

[40] Messner E, Groves JE, Schwartz JH. Autognosis: how psychiatrists analyze themselves. New York: Year Book Medical Publishers; 1989.

[41] Kirk J, Miller ML. Reliability and validity in qualitative research. Beverly Hills (CA): Sage Publications; 1986.

[42] Rich M, Chalfen R. Showing and telling asthma: children teaching physicians with visual narratives. Visual Sociology 1999;14:51–71.

[43] Rich M, Lamola S, Amory C, et al. Asthma in life context: Video Intervention/Prevention Assessment (VIA). Pediatrics 2000;105(3):469–77.

[44] Corrado SP, Patashnick J, Rich M. Factors affecting change among obese adolescents. J Adolesc Health 2004;34(2):112.

[45] Rich M, Patashnick J, Huecker D, et al. Living with obesity: visual narratives of overweight adolescents. J Adolesc Health 2002;30(2):100.

[46] Rich M, Huecker D, Ludwig D. Obesity in the lives of children and adolescents: inquiry through patient-created visual narratives. Pediatr Res 2001;49(4):7A.

[47] Rich M, Patashnick J, Kastelic E. Achieving independence: the role of parental involvement with adolescents with spina bifida. J Adolesc Health 2005;36(2):129.

[48] Buchbinder MH, Detzer MJ, Welsch RL, et al. Assessing adolescents with insulin-dependent diabetes mellitus: a multiple perspective pilot study using visual illness narratives and interviews. J Adolesc Health 2005;36(1):71, e9-13.

[49] Buchbinder MH, Detzer MJ, Welsch RL, et al. Adolescents with type 1 diabetes: video narrative, interview, and provider perspectives. In: Proceedings of the Scientific Session of the 64th American Diabetes Association National Conference. Alexandria (VA): American Diabetes Association; 2004.

ELSEVIER
SAUNDERS

Child Adolesc Psychiatric Clin N Am
14 (2005) 589–602

CHILD AND
ADOLESCENT
PSYCHIATRIC CLINICS
OF NORTH AMERICA

The Use of Film, Literature, and Music in Becoming Culturally Competent in Understanding African Americans

Ardis C. Martin, MD*

West Central Mental Health Center, Canon City, CO 81212, USA

As an African-American physician, I have experienced personally and observed professionally how one's race and ethnicity can affect relationships between colleagues and patients. During my medical school and residency training, on many occasions I observed minority patients being treated differently from their majority counterparts. For example, African-American men often were perceived as more violent and dangerous and given higher doses of antipsychotic medication. They often were expected to have alcohol and substance involvement, gang affiliations, antisocial traits, and poor compliance with recommendations and treatment. These assumptions led to problems with the patient-physician relationship and affected the overall care of the patient.

These observations led me to learn more about the effect of race and ethnicity in psychiatric treatment. They also led me to explore alternative methods of learning about cultural competence and different ways of teaching it to help decrease these occurrences. In this article I explore (1) the persistence of racial and ethnic disparities in health care and expand on the idea that individual practitioners' underlying prejudices and stereotypes may contribute to these disparities; (2) the role that cultural competency and "race consciousness" can play in helping to decrease these disparities; and (3) the potential uses of film, literature, and music as methods of teaching cultural competency about African Americans to help practitioners in psychiatry better treat their patients.

Three seminal reports—by the American College of Physicians [1], the Institute of Medicine [2], and the Surgeon General [3]—discuss the continued

---

* 3765 Cherry Plum Drive, Colorado Springs, CO 80920.
  E-mail address: acmartin99@adelphia.net

1056-4993/05/$ – see front matter © 2005 Elsevier Inc. All rights reserved.
doi:10.1016/j.chc.2005.02.004

existence of racial and ethnic disparities in health care and possible causes for their persistence. In their article, the American College of Physicians reported that "disparities clearly exist in the health care of racial and ethnic minorities...and ample evidence illustrates that minorities do not always receive the same quality of health care, do not have the same access to health care, are less represented in the health professions, and have poorer overall health status than non minorities" [1]. The article also pointed out that these disparities exist even after adjustments are made regarding insurance and socioeconomic status. To improve the delivery of health care, they recommend improving access to affordable health care, practicing culturally competent care, creating a more diverse workforce of health professionals, and increasing the sensitivity of health care providers by helping them to recognize inherent biases that can lead to inequalities in the delivery of care.

In the article "Unequal Treatment," the Institute of Medicine described further that although many sources contribute to these differences, "some evidence suggests that bias, prejudice, and stereotyping on the part of health care providers may contribute to these differences in care" [2]. The authors postulated that these biases may exist in overt, explicit forms or unconsciously, but both may significantly influence how care is guided. Although there has been no direct evidence that provider bias affects the quality of care of minorities, research cited by the American College of Physicians suggested that health care providers' diagnostic decisions and their feelings about their patients are influenced by their patients' race or ethnicity.

The Surgeon General's supplemental report on mental health established the existence of disparities beyond general medicine to mental health. "Ethnic and racial minorities have less access to mental health services, are less likely to receive needed care, and when they receive care, it is poor in quality" [3]. The report points out such factors as cost of care, societal stigma, clinicians' lack of cultural awareness, bias, and client fear and mistrust of treatment as barriers to providing equal treatment. It also points to the fact that these disparities may stem from minorities' day-to-day struggles with discrimination. "Racism and discrimination are stressful events which can directly lead to psychological distress and physiological changes affecting mental health" [4]. For example, Krieger and Sidney [5] found that racism was linked to hypertension in African Americans. Kessler et al [6] found that racism was associated with psychological distress, major depression, and generalized anxiety in African Americans. These findings showed the impact that race and racism may have on patients and providers who are susceptible to the same biases as society. "Clinicians' attitudes often reflect the discriminatory practices of their society" [7].

The role of cultural competency

Understanding the impact of race and racism on society, patients, and providers may help alleviate these problems. Culturally competent care has been introduced as the key to achieving this goal. The Kaiser Family Foundation has documented the various ways that cultural competence has been defined [8]. The Department of Health and Human Services and Health Resources and Services Administration define it simply as "the level of knowledge-based skills required to provide effective clinical care to patients from a particular ethnic or racial group" [9]. Campinha-Bacote [10] goes a step further to define culture competency as a "process in which a nurse [provider] continuously strives to achieve the ability and availability to effectively work within the cultural context of the client, their family, or their community."

The process requires that providers see themselves as "becoming" culturally competent, rather than simply being so. It is misleading to think that just taking a class and hearing a few pieces of information are enough to provide improved care. A provider must play an active role in learning and continuing to learn. Toward this end, Watts [11] suggested the incorporation of the idea of "race consciousness" into this process of cultural competence. She defined race consciousness as "an awareness of the historical journey of the group, knowledge of disparities in health care for the people, and a self appraisal of one's attitudes and biases toward the group." In other words, she emphasized the importance of understanding where our patients come from—their experience of being who they are. Regarding African Americans, "race consciousness" would involve practitioners learning about such topics as slavery, the struggle for civil rights, the experience of discrimination, and the impact that these issues have had on their minority group patients. Practitioners also are encouraged to explore their own cultural background and their personal views about race and racism, to become aware of their own prejudices and stereotypes, no matter how subtle.

A new way to teach: using film, literature, and music

Through my own presentations I have found that the use of film, literature, and music can incorporate effectively the concepts of race consciousness in teaching cultural competence about African Americans. Literature and film often have been used in medical education to help stimulate discussion on such topics as morality, empathy, and ethics. Alexander et al [12] described several reasons for using movie clips in teaching. First, movies capture the attention through words, sight, and sound, which allow the viewer to experience the subject matter totally. Second, movies can expand awareness of diverse lifestyles of which the viewer may have little or no first-hand knowledge. This is important in trying to increase cultural awareness, because direct access to a particular group may not be possible. Third, movies engage the humanistic side of physicians and allow them to experience situations emotionally, which leaves a longer lasting impression. It is analogous to the association of a diagnosis with a person one has treated. Fourth, movies imprint visual images in memory and stimulate the symbolic and imaginative rather than just the linguistic and rational parts of the brain. This enables physicians to draw on the experience when faced with a similar situation in the future, providing a frame of reference for interacting with an ethnic minority patient—or at least reminding physicians to monitor and question their own assumptions so they do not interfere with the process of treatment. Finally, movie clips are time efficient: a short clip can generate many hours of discussion.

There are several examples in the research literature of the effectiveness of movies in medical education. Hyler and Schanzer [13] reported how movie clips were helpful in teaching trainees about borderline personality disorder. Self et al [14,15] emphasized that the practice of medicine is essentially the experience of a story. Their goal of using film was to increase trainees' ethical sensitivity through promotion of introspection (ie, looking at one's own thoughts, feelings, and sensations) and reflection on social issues. They specifically examined issues of reducing prejudice and increasing tolerance of others' differing values. The chosen films (eg, a 10-minute short film called "Walls and Walls") allowed trainees an opportunity to examine the role of caring through a vicarious affective experience and gain a sense of what it is like to walk in someone else's shoes. Based on student discussions and personal reports, the authors concluded that those goals were accomplished. Alexander and Waxman [16] and Blasco [17] explored how using movie clips allowed trainees the opportunity to explore their emotional reactions in a safe environment and helped them gain a better understanding of themselves in relation to their patients.

Music's influence in African-American culture

Although few articles have been written about the use of music to teach medical humanities or ethics, through my own experience I have seen how powerfully music can convey feelings and effectively teach about the African-American experience. Music long has been a source of spiritual strength, free expression, and guidance for the African-American community. During the times of slavery, songs were used to uplift the spirit and provide relief during a time of struggle and pain. Songs also could pass along secret messages and give guidance to persons who wanted to escape from slavery through the Underground Railroad [18]. Because of this history, music can build an emotional connection with and provide insight into the cultural history of African Americans. It also can be used to understand the current issues of African Americans. African Americans have used a wide range of musical genres, including country and western, gospel, R&B, rap, hip-hop, reggae, and blues, to tell their stories. Modern gospel music continues to be a source of strength in the African-American church to deliver praise to God, guidance to followers, and comfort and enlightenment in difficult times. It also reinforces the great importance of religion in the community. In secular culture, especially for African-American youth, hip-hop, R&B, rap, and reggae have provided blacks with an opportunity to express their story of struggle and that of their families, their experience of racism and discrimination, and, in some instances, their triumph against the odds. Many songs in hip-hop and rap express what life is like for persons who live in poverty and are surrounded by violence and how it affects them and those around them. It expresses what it is like to be faced with the issues of prejudice and police harassment and how people deal with these facets of our society. By acknowledging the importance of music in the lives of African-American youths, child and adolescent psychiatrists can be closer to understanding what issues are foremost in their patients' lives and the potential impact on their mental health.

For many young blacks who live in poverty and are exposed to violence and trauma, the discussion of these topics in the songs they listen to can help them feel that they are not alone. Black youths often express their anger and despair in the rap songs that they write. By asking their clients what they listen to and what it means to them, psychiatrists may gain their trust along with a better understanding of how they are coping with the exposure to these traumatic experiences. In my own practice I have seen how powerful the interaction can be when providers step out of their comfort zone to learn something from a client. This interaction also can help improve the self-esteem of the youth and provide an opportunity to show off his or her unique talents and intelligence via the different rhymes and songs. Some artists also voice to the younger generation stories about the accomplishments and achievements of blacks in American history that many African-American youth and their families would otherwise never learn about, which also improves their self-esteem. These artists and their songs also instill the sense of encouragement that dreams can come true and that they can accomplish anything. The following song lyrics provide examples of how music can be used to help practicing physicians learn about the history of African Americans and their struggles, contributions, and triumphs. These themes are evident in Bob Marley's song, "Buffalo Soldier":

> Buffalo Soldier, Dreadlock Rasta: There was a Buffalo Soldier, in the heart of America, Stolen from Africa, brought to America, Fighting on arrival, fighting for survival...If know your history, then you would know where I'm coming from, then you wouldn't have to ask me, who the 'eck do I think I am. I'm just a Buffalo Soldier in the heart of America, stolen from Africa, brought to America,
>> Said he was fighting on arrival, fighting for survival;
>> Said he was a Buffalo Soldier win the war for America... [19]

In Billie Holiday's song, "Strange Fruit," the tragedies and indignities inflicted on African Americans in the South are revealed through this hauntingly and beautifully expressed piece of work:

> Southern trees bear strange fruit, blood on the leaves and blood at the root, black bodies swinging in the southern breeze, strange fruit hanging from the poplar trees. Pastoral scene of the gallant south, the bulging eyes and the twisted mouth, scent of magnolias, sweet and fresh, then the sudden smell of burning flesh... [20]

These images, although remnants of the past, have not been forgotten in the lives of African-American families and their children. I have seen in my own family how these ideas are passed down via stories from elder family members about their fights against oppression and re-experiencing these events vicariously through them, leading to a continued sense of fear and distrust of majority culture at times. These are important points of which practitioners must be aware because they may explain the mistrust that their clients may have about them and the care they provide. It also may account for the sense of paranoia with which many African Americans are constantly faced because of this history, which affects their interactions with society, work, family, and medical/psychiatric treatment. By being aware of these subtle issues in the lives of their clients, practitioners may be more sensitive to clients' needs, not put off by rejecting behaviors (which may be based on their past experiences), and they may be better able to help patients process the pain of these occurrences.

In Louis Armstrong's song, "Black and Blue," he expresses the sense of confusion and pain that is experienced when one is not accepted and left to wonder what one has done to be placed in such a predicament:

> Even the mouse, ran from my house, they laugh at you and all that you do. What did I do to be so black and blue? I'm white inside but that don't help my case...That's life, can't hide what is in my face...How would it end, ain't got a friend, the only sin, is in my skin. What did I do, to be so black and blue? [21]

Stories of poverty, addiction, absentee fathers, living on the streets, violence, and survival are expressed in many of Tupac Shakur's songs, including "Dear Mama":

> Over the years we were poorer than the other kids...even as a crack fiend mama, you always was a black queen mama...no love from my daddy cause the coward wasn't there...seventeen years old kicked out on the streets...everything will be alright if ya hold on, it's a struggle every day, gotta roll on... [22]

Popular songs such as these may help practitioners better understand issues that may affect African-American youth and their families. By acknowledging these various stressors, they can empathize appropriately and help youths and their families more effectively.

A last example is Nas's song, "I Can, " which is an anthem of inspiration for today's youth, a warning about the pitfalls of drugs, sex, and violence, and a lesson on their history:

> I know I can, be what I want to be, If I work hard at it, I'll be where I want to be... you thinkin' life's all about smokin' weed and ice, you don't wanna be my age and can't read and write...be be, 'fore we came to this country we were kings and queens... [23]

Power of the written word

Literature written by African-American writers can help practitioners get a glimpse of the African-American experience. As with the rap songs and lyrics they write, African-American youth may express their feelings through poetry and journal writing, which can be useful in treatment. One of my adolescent patients often wrote rap/poetry as a way to express his feelings of anger, which helped him resist acting out his impulses at home and at school. It gave him an alternative outlet and a way to cope with issues about family and peer relationships. The following examples of acclaimed fiction and poetry by African Americans show different ways with which these artists have dealt with the prejudices and stereotypes of American society.

W.E.B Dubois's book, "The Souls of Black Folks," offers another view of the African-American experience and the effects of slavery on their psyches:

> It is a peculiar sensation, this double consciousness, this sense of always looking at one's self through the eyes of others, of measuring one's soul by the tape of a world that looks on in amused contempt or pity...One ever feels his two-ness— an American, a Negro; two souls, two thoughts, two unreconciled strivings; two warring ideals in one dark body, whose dogged strength alone keeps it from being torn asunder...He wishes simply to make it possible for a man to be both a Negro and an American without being cursed and spit upon by his fellows, without having the doors of opportunity closed roughly in his face. [24]

I personally still struggle with this concept of double consciousness in my daily life. This is a powerful theme that can have many deleterious effects on the self-esteem and identity of African-American youth who still have to struggle to be who they are. Often their race can affect their ability to get a job (eg, being paid less or turned away because of their color), have relationships (eg, interracial dating without family acceptance), go to school (eg, being seen as only an athlete or being ostracized for being smart by other minority students), and do everyday things such as going to the store (and being followed and expected to steal) or simply being unable to hail a taxicab. If practitioners at least can acknowledge how difficult it may be to be black and American, they will be able to listen more effectively to the subtle cues with which their clients may present. It is important for practitioners not to dismiss the issues of slavery and civil rights as belonging to the past and assume that they do not affect the current lives of their minority clients. Although things are better regarding overt racism, their clients still may be affected deeply by the subtler racism that still permeates our society and deserves to be taken seriously. Otherwise, they may risk losing patients in treatment.

Ralph Ellison's famous book, "Invisible Man," draws the reader into the world of the African American as he begins to understand, then accept, the role in which society has placed him:

> I am an invisible man. No, I am not a spook like those who haunted Edgar Allen Poe; nor am I one of your Hollywood movie ectoplasms. I am a man of substance, of flesh and bone, fiber, and liquids—and I might be said to possess a mind. I am invisible, understand, simply because people refuse to see me...you often doubt if you really exist... you ache to convince yourself that you do exist in the real world, that you are part of all the sound and anguish, and you strike out with your fists, you curse, and you swear to make them recognize you, and alas, it's seldom successful. [25]

This moving passage offers insights for practitioners treating African-American adolescents, who may have a greater sense of anger, sense of hopelessness about their futures, and difficulty trusting based on the lives they lead. These feelings affect not only patients who face the hardships of poverty but also patients who are educated, advance in society, and are still often subjected to racist remarks and unable to feel true acceptance. These issues speak to the stress under which African-American youth and their families find themselves, which may lead to increased symptoms of anxiety and depression.

In Maya Angelou's poem, "Still I Rise," one experiences the quest to and victory of overcoming the obstacles placed by society through determination, personal exploration, and faith:

> You may write me down in history, with your bitter, twisted lies, you may trod
> me in the very dirt, but still, like dust, I rise... you may shoot me with your
> words, you may cut me with your eyes, you may kill me with your hatefulness,
> but still, like air, I rise. [26]

As the "Invisible Man" described the difficulties of the African-American man, "The Color Purple," by Alice Walker described the experience of the African-American woman during the postslavery/pre-civil rights era, including the sense of powerlessness and fears about incest and abuse [27]. It also relays the continued struggle that African Americans faced to attain true equality, because despite the end of slavery, racism and inequality persisted. For practitioners it gives insight into the strength of African-American women who, during periods of slavery and even currently, have been forced to be the sole providers for their families. Understanding their many responsibilities helps in giving advice, setting forth treatment options, and understanding possible limitations. It also can remind practitioners to make use of all resources available, including the extended family. Often, aunts, uncles, and grandparents are left with the responsibility of raising children. By involving them, practitioners may have greater success in treatment. Creativity may be needed in instituting treatment, depending on the resources available to the family.

Pictures worth a thousand words

Finally, some films can be used to help practitioners learn about African Americans and about their own underlying assumptions. As with music and literature, movie clips can be used in discussion about cultural issues in psychiatry. Practitioners can take it upon themselves to personally look at different films, movies, and songs by African Americans to broaden their understanding, or it can be applied in a class in which group discussion can occur.

Jonathan Demme's movie, "Beloved," chronicles the story of one woman's escape from slavery [28]. We see the horrors of her experience while enslaved, her experience of freedom, her fears about returning into slavery, and the impact that the institution of slavery had on her and her family. One of the most striking scenes in the movie involves the character, Sethe, played by Oprah Winfrey, telling the story of what happens on her twenty-ninth day of freedom after escaping enslavement. Sethe initially seems happy and safe at her new home but then notices white men coming with chains. She recognizes one of them as her old slave master, School Teacher, and thinks,

> There's a look that white folks get, a righteousness that comes along with the whip and the fist, the burnin', the lie, long before it happens in the open.

Instead of allowing them to take her and her children back, she runs into the shed and tries to kill them one by one, even her infant child, because she would rather see them dead than enslaved. The scene shows School Teacher shedding a tear at what he has seen, which suggests that Sethe's children are biologically his. It also shows the look of astonishment on his face at what has happened and his total lack of understanding of why Sethe would go to that extreme to avoid returning with him. This film allows viewers to see the effects of slavery on African Americans and the effects of slavery as an institution on persons in power.

Alan Parker's movie, "Mississippi Burning," explores the story of three civil rights workers—two Jewish and one African American—who were killed in Mississippi [29]. We get a view of the African-American experience during the civil rights era: the continued struggle and the lives lost by African Americans and others who were working to bring an end to the practices of racism and inequality. The film enables practitioners to witness a continuation of the time line of the African-American experience. This movie also examines themes of religion and its importance. The scene opens with a black congregation singing praise to God in church while Ku Klux Klan members are preparing to ambush them outside. The scene ends with the congregation of men, women, and children being assaulted outside of the church. One young boy who is active in fighting for his civil liberties is kicked in the face by a Klan member while kneeling and praying, and he is told,

> You already been told once, n-gger, now we don't want to have to tell you again... you go making any more trouble by flapping them boot lips off to any of them federal men and we are going to put you in the ground, boy, and that's without a pine box.

Another scene that shows the overt racism that was prevalent involves three white Mississippi residents commenting on the treatment of African Americans. One of them responds to a question about how she thinks the Negroes in Mississippi had been treated:

> They're treated about fair, about as good as they ought to be... they aren't like us, they don't take baths, they stink, they're nasty, they just aren't like white folks...

By contrast, Spike Lee's movie, "School Daze," examines through the lives of African-American college students the divisions that can exist within the African-American community [30]. The movie offers a unique opportunity to see another side of the long-term effects of slavery and racism in the lives of blacks. It delves into the world of African-American self-hatred, intra-racism, and self-identity, and ultimately it helps us examine African-American views of loyalty to the race and what it means to be "black." One scene that beautifully lays out these themes opens when two popular girls on campus, one with lighter skin and the other with darker skin, meet in the hallway of their dormitory and exchange less-than-kind remarks. We are then transported to a fictitious beauty parlor, where a group of women with lighter complexions are seen wearing jerseys with the letter "W" for "Wannabes" and a group of women with darker complexions are wearing jerseys bearing the letter "J" for "Jigabos." The two groups of women then break into song, each deriding the other. The Jigabos, who also have kinkier "bad hair," are described as unattractive and stupid.

You're just a jigabo...trying to find something to do.

The Wannabes, who have straighter "good hair," are described as being ashamed of their race and thinking they are better.

You're just a wannabe...wanna be better than me.

The groups each attempt to express their sense of individual pride but are undermined by their perceived differences. These themes are unfortunate remnants of slavery, when slaves who were mixed (part white/part black) were given better opportunities (eg, education, work in the home versus the field). Some African-American youths still face being called a "white girl/boy" or an "Oreo" (ie, being black on the outside but white on the inside and acting white) and feel forced to prove their "blackness." Practitioners who work with African-American adolescents can be sensitive to the fact that these issues may cause problems with their self-esteem, affect their work ethic in school (being smart may lead to accusations of acting white), and affect the way they dress (wearing popular clothing versus traditional) and the way they speak (speaking slang versus proper English), because they do not want to be outcasts and seen as favoring white society over their black heritage. This understanding is crucial, because in adolescence being included and being part of a group is most important. By understanding the roots of these issues and the terms, practitioners can help their clients through these difficult situations and support them in being whoever they feel comfortable being rather than being what others want them to be.

In Steve Miner's movie, "Soul Man," we see the story of a young white American who is accepted to Harvard Medical School but is unable to go because his father will not pay for his tuition [31]. His solution is to darken his skin chemically to obtain a scholarship intended for an African-American applicant. Through his daily life as an African American, we are able to examine the way that blacks are seen through the eyes of majority society and the stereotypes that persist. Through his experience, the main character, Mark, is forced to face his own stereotypes and he becomes more sensitive to these issues.

One scene that emphasizes these issues involves Mark (played by C. Thomas Howell) going to his new white girlfriend's parents' house for dinner. While he is at their home, the mother, father, and little brother fantasize how they expect him to be. The mother fantasizes that Mark is extremely virile and waits in anticipation to be ravaged by him, and in her dream she hears him say,

> All my life, I've only been able to think about one thing...white women and now at last I'm going to have one.

The father fantasizes about Mark as a pimp and drug addict who will do nothing but abuse his little girl, and he sees his daughter impregnated and being told by the Mark to

> Go get my heroin and my hypodermic needle b-tch and get me some more watermelon while you're at it...white fat a-s slut.

By using comedy, the movie creatively exposes these stereotypes. It may help practitioners face and process their own underlying belief systems, with the goal of preventing these biases from entering into their treatment.

Finally, in Spike Lee's, "Do the Right Thing," the lives of locals in Brooklyn are chronicled as ethnic tensions among its members rise throughout the day and culminate in tragedy [32]. The movie examines different views of the African-American experience: relationships, identity, and activism. It also poignantly shows that everyone is prone to and guilty of acting on and treating others poorly based on underlying stereotypes and prejudices. One of the most powerful scenes begins in Sal's Pizzeria, where Mookie (the main character played by Spike Lee) works. Mookie has had problems with Sal's oldest son, Pino (played by John Turturro), who constantly makes racist remarks such as "How come n-ggers are so stupid?" Tired of this, Mookie pulls Pino aside and asks him to name his favorite musician, basketball player, and movie star. As it turns out, they are all black. Pino then describes how these people aren't "n-ggers." They are more than black.

This exchange draws on the idea of double consciousness and how difficult it is to be denied an individual identity and be maligned as part of a group—except for persons who reach a certain status, escape this mold, and are seen as "better." This is important when treating adolescents, because they are trying to figure out their identity while being faced with how society sees them: as part of their race, or different from their race, but not as a unique person. It is all the more difficult to form a healthy self-image when you and your race are seen in different—and at times demeaning—ways.

The scene ends with everyone in the neighborhood screaming racial slurs about each other. The blacks say about the Italians:

> You dago, wop, guinea, garlic breath, pizza-slinging...

The Italians about the blacks:

> You gold-teeth wearing, fried chicken- and biscuit-eating ape, baboon...

The Latinos about the Asians:

You little slanty-eyed, me-no-speaky the American...

The Asians about the Jews:

It's cheap, I got good price for you, chocolate egg cream, bagel and lox...

The whites about the Latinos:

You goya bean–eating, 15 in a car, 30 in an apartment...

These words remind the practitioner that along with any problems created by his or her own biases, a client's biases may interfere with the therapist-client relationship and affect compliance. They also highlight once more the importance of acknowledging our biases so that we may give our clients equal and excellent care.

Summary

As these examples show, books, films, and music can serve as windows into the experiences of African Americans. By adding a historical context to these experiences, practitioners are able to learn more about how these events affect the lives of their clients and their interactions with the world. Literature, songs, and movies also can help practitioners recognize their own prejudices, which is essential to delivering culturally competent care and may help decrease disparities in health care and health status.

As we seek to improve psychiatric care through cultural competency, there are caveats to keep in mind. First, the goal is not to use cultural competency to make practitioners change the way they see the world. Rather, the goal is to provide practitioners with the opportunity to be well informed, to challenge their beliefs, and to minimize unwarranted assumptions about the people with whom they interact and treat.

Second, although it is important to learn about a minority group's experience, it is crucial to consider and acknowledge each individual's unique experience. Each African American has a different take on his or her own experience as a member of the black race and is affected and interacts with the world differently. If we assume that what applies to one person in a group applies to all its members, we risk creating new harmful stereotypes.

For example, one of my Asian-American classmates learned how over-emphasis on ethnic identity can backfire. In a session with a new patient who was also Asian, she tried to speak to her through their commonality, thinking that the impact of being Asian and adopted into a majority-culture family was her primary issue. Instead, the patient saw that as secondary to concerns about her self-esteem and feelings of depression. This example reminds us to assess from our clients' perspective the pertinent issues that led them to seek treatment—not to assume that information learned about a client's background or an ethnicity or culture shared by therapist and client will lead us in the right direction. If there is a question or curiosity on the practitioner's part about the role that race may play, he or she should ask simply and respectfully, "Do you think some of the problems you are having at school are related to being one of the few African-American students here?" "Does my being [white] make it difficult for you to talk about the discrimination you have experienced?"

In conclusion, the goal of using different forms of media to become culturally competent in understanding African Americans and other minorities is to provide an enjoyable and interesting way to learn about a group's experience while respecting their individuality. Well-chosen media materials are powerful educational tools that can stimulate honest and open discussion. When I incorporate film clips and excerpts from literature and music into presentations on cultural competency, residents and staff report how effectively these words and images enhanced their understanding of African Americans and the issues they face.

> Through her presentations, Dr. Martin reminds us that the roots of psychiatry are a delicate juxtaposition of cultural understanding and resisting knee-jerk assumptions. By using popular film, music, and literature, she removes the controversy from the office and places it squarely in our culture as a whole. In this light, we can tolerate our short comings, and work without shame towards becoming better clinicians. (Steven Schlozman, MD, personal communication, 2004)

References

[1] Groman R, Ginsburg J. Racial and ethnic disparities in health care. Ann Intern Med 2004; 141(3):226–32.

[2] Institute of Medicine. Unequal treatment: what health care providers need to know about racial and ethnic disparities in health care [report brief, March 2002]. Available at: http://www.iom.edu/Object.File/Master/4/175/0.pdf. Accessed September 21, 2004.

[3] Department of Health and Human Services, US Public Health Service. Mental health, culture, race, and ethnicity: a supplement to mental health. A supplement to mental health: a report of the Surgeon General. Available at: http://media.shs.net/ken/pdf/SMA-01-3613/sma-01-3613.pdf. Accessed September 21, 2004.

[4] Williams DR, Williams-Morris R. Racism and mental health: the African American experience. Ethn Health 2000;5(3–4):243–68.

[5] Krieger N, Sidney S. Racial discrimination and blood pressure: the CARDIA study of young black and white adults. Am J Public Health 1996;86(10):1370–8.

[6] Kessler RC, Mickelson KD, Williams DR. The prevalence, distribution, and mental health correlates of perceived discrimination in the United States. J Health Soc Behav 1999;40(3): 208–30.

[7] Whaley AL. Issues of validity in empirical tests of stereotype threat theory. Am Psychol 1998; 5:679–80.

[8] The Henry J. Kaiser Family Foundation. Compendium of cultural competence initiatives in health care [compendium, January 2003]. Available at: http://www.kff.org/uninsured/loader.cfm?url=/commonspot/security/getfile.cfm&pageID=14365. Accessed September 21, 2004.

[9] US Department of Health and Human Services (DHHS). Health resources and services administration (HRSA): definitions of cultural competency. Available at: http://bhpr.hrsa.gov/diversity/cultcomp.htm. Accessed October 2, 2004.

[10] Campinha-Bacote J. Many faces: addressing diversity in health care. Available at: http://www. nursingworld.org/ojin/topic20/tpc20_2.htm. Accessed September 21, 2004.

[11] Watts RJ. Race consciousness and the health of African Americans. Available at: http://www. nursingworld.org/ojin/topic20/tpc20_2.htm. Accessed September 21, 2004.

[12] Alexander M, Hall MN, Pettice YJ. Cinemeducation: an innovative approach to teaching psychosocial medical care. Fam Med 1994;26(7):430–3.

[13] Hyler SE, Schanzer B. Using commercially available films to teach about borderline personality disorder. Bull Menninger Clin 1997;61(4):458–68.

[14] Self DJ, Baldwin Jr DC, Olivarez M. Teaching medical ethics to first-year students by using film discussion to develop their moral reasoning. Acad Med 1993;68(5):383–5.

[15] Self DJ, Baldwin Jr DC. Teaching medical humanities through film discussions. J Med Humanit 1990;11(1):23–9.

[16] Alexander M, Waxman D. Cinemeducation: teaching family systems through the movies. Fam Syst Med 2000;18:455–66.

[17] Blasco PG. Literature and movies for medical students. Fam Med 2001;33(6):426–8.

[18] National Geographic. The underground railroad. Available at: http://www.nationalgeographic. com/railroad/. Accessed September 25, 2004.

[19] Marley B. Buffalo soldier [song lyrics, 1984]. On: Legend [compact disc]; Polygram Records (USA). Song lyrics available at: http://www.oldielyrics.com. Accessed September 11, 2004.

[20] Allan L. Strange fruit [song lyrics, 1991; recorded by Billie Holiday]. On: Lady in autumn: the best of the verve years [compact disc]; Polygram Records (USA). Song lyrics available at: http://www.songlyrics.com. Accessed September 11, 2004.

[21] Razaf A. Black and blue [song lyrics, 1929; recorded by Louis Armstrong]. On: 16 most requested songs [compact disc]; Sony (USA). Song lyrics available at: http://www.lyrics007.com. Accessed October 2, 2004.

[22] Shakur T. Dear mama [song lyrics, 1998]. On: 2Pac greatest hits [compact disc]; Interscope Records (USA). Song lyrics available at: http://www.azlyrics.com. Accessed September 11, 2004.

[23] Nas. I can [song lyrics, 2002]. On: God's son [compact disc]; Sony (USA). Song lyrics available at: http://www.azlyrics.com. Accessed September 11, 2004.

[24] DuBois WEB, Gibson D, Elbert M. The souls of black folk. New York: Penguin Books; 1996.

[25] Ellison R. The invisible man. New York: Modern Library; 1992.

[26] Angelou M. And still I rise. New York: Random House; 1978.

[27] Walker A. The color purple. Orlando (FL): Harvest Edition; 2003.

[28] Saxon E, Demme J, Goetzman G, et al. Beloved [motion picture]. Burbank (CA): Touchstone Pictures; 1998.

[29] Zollo F, Colesberry RF, Parker J. Mississippi burning [motion picture]. Santa Monica (CA): Metro Goldwyn Mayer; 1989.

[30] Lee S, Lee S. School daze [motion picture]. Culver City (CA): Columbia Pictures; 1988.

[31] Tisch S, Miner S. Soul man [motion picture]. Troy (MI): New World Pictures; 1986.

[32] Lee S, Lee S. Do the right thing [motion picture]. Universal City (CA): MCA/Universal Pictures; 1989.

ELSEVIER
SAUNDERS

Child Adolesc Psychiatric Clin N Am
14 (2005) 603–612

CHILD AND
ADOLESCENT
PSYCHIATRIC CLINICS
OF NORTH AMERICA

How and Why for the Camera-Shy: Using Digital Video in Psychiatry

Richard L. Falzone, MD[a,b,*], Sarah Hall, BS[a,b],
Eugene V. Beresin, MD[a,b,c]

[a]*Division of Child and Adolescent Psychiatry, Department of Psychiatry,
Massachusetts General/McLean Hospitals, 15 Parkman Street, Boston, MA 02114, USA*
[b]*Department of Psychiatry, Harvard Medical School, 25 Shattuck Street, Boston, MA 02115, USA*
[c]*Harvard Medical School Center for Mental Health and Media, Massachusetts General Hospital,
Boston, MA 02114, USA*

Even when optimally attentive, we can only register, much less recall, a small fraction of what transpires during therapy sessions. We leave the office with the sense that we understood our patients, that we were reasonably empathically attuned, made useful responses, and more or less helped the patients. What might we do differently if we had the chance to roll back the hour and watch ourselves doing therapy? What might we discover about our patients and how we are relating to them? What might our patients discover about themselves and how they come across to others?

Our purpose in writing this article is to demonstrate that desktop video is well suited to the work of psychotherapy and is accessible to the interested clinician. It may prove especially helpful in working with children and families, for whom a wealth of observable material is nonverbal. First, we survey the use of video by several clinicians from different disciplines in psychotherapy. Next, we review a study that evaluates the effect of videotaping on therapist performance. We then examine the issues of confidentiality and informed consent relevant to videotaping psychotherapy. Finally, we offer a basic primer on videotaping psychotherapy and an introduction to digital video editing.

* Corresponding author. Division of Child and Adolescent Psychiatry, Department of Psychiatry, Massachusetts General/McLean Hospitals, WACC 725, 15 Parkman Street, Boston, MA 02114.
E-mail address: mail@rfalzone.info (R.L. Falzone).

1056-4993/05/$ – see front matter © 2005 Elsevier Inc. All rights reserved.
doi:10.1016/j.chc.2005.02.006 *childpsych.theclinics.com*

As noted by the Boston Change Process Study Group [1]:

> The usual way of discussing analytic material is in narratives reconstructed by the analyst from memory or with the aid of notes taken during the session. However, videotape observations reveal that these narratives fail to capture many of the micro-events of the complex, multilayered interactive process.

By harnessing the persuasive power of self-observation, video technology provides a scalpel for cutting through denial and a clarifying lens for correcting distorted perceptions. During a psychotherapy session the video camera acts as a silent scribe, tirelessly recording the myriad communications—verbal and non-verbal, conscious and unconscious, perceived and unnoticed—that pass between the human actors. Video provides a nonjudgmental mirror and helps to illuminate blind spots and identify missteps and missed opportunities. For teaching and presentation, concisely edited video vignettes provide clarity and hold an audience's attention.

In discussions with colleagues we noted several themes regarding the use of taping in our child psychiatry service. One analytic supervisor marveled at the efficiency of watching session tapes, noting that usually many weeks must pass before a supervisor has a feel for what is happening between patient and trainee (Martin Miller, MD, personal communication, 2004). Another senior supervisor commented on the amount and variety of nonverbal material available for exploration and review: how the patient looked, moved, and expressed affect; how the therapist attended, responded, and so on (Jacqueline Olds, MD, personal communication, 2004).

Video and therapist development

Videotaping has proved useful within and beyond the formal training period. In a review of the status of short-term dynamic psychotherapy, Peter Sifneos [2] lauds the benefits of videotaping:

> The advent of the videotape has revolutionized evaluation, technique, and outcome research in the whole field of psychotherapy...I furthermore have emphasized that the videotape has become "the microscope" which psychiatry has lacked in the past and have used it extensively in my workshops throughout Europe and North America.
>
> For the education of trainees there is no better teaching tool for the study of the process of short-term dynamic psychotherapy and for the follow-up research. Nothing can be more impressive to students than to look at their teachers interviewing or treating patients both live and on videotape. The tapes can be scrutinized repeatedly and can also be shown on a continuous basis to demonstrate the process of the therapy.

Sifneos believes so strongly that videotaping is useful and suited to psychotherapy that he describes the lack of enthusiasm for videotaping by some workers in the field as peculiar.

Daniel Sweeney [3] advocates for the use of video in play therapy and comments on its importance for clinical supervision and professional growth. He encourages clinicians to continue videotaping beyond training to maintain a "professional edge":

> ...there is simply no better way in which to review play therapy skills and therapeutic progress than taping and reviewing sessions. Simply knowing that a play therapy session is being taped tends to heighten the therapist's awareness and dedication to the process.

Video as a therapeutic tool

Although enhancing therapist development indirectly benefits patients, video also has been used directly with patients and families as a novel and effective therapeutic tool. The power of self-observation is illustrated in a study in which the authors describe their use of videotaping while working with a particularly challenging population of chemically dependent patients [4]. In the context of a structured cognitive-behavioral cocaine treatment program, patients, after being taught how to operate a video camera, recorded three individual sessions that represented the beginning, middle, and end phases of a 6-month therapy period. In individual sessions after each of the taping sessions, participants watched themselves on tape and were asked open-ended questions that encouraged self-reflection. This therapy format provided numerous opportunities for patients to express strong feelings in a contained, supportive, nonjudgmental setting. The authors found video particularly useful for engaging this difficult population and noted that these patients are often defensive and resistant to attempts at helping them see the destructive nature of their behavior.

> We have found that video feedback is experienced by patients as intense yet neutral and nonjudgmental. Through the distance it allows, patients are helped to begin the process of commenting on themselves. The value in having patients comment on themselves spontaneously is that it allows for less defensiveness and less rejection of the therapist's observations. As the observation comes first from the patient, this technique spares the therapist from being seen as critical.

The authors observed that videotaping is particularly useful for patients with a limited capacity for self-observation, and they speculated that cognitive restructuring occurs through helping patients adopt a more objective, observing stance. They emphasized the importance of therapist attunement and highlighted that it is the therapist's responsibility to contain the emotion generated as patients view and begin to accept unsavory aspects of their behavior. As therapist and patient review the taped sessions together, the therapist is advised to watch for opportunities to offer positive observations to balance a patient's self-deprecatory tendencies.

In another study that involved video feedback, investigators recorded youths with mild mental retardation and behavior problems and then reviewed the tapes with them [5]. Participants were rewarded for identifying their behaviors and classifying them as appropriate or inappropriate. After seeing themselves on tape, the clients' capacity to self-monitor improved and the frequency of inappropriate behaviors decreased. Importantly, these improvements generalized across settings. The authors speculated on what factors specific to videotaping may have contributed to the behavioral improvements observed in the study.

> Several reasons may explain the effectiveness of the present procedure. First, video feedback and self-management procedures may have operated as a positive reinforcement for appropriate behavior of the participants during lunch, dinner, and group meetings. Second, participants may have decreased their target behavior because the presentation of feedback served as a punisher.

Beatrice Beebe [6] has written extensively on the microanalysis (detailed frame-by-frame review) of videotaped mother-infant interactions from a psychoanalytic perspective. Using dual cameras, one focused on the mother and the other on her baby, a face-to-face split screen recording of the interaction is obtained. Later, mother and therapist together review segments of the tape in minute detail to understand and correct disturbed interaction patterns between mother and infant.

> Microanalysis of behavior operates at a level of detail and specificity that is richly useful to the mother-infant clinician, moving the treatment out of vague complaints (my baby does not like me) into exact behaviors, and how they are interactively as well as self-regulated. The advantage of watching the videotape with the mother, informed by interaction sequences revealed by microanalysis, is that the behavioral details then become the springboard for associations, reflections, memories, and insights into the meanings of these behaviors...There is no time to waste in a mother-infant disturbance, and this method goes directly to the core interactional dynamic.

Beebe identified positive reinforcement, modeling, information giving, and interpretation as key elements of learning, which are facilitated by watching the videotape with the therapist.

Terry S. Trepper [7] has written extensively in the field of marriage and family therapy. In a paragraph entitled "A videotape is worth a thousand words," he wrote:

> I believe that the critical incident—the showing of a videotape of a recent therapy session—indeed was a serendipitous turning point in therapy. Showing the family the videotape was an insight-oriented intervention presented in a way that they could 'hear.'

Trepper discussed the role of videotape in enhancing the spectator's role [7].

> ...after-session videotapes also can let people see how they affect others in a way that is not possible during the in vivo interaction itself. The reality of the current age of technology shared by most clients: an experience is more powerful, more 'valid,' and ironically more 'real' if it is seen on a television screen. This may be particularly true for children and adolescents, whose attention definitely will be far more focused when watching their family on a video monitor than it would be were it occurring 'live.'

Working from an educational counseling perspective, Getz and Nininger [8] emphasize the importance of responsibility assumption in therapeutic change. Citing several other family therapists, they noted that patients who see their own dysfunctional communication patterns on videotape are more willing to take responsibility for their contribution to the problem. In one family case they described how "videotaping appeared to be the key to unlock the blocked-communication patterns" between a mother and her grade school–aged son.

Irvin Yalom [9], who has written extensively on individual and group psychotherapy and who has published teaching videos on group process, described the benefit of providing patients in individual therapy with audiotapes, which enabled them to review the previous session [10]. This is one method he uses to keep therapy moving forward, true to his belief that "therapy works best if it approximates a continuous session."

Effect on the therapist

How does videotaping affect the therapy session? In our experience we have found that in early sessions both parties are acutely aware of the camera, but this awareness passes quickly as they "consciously forget" that the camera is present.

Ellis et al [11] wanted to know whether videotaping adversely affected therapist performance in a supervisory setting, noting that prior studies had yielded equivocal results. In a carefully controlled experiment, the authors found that videotaping an initial counseling session (when anxiety could be expected to be highest) did not significantly increase therapist anxiety or decrease performance. It was hypothesized that the counselor is motivated to avoid self-focusing stimuli and attend more fully to the patient. The authors speculated that relationship-building activities and demands overpower the potential distraction of videotaping.

Consent and confidentiality

Before videotaping is undertaken, therapist and patient must be clear about the reasons for recording the sessions. When ambiguity exists about who will view the tapes, whether the patient will see the tapes, or who ultimately will have possession of them, it is more difficult to regain spontaneity and further the work of therapy. This issue is related closely to the question of patient selection for videotaping. Although it is permissible to videotape any competent patient who consents to being recorded, in some cases it is not a good idea. For example, patients with paranoia, psychosis, or personality disorders may not be suitable for videotaping early on, although many of these patients might become suitable for—and benefit from—videotaping later in therapy. In short, bringing a camera into the room presents an additional challenge in building a therapeutic alliance.

The process of obtaining informed consent occurs over time and involves discussions about the purpose, risks, and benefits of videotaping. These discussions are noted in the patient's progress notes. A signed consent form should be placed in the patient's record and should specify (1) how the tapes will be used (eg, supervision and clinical training, academic lectures, marketing and public relations, therapeutic review with the patient), (2) what audiences will view the tapes, (3) whether the tapes are considered part of the medical record, (4) whether and when the tapes will be destroyed, (5) how the tapes will be stored (eg, in a locked cabinet in a secured area of the clinic), (6) what personal and clinical data may be revealed in the tapes, and (7) the fact that the patient may withdraw consent for taping or for one or more uses of the tapes and request that the tapes be destroyed at any time. It is a good idea to review consent forms with legal counsel or other administrative leader in one's home institution.

In the case of videotaping therapy with children, assent from a child is as important as consent from the parents. Respect for confidentiality mandates that a child must understand and agree with the purpose for videotaping, as with adult patients. The parents must agree that they will not be allowed to view the tapes unless the child gives permission to do so.

Videotaping provides the competent, ethical therapist with more protection than liability because the videotape is a durable record of what transpired during the session. Daniel Sweeney is a psychotherapist who often works with physically and sexually traumatized children. He notes that it is easy to imagine a scenario in which a child, in describing sexualized play during a session, could be misunderstood and that "a videotaped record of the session would circumvent the question of unprofessional behavior, and avoid the risk of damage to professional reputation and licensure" [3].

Videotaping psychotherapy

Minimally, all that is required to record a diagnostic interview or a therapy session are a video camera, tripod, and television for playback. Video cameras have dropped significantly in price in recent years. Current digital technology offers several advantages over older analog formats, such as VHS, which has fewer lines of resolution and degrades significantly in quality when copied. In contrast, digital information can be recorded, copied, compressed, stored, transmitted, and played back with little distortion or degradation.

Modern video cameras record well in typical office lighting situations. One should keep table lamps and other bright sources of light out of the shot. The camera's automatic functions—focus, white balance, shutter speed, and exposure—are useful for recording in rapidly changing environments, such as birthday parties or soccer games. Although psychotherapy is often dynamic, it is not usually kinetic (play therapy excepted), and for this reason it is preferable to use the camera's manual settings. This method prevents the annoying "swimming" effect that occurs as the camera hunts for the proper focus and light level whenever there is movement in front of the lens. This also applies to the camera's white balance function, which compensates for the color temperature of the ambient light. (Although our brains automatically adjust to different color temperatures of light, video cameras do not. Compared to each other, incandescent lamps have a reddish tinge, daylight has a bluish tinge, and fluorescent lamps have a greenish tinge.) Once the camera is turned on and allowed to adjust, the automatic functions are switched to manual to ensure image consistency while taping during the hour.

The therapist should experiment with placing the camera in different locations in the office. Looking through the viewfinder, one should frame an individual (patient or therapist) so there is a comfortable amount of space, or "nose-room," between the subject's head and the edge of the screen. Depending on the space available, and especially if one is trying to film the therapist and patient, it may be necessary to use a camera equipped with a wide-angle lens.

Attention to sound quality is important for picking up verbal nuances. The camera's built-in microphone works well in a quiet office when the subject is facing the camera. Many mid-range video cameras have input jacks for external microphones, which can improve sensitivity. A shotgun microphone is useful for focusing on an area in play therapy situations. Lapel-mounted lavaliere microphones offer excellent sound quality but may remind patients that they are on camera. Boundary or pressure-zone microphones are designed to sit on or be mounted to flat surfaces, such as tables or wall panels. They can be placed discreetly and capture speech well. The key recommendation is to bring the microphone as close to the subject's mouth as feasible, because sound level drops exponentially as a function of distance from the source.

Introduction to digital editing

Whether reviewing tapes for supervision or therapeutic treatment with patients, editing allows for the removal of tedious or irrelevant segments to improve efficiency and maintain interest. For teaching and professional presentation, concisely edited vignettes can convey complex, subtle clinical details far more effectively than static slides.

Personal computers have advanced to the point that an individual can produce videos that rival what would have required a $100,000 production studio just 10 years ago. Until recently, video and film production was done in a step-wise, linear fashion, working from the beginning of a project to the end. Specialized tape decks were used to edit segments together, and extra equipment was needed for transitions such as dissolves from one scene to another or digital effects. This process required much planning and expense and made modification of a project more time consuming.

In contrast, digital video editing, or desktop video, is "nonlinear." It allows the editor to trim, move, and rearrange the order of video segments as easily as a writer moves sentences and paragraphs around in a word processor document.

The basic process of desktop video involves connecting the video camera to a computer using a high-speed data cable and transferring the data to the computer's hard drive. (FireWire or USB-2 connections allow for high-speed streaming data transfer. FireWire is Apple Corporation's name for the IEEE-1394 protocol, which is called iLink by Sony Corporation. FireWire supports data transfer rates up to 400 megabytes per second (Mbps); Firewire-2 supports up to 800Mbps. USB (universal serial bus) supports rates up to 12Mbps (too slow for some video applications); USB-2.0 supports up to 480Mbps.) Many excellent video editing programs are available for Windows-based and Macintosh personal computers, and they all work similarly. DVD authoring takes this one step further and allows the therapist to create sophisticated, menu-driven, interactive presentations. Most popular bookstores have a section dedicated to desktop video, and many good introductory books are available [12,13].

The power of editing is tremendous, as it allows for the distillation of key information and the removal of distracting or extraneous material. The purpose for taping dictates what is of interest. For example, from a collection of taped sessions one could put together clips of the opening or closing moments to focus on patient (or therapist) behavior at the time boundaries. Other areas of focus might include the tracking of eye contact, approach/avoidance behavior, periods of affective arousal, response to interpretations, and evidence of synchronicity with the therapist. The list is endless.

Future directions and challenges

As we have demonstrated, digital video can be a remarkably useful tool in psychiatry. Given the complexity of human behavior, more attention must be directed at codifying and classifying interpersonal interactions in this medium. Although it has been done for research purposes, few attempts have been made to define techniques that allow for valid and reliable observations by clinicians, patients, and students. There are many reasons to pursue efforts to achieve these goals. We see the use of digital video as an exceptional tool for treatment, research, performance evaluation, and clinical training. Some uses in the context of therapy have been mentioned. The potential uses of digital videotaping for research are myriad and beyond the scope of this article. We offer some thoughts about the use of video in evaluation of clinical skills and in education, however.

In recent years, increasing attention has been given to the assessment of competencies in medicine. Progressive growth in knowledge, skills, and attitudes is mandated for medical school curricula, graduate medical education, and postgraduate life-long learning. Six broadly defined core competencies of patient care, medical knowledge, professionalism, interpersonal and communication skills, practice-based learning, and systems-based practice have been instituted for all accredited graduate medical programs [14], and this model is being considered by numerous medical schools. In psychiatry residencies, demonstrated competency in psychotherapies is a current requirement [15]. Digital video can be a superb medium for the assessment of a wide range of competencies in psychiatry, including skills in patient care, interviewing, application of the various therapeutic modalities, and assessment of case presentations. The American Board of Psychiatry and Neurology has used videotapes of clinical interviews for certification examinations. Medical schools have a long history of using videotape for teaching students about clinical interviewing. Despite these current and potential uses, there are few standardized ways of viewing and evaluating tapes. Research is needed in developing systems of observation that can be generalized across institutions and for different evaluation purposes.

As evidence-based medicine widens and deepens, digital video, properly used, may be another way of accumulating and disseminating evidence about best practices. Although the American Psychiatric Association and the American Academy of Child and Adolescent Psychiatry have produced practice guidelines and practice parameters, respectively, in the evaluation and treatment of many psychiatric disorders, they have not used video as a means to assist the profession in interviewing, diagnosing, and treating. One potential addition to the literature on clinical standards of care—supplementing print media—may be digital video demonstrations of best clinical practices.

Virtually all medical institutions are required to administer annual performance evaluations of clinicians as a part of quality assurance and improvement and credentialing. These evaluations are intended to give practitioners feedback about their strengths and weaknesses and to ensure that competent, professional care is being provided. That is another situation in which digital video may be useful.

Finally, there is a wealth of opportunities for using digital video in clinical education. Using this technology, many academic centers are able to create teaching libraries for use in clinical seminars. Faculty supervisors from diverse fields (eg, psychopharmacology and family therapy) can select from a menu of clinical vignettes, view segments with trainees, and comment from the perspectives of their various disciplines. This allows trainees to ask questions and integrate complementary (and sometimes conflicting!) information in a way not easily achieved before this technology was available. Digital video is easily integrated with commonly used digital graphic slide presentations (eg, Powerpoint). Many universities have Websites on which articles, lectures, and digital video are accessible to students, residents, faculty, and staff. Given the current universal accessibility of digital media through personal desktop computers, wireless laptop computers, and personal hand-held devices, the scope of clinical education is limitless.

Acknowledgments

The authors wish to express their gratitude to Dr. Larry Kutner for his thoughtful comments and review of the technical section of the article; to Dr.

Steve Schlozman for his support and guidance; and to videographer Dave Peterson for his technical advice.

References

[1] The Boston Change Process Study Group. Explicating the implicit: the local level and the microprocess of change in the analytic situation. Int J Psychoanal 2002;83:1052–62.

[2] Sifneos P. The current status of individual short-term dynamic psychotherapy and its future: an overview. Am J Psychother 1984;38(4):472–83.

[3] Sweeney D. Legal and ethical issues and play therapy. In: Landreth G, editor. Innovations in play therapy. New York: Brunner-Routledge; 2001. p. 65–81.

[4] Seligman M, Foote J, Magura S, et al. Video techniques with chemically-dependent patients. Subst Use Misuse 1996;31(8):965–1000.

[5] Embregts P. Effectiveness of video feedback and self-management on inappropriate social behavior of youth with mild mental retardation. Res Dev Disabil 2000;21:409–23.

[6] Beebe B. Brief mother-infant treatment: psychoanalytically informed video feedback. Infant Ment Health J 2003;24(1):24–52.

[7] Trepper T. Commentary: show me one more time. In: Baptiste D, editor. Clinical epiphanies in marital and family therapy. New York: Haworth Press; 2002. p. 217–20.

[8] Getz H, Nininger K. Videotaping as a counseling technique with families. Family Journal 1999;7(4):395–8.

[9] Wyatt R, Yalom I. Understanding group psychotherapy [videotape]. Pacific Grove (CA): Brooks Cole Publishing; 1991.

[10] Yalom I. The gift of therapy: an open letter to a new generation of therapists and their patients. New York: HarperCollins; 2002.

[11] Ellis M, Beck M, Krengel M. Testing self-focused attention theory in clinical supervision: effects on supervisee anxiety and performance. J Couns Psychol 2002;49(1):101–16.

[12] Gaskel E. The complete guide to digital video. Boston: Muska and Lipman Publishing; 2003.

[13] Rice J, McKernan B. Editing digital video: the complete creative and technical guide. New York: McGraw Hill; 2003.

[14] Beresin E, Mellman L. Competencies in psychiatry: the new outcomes-based approach to medical training and education. Harv Rev Psychiatry 2002;10(3):185–91.

[15] Mellman LA, Beresin E. Psychotherapy competencies: development and implementation. Acad Psychiatry 2003;27(3):149–53.

ELSEVIER
SAUNDERS

Child Adolesc Psychiatric Clin N Am
14 (2005) 613–622

CHILD AND
ADOLESCENT
PSYCHIATRIC CLINICS
OF NORTH AMERICA

Media Outreach for Child Psychiatrists

Cheryl K. Olson, SD[a,b,*], Lawrence A. Kutner, PhD[a,b]

[a]Harvard Medical School Center for Mental Health and Media, Department of Psychiatry,
Massachusetts General Hospital, 271 Waverley Oaks Road, Suite 204, Waltham, MA 02452, USA
[b]Department of Psychiatry, Harvard Medical School, Boston, MA, USA

In July, 1899, an editorial in the *Journal of the American Medical Association* bemoaned the difficulty of "instilling correct ideas of insanity into the public mind" [1]:

> There is such an opportunity for sensationalism that newspaper reporters in particular are rarely able to keep their imagination in restraint and the average literature they produce on the subject is about as thoroughly untrustworthy as it can well be. The physician who unguardedly allows himself to be interviewed on any remarkable incident or phase of the subject [of insanity] is liable to have to repent it. . ...

As this century-old quote shows, physicians long have been aware of the potential of mass media for public education, but also (often rightly) have been critical of inaccuracies and sensationalism in media reports.

Child and adolescent psychiatrists may see little reason to get involved with media reporters or producers, and plenty of reasons to avoid them. There is the fear of being viewed as a self-promoting popularizer rather than a serious clinician or researcher. There is concern about being misquoted or having statements taken out of context, to the detriment of their reputation and the public's education. Uncertainty about the expectations, methods, and motivations of media professionals creates uncomfortable feelings of confusion and lack of control [2].

In this article we suggest several reasons why psychiatrists should get involved with the media. We demystify some of the workings of the news media,

---

* Corresponding author. Harvard Medical School Center for Mental Health and Media, 271 Waverley Oaks Road, Suite 204, Waltham, MA 02452.

E-mail address: colson@hms.harvard.edu (C.K. Olson).

1056-4993/05/$ – see front matter © 2005 Elsevier Inc. All rights reserved.
doi:10.1016/j.chc.2005.02.011   *childpsych.theclinics.com*

so that when a reporter calls, you can be better prepared and increase the odds of a positive outcome. We describe ways to reach out proactively to media professionals to educate the public or support improved mental health policies. Finally, we examine more sophisticated uses of media, including public education campaigns.

Why get involved with the media?

The need to raise public awareness about mental illness and effective treatment

Surveys in the United States and other countries have found that many people have little understanding of what mental illness looks like, what symptoms characterize different illnesses, and what is meant by labels such as "schizophrenia" and "mania" [3]. Given these misunderstandings about the nature of mental illness, it is likely that upsetting but normal child behaviors are often misconstrued as symptoms of pathology, while true symptoms may be missed.

Despite some progress in recent years, stigmatizing myths about causality persist. For example, many members of the public believe that schizophrenia and depression are caused by "the way a person was raised" or "one's own bad character" [4]; the contribution of biologic factors is underrated [3]. There are also misconceptions about the nature and value of psychiatric treatment. Although surveys show generally positive views of psychotherapy, misconceptions about medication are rampant, including exaggerated concerns about side effects and a belief that drugs merely cover up symptoms [5].

The need to reduce stigma and other barriers to care

Although the cost of and access to services affect whether a child receives treatment, research suggests that beliefs about mental health problems and treatment may be even greater obstacles to care [6]. These beliefs include parents' knowledge about symptoms of mental illness and parents' beliefs about the seriousness of the symptoms, the need for treatment, and the likely effectiveness of mental health services. Parents' expectations about their children's treatment also predict the level of parental involvement in therapy and whether treatment is terminated prematurely [7]. Given that more than three-fourths of children with mental health needs are not receiving treatment [8], removing barriers to care is a critical priority.

The need to counteract media misinformation that contributes to stigma

Unfortunately, a significant amount of current health-related media content is confusing, misleading, or downright wrong. Poor reporting can, for example, lead viewers to misconstrue research results, dangerously halt medical treatment, or turn to unproven "cures" [9]. Selective reporting also can reinforce myths, such as the belief that mentally ill persons are dangerous [10]. In fact, perceptions of the dangerousness of mentally ill people, particularly persons with schizophrenia, actually have increased in recent decades [4]. Reviews of press coverage in the United States, United Kingdom, Canada, and New Zealand have found that mental illness is frequently linked with violence [11]. In one US study of major newspapers' reporting of mental illness, crime or violence perpetrated by a mentally ill person was the focus of 26% of such stories and was by far the most common theme [12]. Perceptions such as these make people wary of contact with mentally ill individuals and may increase support for coercive or counterproductive policies [13].

Entertainment media also can perpetrate harmful stereotypes. A review of Disney animated films found a surprisingly high number of stigmatizing comments, including "crazy" thoughts, ideas, behaviors, or clothing, with the implication that these traits were irrational and inferior [14]. A study of television programs aimed at young children also found frequent negative stereotypes, especially in cartoon programs; "twisted" or "nuts" characters were portrayed as evil or funny [15]. The authors were concerned that these shows may increase stigma and verbal harassment in real life.

Mental illness is a common theme in movies, including horror films. They not only present mentally ill persons as scary and dangerous but also can affect the image of psychiatrists and the expectations that children and their parents have about the nature and outcome of therapy. (See the article by Butler and Hyler elsewhere in this issue.) Media portrayals of electroconvulsive therapy have been particularly horrifying and distorted [16].

The need to counterbalance information from special interests

Much of the health information presented to the public is put forward by special interests, such as pharmaceutical companies. Special interest advertising and promotion have the potential to be helpful, as when therapies widely viewed as effective for undertreated conditions are advertised [17]. When celebrities are paid to make the rounds of talk shows to promote medications [18], news stories are based on corporate press releases or conference abstracts, and the benefits of new medications are exaggerated and risks overlooked [19], disinterested physicians must come forward to balance the picture.

The potential of mass media to teach and counteract stigma

If we wish to educate the public, it is far easier to reach them through their usual channels of information, which means reaching out through the mass media. In a 2001 survey [20], 51% of respondents said that television was their most important source of news and information about health issues, especially television news programs. This is not necessarily a bad thing. Intelligent news coverage has led to needed changes in health and research policies and legislation

[21], and television programs repeatedly have shown themselves—intentionally or accidentally—to be highly effective health and science public education tools. Even entertainment programming content has been shown to influence health-related knowledge and behaviors, such as family discussions and choices about health care, deciding to visit a doctor or clinic, or encouraging others to seek help [22,23].

How to work with the media

Although clinicians and researchers may acknowledge the power of mass media as public health and education tools for mental health promotion, primary prevention, and stigma reduction, few psychiatrists receive any formal training in how to use those tools. Many psychiatrists are concerned that attempts to work with the media will be viewed by colleagues as little more than self-aggrandizement. To counteract these problems, we have incorporated formal and informal media training into the curriculum of the child and adolescent psychiatry training program at Massachusetts General Hospital/McLean Hospital. Training includes seminars in health communication, structured practice sessions such as mock broadcast and print interviews, and opportunities to work on media-based outreach projects. Several of the points emphasized in these sessions can be used readily by experienced psychiatrists who wish to explore the use of mass media as extensions of their clinical practice or research.

There are three general types of "triggers" for contact with mass media: (1) Contact by a reporter or producer about a specific story. This is probably the most common first interaction between physicians and the press. For example, one may receive a telephone call from a journalist who is writing a news story about local children who were sexually abused, or who is producing a television feature story on the supposed increase in autism over the past few generations. (2) Promotion of a story idea that you have developed. This includes promotion of new clinical services or a book, interpretation of research findings for the general public or for public policy makers, and even an organized mental health-related media campaign. (3) The use of natural opportunities, such as breaking national news, to help guide coverage of that news and related topics. For example, recent concerns and publicity over the use of antidepressant medications by children provided child psychiatrists with opportunities to reach out to the press not only on that specific topic but also on the nature of childhood mood disorders, the purpose and limits of these types of studies, and the predicaments of parents who seek help for children who have mental illnesses.

When a reporter calls

When you receive a telephone call from a reporter asking for your comments or insights into a story, your first response should be to ask a few questions of your own. (Psychiatrists who work for academic medical centers may find that their employers have a policy of channeling all such calls through a public affairs office, where the staff should do this.) For example: (1) What is the name of the publication or the broadcast program? A reporter who says he or she is with the *Enquirer* may mean the venerable *Cincinnati Enquirer* or the tabloid *National Enquirer*. (2) What is the focus of the story? Knowing this before you start can help you structure what you say and help ensure that your statements are taken in context. (3) What is the deadline? Reporters who work for daily publications or news broadcasts often have only hours to put together a story. If you cannot meet the reporter's deadline, simply say so.

Reporters, radio talk show hosts, and others who may call for an interview have a wide range of experience and expertise that may color their coverage of a topic. A few have doctoral degrees in medicine, psychology, or a related subject; others have not set foot in a science classroom since high school and may spend most of their workday reporting on fires and local politics. No matter what their background, most journalists are simply trying to get their facts straight, put issues into perspective, and present them in a way that is interesting and attractive to their audience. The challenge for psychiatrists who present information on mental health is to help reporters achieve their goals in ways that also help us achieve ours.

This challenge is sometimes made more difficult because the priorities of the media can stand in stark contrast to the priorities of mental health professionals [24]. For example, say you are contacted by a reporter who is writing a story in response to the suicide of a local and popular high school athlete. The reporter's focus for the story—especially if that reporter is relatively unsophisticated—may be different from what you might wish to get across to the public about the underlying issues. If your voice is to be heard, you must gently guide the reporter and shape or "frame" the story. Address the reporter's assumptions about the nature of the problem or issue, the causes of the problem, moral or value judgments associated with those perceived causes, and potential remedies for the problem [25]. The following questions are examples of what a reporter may ask:

1. *Why did the child kill himself?* You should decline to answer that question; however, you can use it to segue to the larger issue. For example, you might begin your response with, "I cannot comment on this specific child because I did not know him. However, we do know that the large majority of young people who kill themselves are depressed; but their depression can look different than depression in adults."
2. *We know that most of these kids who shoot other people and themselves— like the kids at Columbine and that DC sniper—play a lot of violent computer games. Do you think this kid played those games? Shouldn't we just ban them?* Always correct a false premise before attempting to answer any question. Otherwise, your silence acts as a tacit endorsement of the premise. "I think that you (and many other people) are making some

assumptions that are not supported by research. Let's look at them one at a time."

3. *This kid had everything going for him. He was smart and popular. What happened?* Again, you can use this to help shape the reporter's story by talking about the myths of depression and suicide and the need for treatment. "Depression is a brain disorder. One of the things it does is give a person a distorted picture of his or her life. Although other people may say he is doing well, he may feel hopeless and doomed. Medication and talk therapy can help. The big problem is getting teenagers to go for that help."

By acknowledging the reporter's questions, correcting false premises, and segueing to relevant materials that lend insight to the story, you are helping shape it so that it is more likely to address the following important issues that might otherwise have been missed: (1) Perspective on the epidemiology of suicide and adolescent depression. (2) Identification of children at risk. What are the symptoms of depression among adolescents? Why are these symptoms sometimes missed, even by family, friends, and teachers? How does adolescent depression present differently than adult depression? (3) Primary prevention. What can schools and parents do to help these children before they become suicidal? What can be done to help prevent additional suicide attempts ("contagion") by teenagers in the community? (4) Posttrauma intervention. What can parents and teachers say to teenagers and younger children who are frightened or upset by an adolescent's suicide?

As you plan your response, remember that your goal is to get just a few key points across. This is especially true in a television news story, which may be just 75 to 90 seconds long.

Reaching out to the media to influence behaviors or policies

These same techniques can be used in a proactive rather than a reactive manner. Whether you are promoting the expansion of services at a community mental health center or working on a national stigma reduction initiative, you will be much more effective if you start with a detailed plan for strategy and implementation. Key issues that the plan must address include the following:

• Whom are you trying to reach with your message? Be as specific as you can (eg, parents of children who are making the transition to middle school). Think about the types of media the members of your target audience regularly listen to, watch, or read. There are times when you can use mass media effectively to influence a small but critical group of individuals, such as state legislators who are about to vote on a particular bill. The political media specialist Tony Schwartz used low-cost targeted radio advertising to great effect [26].

- What exactly is your message? Media interviews do not offer time or space for complex arguments. Focus on one to three clear points you would like to make. If you find yourself thinking in vague terms ("My goal is to tell parents about childhood stress"), you must rethink your approach.
- What are the specific responses you want from your target audience when they receive your information? Too often, mental health professionals focus exclusively on conveying detailed information, such as the symptoms of posttraumatic stress disorder. In many situations, other types of responses are at least as important. How should a person feel upon seeing, hearing, or reading your message? (Reassured? Empowered? Ashamed?) What specific behaviors do you want from that person? (To speak with their child or spouse about the topic? To call a clinic to set up an appointment?)
- How will you know if your efforts are successful? Did readers contact you for more information? Did clinical appointments increase? Was a bill passed in the legislature? Defining your criteria for success ahead of time sometimes leads you to re-examine whether you are offering the information your target audience needs to give the specific responses you hope for.

Although more published studies are needed, there is evidence that reaching out to reporters with accurate background information and ideas for positive stories can improve the amount and tone of mental health coverage [27].

Taking advantage of events to educate the public

Predictable (eg, the holiday season) and unpredictable (the 2004 tsunami in Asia) events can provide opportunities to reach out to the media on children's mental health issues. Although the window of opportunity may be brief, the key issues listed above still apply. For example, a school shooting in a different state might make reporters more interested in the issue of posttraumatic stress disorder among school-aged children. Before you speak with a reporter about a topic, you should define clearly your target audience, your message, the behavioral responses you want, and your criteria for success. If the story is based on newly published research, it is important to provide information that helps reporters put those findings into perspective. For example, a mention in one small study that one-fourth of patients with schizophrenia had carried weapons during psychotic episodes led to hysterical headlines about dangerous mental patients [28].

Be explicit about what the data mean, what they do not tell us, and what the practical implications might be. Try to put the data into a real-world context. If your goal is to increase the recognition of depression, it is more compelling to state that every high school classroom has at least one student with undiagnosed depression and to give examples of what untreated depression might mean for that child's future, than to recite statistics. Thinking in terms of examples also helps you put information into lay language and avoid medical jargon.

Take advantage of the power of imagery—whether a video image, or photograph, or images created by phrases or metaphors—to get your points across. When a person who looks like your next-door neighbor describes her struggle with schizophrenia, the visual impression she makes (so different from the iconic image of a violent, disheveled "crazy" person) may convey a stronger and more memorable message than any of her words.

What others have done to educate the public about mental illness

Because little is known about what works to educate the public about mental illness (and disorders of children and adolescents in particular), it is important to share information on what has been tried and what approaches seem most effective [29]. The World Psychiatric Association has collected information on programs from 11 countries, including the United States, designed to reduce stigma and discrimination related to schizophrenia and other mental illnesses. Some of these programs involve the distribution of media materials such as videotapes, efforts to work with reporters, critiques of poor news coverage, and awards for good reporting. (This compendium as of 2002 can be viewed or downloaded at http://www.openthedoors.com/english/01_02.html.) Unfortunately, few of these programs include the evaluation of educational media materials or the campaigns that use these materials. They typically rely on informal measures, such as feedback from conference participants or counts of requests for materials.

A notable exception is the "Like Minds, Like Mine" campaign initiated by the New Zealand Ministry of Health in 1996 [30]. This research-based campaign includes strategically placed television, radio, and cinema advertisements (some of which feature nationally known and respected people who had experience with mental illness), public relations activities to support the advertising messages (including media interviews and placed articles), and more-targeted locally based education and grassroots activities. National tracking surveys found high awareness of campaign messages and significant changes in attitudes and behavior. For example, 62% of persons surveyed reported discussing the advertising one or more times with someone else. Most important, there were reports of reduced stigma and discrimination related to family, the public, mental health services, media content, police, and housing. More information on the ongoing campaign, including the National Plan [31], can be found at http://www.likeminds.govt.nz.

Also worth noting are the public education campaigns developed by the Royal College of Psychiatrists in Great Britain, including "Defeat Depression" from 1992 to 1996 [32] and "Changing Minds" from 1998 to 2003 [33,34]. The goal of "Defeat Depression" was to decrease stigma in order to encourage earlier treatment seeking. "Changing Minds" broadened the effort to include anxiety, schizophrenia, dementias, alcohol and other drug misuse, and eating disorders. In addition to exhorting the public "to stop and think about their own attitudes and behaviour in relation to mental disorders...and become more tolerant of people with mental health problems," the campaign's designers sought to reduce discrimination against people who suffer from these problems. Surveys suggested that these campaigns may have contributed to encouraging but small shifts in attitudes (eg, regarding perceptions of dangerousness and whether a mentally ill person is to blame for his or her condition), but it is not clear whether discriminatory behaviors were affected. Survey data tables, campaign materials, and information on the current "Partners in Care" campaign (which addresses the needs of families caring for someone who is mentally ill) can be found at http://www.rcpsych.ac.uk/campaigns/index.htm.

Summary

If psychiatrists can overcome their discomfort and develop realistic expectations and clear goals, working with the media often can be a positive experience. For clinicians, it provides opportunities to counter misinformation and stereotypes, to remove barriers to seeking diagnosis and treatment, to improve therapeutic relationships, compliance with treatment, and treatment outcomes, and to increase social and political support for families who struggle with mental illness. It is also important to network with colleagues locally and internationally to build our limited knowledge base of innovative and effective ways to use mass media for the benefit of the public's mental health.

References

[1] Reiling J. Psychiatry and sensationalism (JAMA 100 Years Ago: July 29, 1899). JAMA 1999; 282(4):308F.
[2] Kutner L, Beresin EV. Media training for psychiatry residents. Acad Psychiatry 1999;23: 227–32.
[3] Jorm AF. Mental health literacy: public knowledge and beliefs about mental disorders [review]. Br J Psychiatry 2000;177:396–401.
[4] Link BG, Phelan JC, Bresnahan M, et al. Public conceptions of mental illness: labels, causes, dangerousness, and social distance. Am J Public Health 1999;89:1328–33.
[5] Priest RG, Vize C, Roberts A, et al. Lay people's attitudes to treatment of depression: results of opinion poll for Defeat Depression Campaign just before its launch. BMJ 1996;313(7061): 858–9.
[6] Owens PL, Hoagwood K, Horwitz SM, et al. Barriers to children's mental health services. J Am Acad Child Adolesc Psychiatry 2002;41(6):731–8.
[7] Nock MK, Kazdin AE. Parent expectancies for child therapy: assessment and relation to participation in treatment. J Child Fam Stud 2001;10(2):155–80.
[8] Coyle JT, Pine DS, Charney SD, et al. Depression and bipolar support alliance consensus statement on the unmet needs in diagnosis and treatment of mood disorders in children and adolescents. J Am Acad Child Adolesc Psychiatry 2003;42(12):1494–503.
[9] Shuchman M, Wilkes MS. Medical scientists and health news reporting: a case of miscommunication. Ann Intern Med 1997;126(12):976–82.

[10] Angermeyer MC, Matschinger H. The effect of violent attacks by schizophrenic persons on the attitude of the public towards the mentally ill. Soc Sci Med 1996;43(12):1721–8.

[11] Wahl OF. News media portrayal of mental illness: implications for public policy. Am Behav Sci 2003;46(12):1594–600.

[12] Wahl OF, Wood A, Richards R. Newspaper coverage of mental illness: is it changing? Psychiatric Rehabilitation Skills 2002;6(1):9–31.

[13] Taylor PJ, Gunn J. Homicides by people with mental illness: myth and reality. Br J Psychiatry 1999;174(1):9–14.

[14] Lawson A, Fouts G. Mental illness in Disney animated films. Can J Psychiatry 2004;49:310–4.

[15] Wilson C, Nairn R, Coverdale J, et al. How mental illness is portrayed in children's television: a prospective study. Br J Psychiatry 2000;176:440–3.

[16] Walter G, McDonald A. About to have ECT? Fine, but don't watch it in the movies. Psychiatric Times 2004;21(7):65–8.

[17] Dubois RW. Pharmaceutical promotion: don't throw the baby out with the bath water (February 26, 2003). Available at: http://content.healthaffairs.org/cgi/content/full/hlthaff.w3.96v1/DC1. Accessed March 15, 2005.

[18] Moynihan R. Celebrity selling: part two. BMJ 2002;325:286.

[19] Moynihan R. Making medical journalism healthier. Lancet 2003;361:2097–8.

[20] Kaiser/Harvard School of Public Health Program on the Public and Health Policy. Sources of health news and information. Kaiser/Harvard Health News Index 2001;6(5):2. Available at: http://www.kff.org/kaiserpolls/3189-index.cfm. Accessed March 15, 2005.

[21] Shuchman M. Journalists as change agents in medicine and health care. JAMA 2002;287(6):776.

[22] Centers for Disease Control and Prevention Entertainment Education Program. 1999 Porter Novelli Healthstyles survey: soap opera viewers and health information. Presented at the Annual Meeting of the American Public Health Association. Boston, November 15, 2000. Available at: http://www.cdc.gov/communication/surveys/surv1999.htm. Accessed March 15, 2005.

[23] Brodie M, Foehr U, Rideout V, et al. Communicating health information through the entertainment media. Health Aff 2001;20(1):192–9.

[24] Kutner L, Beresin EV. Reaching out: mass media techniques for child and adolescent psychiatrists. J Am Acad Child Adolesc Psychiatry 2000;39(11):1452–4.

[25] Sieff EM. Media frames of mental illness: the potential impact of negative frames. J Ment Health 2003;12(3):259–69.

[26] Schwartz T. Media: the second god. Garden City (NY): Anchor Press/Doubleday; 1983. p. 97–9.

[27] Stuart H. Stigma and the daily news: evaluation of a newspaper intervention. Can J Psychiatry 2003;48:651–6.

[28] Ferriman A. The stigma of schizophrenia. BMJ 2000;320(7233):522.

[29] Sartorius N. Stigma: what can psychiatrists do about it? Lancet 1998;352:1058–9.

[30] Vaughan G, Hansen C. Like minds, like mine: a New Zealand project to counter the stigma and discrimination associated with mental illness. Australas Psychiatry 2004;12(2):113–7.

[31] New Zealand Ministry of Health. Like minds, like mine national plan 2003–2005. Wellington (New Zealand): New Zealand Ministry of Health; 2003.

[32] Paykel ES, Hart D, Priest RG. Changes in public attitudes to depression during the Defeat Depression Campaign. Br J Psychiatry 1998;173(12):519–22.

[33] Byrne P. Stigma of mental illness and ways of diminishing it. Advances in Psychiatric Treatment 2000;6:65–72.

[34] Crisp AH, Gelder MG, Rix S, et al. Stigmatisation of people with mental illness. Br J Psychiatry 2000;177:4–7.

ELSEVIER
SAUNDERS

Child Adolesc Psychiatric Clin N Am
14 (2005) 623–629

CHILD AND
ADOLESCENT
PSYCHIATRIC CLINICS
OF NORTH AMERICA

Index

Note: Page numbers of article titles are in **boldface** type.

1056-4993/05/$ – see front matter © 2005 Elsevier Inc. All rights reserved.
doi:10.1016/S1056-4993(05)00047-7
childpsych.theclinics.com

Changing Your Address?

Make sure your subscription changes too! When you notify us of your new address, you can help make our job easier by including an exact copy of your Clinics label number with your old address (see illustration below.) This number identifies you to our computer system and will speed the processing of your address change. Please be sure this label number accompanies your old address and your corrected address—you can send an old Clinics label with your number on it or just copy it exactly and send it to the address listed below.

We appreciate your help in our attempt to give you continuous coverage. Thank you.

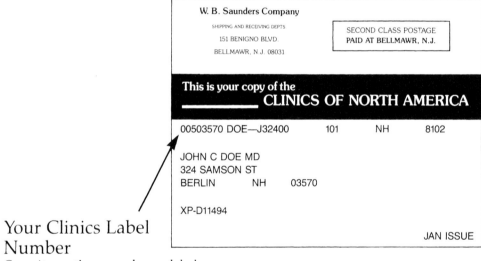

W. B. Saunders Company

SHIPPING AND RECEIVING DEPTS
151 BENIGNO BLVD.
BELLMAWR, N.J. 08031

SECOND CLASS POSTAGE
PAID AT BELLMAWR, N.J.

This is your copy of the
_____ CLINICS OF NORTH AMERICA

00503570 DOE—J32400   101   NH   8102

JOHN C DOE MD
324 SAMSON ST
BERLIN   NH   03570

XP-D11494

JAN ISSUE

Your Clinics Label Number

Copy it exactly or send your label
along with your address to:
W.B. Saunders Company, Customer Service
Orlando, FL 32887-4800
Call Toll Free 1-800-654-2452

Please allow four to six weeks for delivery of new subscriptions and for processing address changes.

Order your subscription today. Simply complete and detach this card and drop it in the mail to receive the best clinical information in your field.

Please Print:

Name _____

Address _____

City _____ State _____ ZIP _____

Method of Payment

❏ Check (payable to **Elsevier**; add the applicable sales tax for your area)

❏ VISA   ❏ MasterCard   ❏ AmEx   ❏ Bill me

Card number _____ Exp. date _____

Signature _____

Staple this to your purchase order to expedite delivery

Adolescent Medicine Clinics
❏ Individual $95
❏ Institutions $133
❏ *In-training $48

Anesthesiology
❏ Individual $175
❏ Institutions $270
❏ *In-training $88

Cardiology
❏ Individual $170
❏ Institutions $266
❏ *In-training $85

Chest Medicine
❏ Individual $185
❏ Institutions $285

Child and Adolescent Psychiatry
❏ Individual $175
❏ Institutions $265
❏ *In-training $88

Critical Care
❏ Individual $165
❏ Institutions $266
❏ *In-training $83

Dental
❏ Individual $150
❏ Institutions $242

Emergency Medicine
❏ Individual $170
❏ Institutions $263
❏ *In-training $85
   ❏ Send CME info

Facial Plastic Surgery
❏ Individual $199
❏ Institutions $300

Foot and Ankle
Individual $160
Institutions $232

Gastroenterology
❏ Individual $190
❏ Institutions $276

Gastrointestinal Endoscopy
❏ Individual $190
❏ Institutions $276

Hand
❏ Individual $205
❏ Institutions $319

Heart Failure (NEW in 2005!)
❏ Individual $99
❏ Institutions $149
❏ *In-training $49

Hematology/ Oncology
❏ Individual $210
❏ Institutions $315

Immunology & Allergy
❏ Individual $165
❏ Institutions $266

Infectious Disease
❏ Individual $165
❏ Institutions $272

Clinics in Liver Disease
❏ Individual $165
❏ Institutions $234

Medical
❏ Individual $140
❏ Institutions $244
❏ *In-training $70
   ❏ Send CME info

MRI
❏ Individual $190
❏ Institutions $290
❏ *In-training $95
   ❏ Send CME info

Neuroimaging
❏ Individual $190
❏ Institutions $290
❏ *In-training $95
   ❏ Send CME inf0

Neurologic
❏ Individual $175
❏ Institutions $275

Obstetrics & Gynecology
❏ Individual $175
❏ Institutions $288

Occupational and Environmental Medicine
❏ Individual $120
❏ Institutions $166
❏ *In-training $60

Ophthalmology
❏ Individual $190
❏ Institutions $325

Oral & Maxillofacial Surgery
❏ Individual $180
❏ Institutions $280
❏ *In-training $90

Orthopedic
❏ Individual $180
❏ Institutions $295
❏ *In-training $90

Otolaryngologic
❏ Individual $199
❏ Institutions $350

Pediatric
❏ Individual $135
❏ Institutions $246
❏ *In-training $68
   ❏ Send CME info

Perinatology
❏ Individual $155
❏ Institutions $237
❏ *In-training $78
   ❏ Send CME inf0

Plastic Surgery
❏ Individual $245
❏ Institutions $370

Podiatric Medicine & Surgery
❏ Individual $170
❏ Institutions $266

Primary Care
❏ Individual $135
❏ Institutions $223

Psychiatric
❏ Individual $170
❏ Institutions $288

Radiologic
❏ Individual $220
❏ Institutions $331
❏ *In-training $110
   ❏ Send CME info

Sports Medicine
❏ Individual $180
❏ Institutions $277

Surgical
❏ Individual $190
❏ Institutions $299
❏ *In-training $95

Thoracic Surgery (formerly Chest Surgery)
❏ Individual $175
❏ Institutions $255
❏ *In-training $88

Urologic
❏ Individual $195
❏ Institutions $307
❏ *In-training $98
   ❏ Send CME info

*To receive in-training rate, orders must be accompanied by the name of affiliated institution, dates of residency and signature of coordinator on institution letterhead. Orders will be billed at the individual rate until proof of resident status is received.

BUSINESS REPLY MAIL

FIRST-CLASS MAIL   PERMIT NO 7135   ORLANDO FL

POSTAGE WILL BE PAID BY ADDRESSEE

PERIODICALS ORDER FULFILLMENT DEPT
ELSEVIER
6277 SEA HARBOR DR
ORLANDO FL 32821-9816